Blockchain-Based Healthcare Management in the Metaverse

Mohammed Shuaib
Jazan University, Saudi Arabia

Shadab Alam
Jazan University, Saudi Arabia

A. Rajaram
E.G.S. Pillay Engineering College, India

IGI Global
Scientific Publishing
Publishing Tomorrow's Research Today

Vice President of Editorial Melissa Wagner
Director of Acquisitions Mikaela Felty
Director of Book Development Jocelynn Hessler
Production Manager Mike Brehm
Cover Design Jose Rosado

Published in the United States of America by
IGI Global Scientific Publishing
701 East Chocolate Avenue
Hershey, PA, 17033, USA
Tel: 717-533-8845 | Fax: 717-533-7115
Website: https://www.igi-global.com E-mail: cust@igi-global.com

Library of Congress Cataloging-in-Publication Data

Names: Shuaib, Mohammed, 1989- editor http://id.loc.gov/rwo/agents/n2025014113 | Alam, Shadab, 1985- editor http://id.loc.gov/rwo/agents/n2025014115 | Ayyasamy, Rajaram, 1982- editor http://id.loc.gov/rwo/agents/n2025014116
Title: Blockchain-based healthcare management in the metaverse / edited by Mohammed Shuaib, Shadab Alam, Rajaram Ayyasamy.
Description: Hershey, PA : IGI Global Scientific Publishing, [2026] | Includes bibliographical references and index. | Summary: "The book aims to highlight how blockchain technology can overcome limitations in current healthcare systems by ensuring data privacy, enhancing interoperability, and creating secure virtual healthcare environments. Its purpose is to showcase the transformative role blockchain plays in redefining healthcare interactions within the metaverse"-- Provided by publisher.
Identifiers: LCCN 2025000128 (print) | LCCN 2025000129 (ebook) | ISBN 9798337312255 hardcover | ISBN 9798337312262 paperback | ISBN 9798337312279 ebook
Subjects: LCSH: Blockchains (Databases)--Medical applications http://id.loc.gov/authorities/subjects/sh2023002955 | Metaverse http://id.loc.gov/authorities/subjects/sh2022006294
Classification: LCC R859.7.B56 B558 2025 (print) | LCC R859.7.B56 (ebook) | DDC 610.285/7588--dc23/eng/20250328
LC record available at https://lccn.loc.gov/2025000128
LC ebook record available at https://lccn.loc.gov/2025000129

British Cataloguing in Publication Data
A Cataloguing in Publication record for this book is available from the British Library.

Table of Contents

Detailed Table of Contents

As one of the most disruptive forces across industries, blockchain technology holds immense promise for the healthcare sector. In this chapter, we will discuss the advantages, applications, and challenges of integrating blockchain into healthcare systems. The chapter opens by outlining the key features of blockchain technology, highlighting its decentralization, immutability, and transparency. It then looks at individual use cases in health care, such as patient data management, drug traceability, and supply chain logistics. The ethical and legal implications of using blockchain in healthcare with a particular emphasis on patient confidentiality and consent. Case studies from real life and existing efforts are utilized to show the potential of blockchain-based solutions in healthcare. This chapter aims to provide researchers, medical professionals, and policymakers with a comprehensive understanding of blockchain's potential to improve the management of healthcare information and security, as well as insights into the challenges and concerns associated with its implementation.

Blockchain technology, renowned for its decentralized and immutable nature, is poised to revolutionize the landscape of smart healthcare. In this transformative paradigm, patient data becomes securely stored and efficiently managed, fostering unprecedented levels of trust, transparency, and interoperability among healthcare stakeholders. By leveraging blockchain, institutions can ensure the integrity and confidentiality of medical records, mitigating the risk of data breaches. Smart contracts embedded within the blockchain facilitate automated execution of agreements, streamlining processes such as insurance claims, medication adherence monitoring, and patient consent management. Moreover, it enables the creation of comprehensive patient-centric networks, facilitating seamless data sharing across disparate healthcare systems while maintaining patient privacy. This technology holds immense promise for reforming smart healthcare, fostering a future where data is securely shared, patient outcomes are optimized, and the delivery of healthcare services is truly patient-centric.

Data are necessary for learning health systems, but feedback loops of knowledge into revised behaviour. This is dependent on knowledge application and management, both of which are reliant on efficient system development. The multidisciplinary area that covers the complete spectrum of health science, social science, information science, and technology is known as biomedical informatics. IssuesConclusions Policy makers and research funders must acknowledge the gap between the "two cultures" that currently exists and understand that in order to fully reap the social and economic benefits of data science and digital health, it is necessary to accept the interdisciplinary nature of biomedical informatics and to support a significant expansion of clinical informatics capacity and capability

All the healthcare sector problems of the past, including security, privacy, interoperability, and transparency, are addressable with blockchain technology. Because of the decentralized, tamper-resistant, and transparent nature of blockchain, it is highly appropriate to facilitate secure and effective sharing of information between healthcare professionals, patients, and stakeholders. This document details the place blockchain must occupy in enhancing the digital health system, its applications for rendering patient data secure, interoperability, ownership of health data by patients, and efficient management of healthcare supply chains. Blockchain's function in clinical trials, medical billing, eradication of fraud, and emergency response is discussed as well. While it has tremendous potential, healthcare brings to it challenges inherent in the utilization of blockchain technology, such as cost, scalability, and legality. Future development will be towards eliminating the barriers to the utilization of blockchain technology in widespread use in the health sector globally.

This chapter describes the integration of AI, IoT, and blockchain with healthcare, with a focus on transformative impact. AI supports predictive analytics, data security, and workflow automation, whereas IoT enables real-time monitoring of patients and data transmission without interruption. Blockchain focuses on data integrity, transparency, and security and thereby addresses issues such as interoperability and scalability. Remote monitoring, decentralized clinical trials, and drug supply chain management will improve safety and efficiency. It will discuss the challenge of data privacy, ethical concerns, and regulatory complexities while calling for responsible implementation. The envisioned next-generation healthcare system would leverage such technologies to make care efficient, secure, and centered on the patient, supporting global collaboration and innovation to build a more equitable healthcare ecosystem.

Healthcare is in a paradigm shift with technology adoption like Artificial Intelligence (AI), Explainable AI (XAI), and Blockchain (BC) in the metaverse. The article presented the use, limitation, and effect of adoption of these technologies to bring about a transformation in healthcare delivery. Blockchain and XAI based health metaverse is an emerging paradigm to improve patient treatment, secure data, and optimize. XAI improves the interpretability and explainability of AI-based health decisions, while blockchain allows for distributed control of patient data securely. Healthcare in the Metaverse can be provided within virtual space, thus allowing remote visits, treatment plans customized to individual patients, and secure sharing of medical data. All these technologies together create new possibilities of health delivery innovation regarding accessibility, efficiency, and trust. There are numerous issues still to be addressed, though, such as ethics, regulation, and how doctors will take advantage of new technology. This report ends with some analysis of how the technologies as a whole will shape the future of healthcare.

Preface

The rapid convergence of blockchain technology and the metaverse is poised to redefine the landscape of healthcare management. Traditionally, healthcare has relied on centralized infrastructures, fragmented records, and vulnerable data systems. Blockchain addresses these limitations by ensuring immutability, decentralized trust, and verifiable transactions, while the metaverse contributes immersive and interactive environments for virtual consultations, rehabilitation, and personalized medicine. Together, these technologies are redefining how data is managed, how care is delivered, and how patients engage with healthcare systems. This edited volume, *Blockchain-Based Healthcare Management in the Metaverse*, offers an in-depth exploration of how these cutting-edge technologies combine to create secure, immersive, and efficient healthcare systems within virtual environments.

Unlike existing literature that often treats blockchain and metaverse applications separately, this book uniquely bridges the two, providing a forward-looking perspective on the digital transformation of healthcare. Through comprehensive analysis, the chapters delve into critical topics such as secure patient data management, decentralized identity frameworks, interoperability challenges, and the deployment of smart contracts for health-related transactions. Furthermore, the volume addresses practical applications including digital therapeutics, telemedicine, and personalized medicine—all within the evolving metaverse context.

Our goal is to highlight blockchain's transformative potential to overcome limitations of traditional healthcare systems by ensuring robust data privacy, fostering seamless interoperability, and enabling secure virtual healthcare interactions. Readers will gain valuable insights into the implementation of blockchain solutions for patient privacy, the operational efficiencies introduced by blockchain-enabled digital identities and smart contracts, and the broader implications for healthcare delivery in virtual spaces.

This book is intended primarily for academics and researchers in computer science, healthcare technology, and data science who seek to deepen their understanding of blockchain's role in virtual healthcare. Healthcare professionals interested in emerging technological applications will also find this volume instructive and timely. Additionally, technology developers working at the intersection of healthcare, blockchain, and artificial intelligence, as well as advanced students in these fields, will benefit from the practical examples, case studies, and future research directions presented throughout.

We believe this book serves as an essential resource for anyone seeking to navigate and contribute to the rapidly evolving domain of blockchain-powered healthcare management within the metaverse, and we hope it inspires further innovation and scholarship in this exciting frontier.

CHAPTER OVERVIEW

Chapter 1: A Survey on Blockchain and the Metaverse in Healthcare: Opportunities, Challenges, and Emerging Trends

This opening chapter lays the foundation by examining how the convergence of blockchain technology and the metaverse has the potential to revolutionize healthcare delivery. It highlights key innovations such as secure data management, self-sovereign identity, telemedicine, and decentralized clinical trials, while also discussing unresolved challenges related to scalability, legal frameworks, and ethics.

Chapter 2: Blockchain Technology in Healthcare: Transforming Data Management and Security

Building on this foundation, Chapter 2 explores the core advantages of blockchain—its decentralization, immutability, and transparency—and investigates how these features enhance data transmission, security, and fraud reduction in healthcare. The chapter also addresses ethical and regulatory complexities surrounding blockchain adoption.

Chapter 3: Blockchain Technology for Smart Healthcare

This chapter focuses on the transformative potential of blockchain to create secure, interoperable, and patient-centric healthcare ecosystems. It discusses the role of smart contracts in automating healthcare processes, enhancing transparency, and improving patient data integrity across diverse healthcare stakeholders.

Chapter 4: Recent Trends in Healthcare: Computational Intelligence, Challenges, and Opportunities

Placing blockchain-metaverse integration within a broader context, this chapter reviews computational intelligence applications in healthcare. It highlights advances in AI-driven diagnostics, decision-support systems, and digital therapeutics while mapping ongoing challenges and future opportunities.

Chapter 5: A Blockchain-Based Framework for Secure Data Sharing in Healthcare

Chapter 4 examines blockchain's capabilities in addressing longstanding challenges such as data privacy, interoperability, and supply chain management. It highlights blockchain's impact on clinical trials, billing, and fraud mitigation, while acknowledging implementation challenges like scalability and regulatory compliance.

Chapter 6: Application of AI and IoT in Blockchain-Based Healthcare

The integration of emerging technologies is central to Chapter 5, which details how artificial intelligence and the Internet of Things synergize with blockchain to enable predictive analytics, real-time patient monitoring, and secure data management. The chapter also discusses ethical concerns and calls for responsible deployment to create equitable healthcare systems.

Chapter 7: Virtual Healthcare in the Metaverse Leveraging XAI and Blockchain for Secure and Personalized Care

This chapter examines the transformative potential of explainable AI in conjunction with blockchain for virtual healthcare. It emphasizes how transparency and trust are enhanced in AI decision-making, facilitating remote consultations and personalized care in secure metaverse settings.

Chapter 8: Blockchain and Metaverse Revolutionizing Healthcare Systems: Transforming Healthcare for a Secure and Patient-Centric Future

Chapter 7 provides a comprehensive look at how blockchain and the metaverse converge to address critical challenges such as data security, patient privacy, and decentralized identity management. It also discusses emerging applications such as

NFTs and the Internet of Medical Things (IoMT), underscoring the need for sustainable and ethical solutions.

Chapter 9: Navigating the Ethical and Legal Landscape of Blockchain in Healthcare: A Critical Analysis

This chapter critically reviews the ethical, legal, and regulatory issues inherent to blockchain's healthcare applications. Topics such as informed consent, algorithmic bias, data ownership, and global regulatory frameworks are explored, emphasizing the importance of multi-stakeholder collaboration.

Chapter 10: Future Research Directions for Blockchain in Metaverse Healthcare Management

The final chapter extends the discussion to healthcare management. It addresses adoption challenges, institutional readiness, and governance strategies, presenting a holistic research agenda for future blockchain-metaverse healthcare systems.

Chapter 11: Future Research Directions for Blockchain in Metaverse Healthcare

Looking ahead, Chapter 10 outlines promising avenues for research and development. It highlights blockchain's role in global privacy compliance, digital identity verification, and smart contract-based administration, emphasizing the synergy between blockchain and AI for personalized metaverse healthcare.

As editors, we believe this volume offers a timely and comprehensive exploration of the powerful intersection between blockchain technology and the metaverse in healthcare management. The chapters collectively illuminate how these emerging technologies can address critical challenges around data security, interoperability, patient privacy, and decentralized care, while fostering innovation in virtual healthcare delivery. At the same time, the book does not shy away from the complex ethical, legal, and technical hurdles that must be overcome to realize this vision. By bringing together cutting-edge research, practical applications, and forward-looking insights, this work aims to serve as an essential resource for academics, healthcare professionals, technology developers, and policymakers alike. We hope it will inspire ongoing interdisciplinary collaboration and encourage the development of responsible, scalable solutions that ultimately empower patients and transform healthcare systems worldwide. In embracing the promise of blockchain and the metaverse, the future of healthcare management is poised to become more secure, patient-centric, and inclusive—paving the way for a digital health ecosystem that is both innovative and equitable.

Chapter 1

A Survey on Blockchain and the Metaverse in Healthcare: Opportunities, Challenges, and Emerging Trends

R. Siva Subramanian
SRM Institute of Science and Technology, India

J. Elavarasi
Vel Tech High Tech Dr. Rangarajan Dr. Sakunthala Engineering College, India

T. Venketbabu
https://orcid.org/0000-0002-0488-9332
Vel Tech Rangarajan Dr. Sagunthala R&D Institute of Science and Technology, India

L. A. Anto Gracious
https://orcid.org/0000-0003-2386-9182
R.M.K. College of Engineering and Technology, India

N. Pavithra
Jeppiaar Institute of Technology, India

M. Ezhilvendan
https://orcid.org/0009-0003-3213-1304
Panimalar Engineering College, India

R. Anand Babu
Panimalar Engineering College, India

ABSTRACT

This chapter explores the transformative potential of Blockchain technology and the Metaverse in revolutionizing healthcare. Blockchain's decentralized, secure, and transparent framework addresses critical healthcare challenges, such as data privacy, security, and patient management. The Metaverse, with its immersive virtual environments, enhances patient engagement, telemedicine, and remote healthcare delivery. The convergence of these technologies offers innovative solutions,

DOI: 10.4018/979-8-3373-1225-5.ch001

including secure data sharing, self-sovereign identity (SSI), virtual consultations, and decentralized clinical research. Key use cases, such as digital therapeutics, smart contracts, and interoperability, are discussed along with their implications for improving healthcare efficiency, trust, and transparency. This chapter concludes with a vision for the future of virtual healthcare, emphasizing the need for further research to overcome barriers and fully harness the potential of Blockchain and the Metaverse in shaping the future of global healthcare.

1. INTRODUCTION

1.1 Background

Blockchain and Metaverse technologies are among the most effective innovative technologies that are revolutionizing several sectors, including healthcare. Blockchain is an open database that provides decentralization, data integrity, security, and no possibility of data manipulation. Such characteristics make it possible to use it for delicate data that include EHRs, patient data, and medical transactions. On the other hand, the Metaverse is a virtual reality that emulates or reproduces real life activities or provides an opportunity to redesign them. This three-dimensional digital environment can change the face of healthcare by allowing live consults, engaging patient counselling and cooperate researches. As the research shows Blockchain and the Metaverse are complementary technologies that solve some of the most important issues of present-day healthcare.

1.2 Healthcare Challenges

Health care systems continue to experience some of the biggest problems such as data privacy violations, problems of data sharing and data accessibility, lack of access to health care and complex management of patients. Typical healthcare systems face problems regarding siloed data structures therefore, the patients' data remain insecure. Security threats like unauthorised access and cyber insecurity undermine patient's confidence. (Ali et al 2023) In addition, the access to quality care is still a problem around the world and especially in rural and underdeveloped regions. The issue becomes worse because of limited integration between healthcare systems, which results in poor communication, hence straining the healthcare delivery system and medical decision information systems. Solving these problems can only be achieved by finding out new methods of addressing security, openness, and fairness in accessing these facilities(Ponnuviji, N. P., et al., 2024).

1.3 Scope of the Survey

This study aims at analyzing how Blockchain and the Metaverse intersect in order to solve some of the most important healthcare issues. Through the use of Blockchain's secure framework, and Metaverse's virtual environments, the healthcare industry can go from a fragmented model and be patient-centric instead. The paper looks at the real-world applications including secure patient data handling, virtual care, and an SSI approach to privacy and ownership of Personal Health Records (PHRs). Other topics covered include digital therapeutics, AI in diagnostics, and Decentralized Clinical Trials. Furthermore, this survey seeks to understand how AI and ML combine with Blockchain and the Metaverse to provide personalised care and improve decision making. A brief examination is given to the ethical issues, legal requirements and concerns, and implementation barriers. Last, future research directions are provided to present the potential for expanding this convergence to foster a more robust, productive, and equitable health care system. Realizing this future, Blockchain and the Metaverse are expected to revolutionalise the delivery and management of healthcare by examining opportunities and challenges.

2. BLOCKCHAIN AND THE METAVERSE IN HEALTHCARE

2.1 Blockchain Overview

Blockchain is a method of storing transactions on an open database that exists simultaneously on all the network participants. It has low central authority hence does not require concentration of authorities which is very important in industries like healthcare. Blockchain makes it possible to store the medical data without the risk of someone hacking it or even changing any information. It can be stated that Blockchain increases trust between different health actors, such as patients, providers, and insurers due to an immutable record. Blockchain has the following advantages in the healthcare sector namely safer EHR transfers, better accountability in supply systems, and smart contracts. These attribute makes Blockchain a strategic tool for enhancing the healthcare sector through dealing with problems such as data compartmentalization, fraud, and poor organizational flow.

2.2 Metaverse in Healthcare

The Metaverse is a virtual world in which people are able to live and communicate in real time, primarily using avatars and can participate in fully realized three-dimensional environments. Metaverse in healthcare can be a radical shift in the way patients and their families are approached, educated, and engaged. In this context, enlarging the effectiveness and engagement of patients' experiences and supporting the skill development and collaboration of healthcare workers is the Metaverse. In addition, it also brings geographical and accessibility divides and helps the large population, as well as unites medical practitioners across the world(Bansal, G et al 2022; Dhinakaran, D et al., 2025).

2.3 Convergence of Blockchain and Metaverse

Blockchain integration into the Metaverse is therefore crucial in solving issues such as data security, privacy, and ownership, within virtual healthcare scenarios. To this end, the decentralized nature of the blockchain means that any sensitive patient data within the Metaverse space is well protected and only shareable with the right people. For instance, Blockchain can securely record and authenticate the health records of the patient seen during a teleconsultation while protecting patients' data. Blockchain also supports self-sovereign identity (SSI) whereby patients dictate their health identities in the Metaverse. Moreover, the smart contract in the blockchain system is responsible for the smooth purchase of the Metaverse services like payment for teleconsultation or virtual therapies. The integration of these technologies opens a paradigm in healthcare where the Metaverse's reality is complemented by the Blockchain's security and decentralization. Altogether, they create a solid foundation for the patient-centered, efficient, and equality-based healthcare system making the further progressive change for the delivery and experience of the services.

3. PATIENT DATA MANAGEMENT AND PRIVACY IN VIRTUAL SPACES

3.1 Challenges of Managing Patient Data

The process of managing patient information has for instance been an age old problem within conventional healthcare organizations. Much of personal health data is amassed in data stores centrally, and therefore are prone to hackers, intruders, and data leaks. This means that there is a lot of fragmented data, not well integrated to allow for effective sharing and efficient interoperability essential for the provision of appropriate and well-coordinated care. Security is a major issue here since the healthcare providers are hard pressed to meet the laws for maintaining patient data security while providing services online. Secondly, delays in data interface erode the confidence that patients and providers have in the results since they were unable to get the information they needed when they needed it (Rosaline et al., 2023).

3.2 Blockchain Solutions

These challenges are met by blockchain technology by providing a decentralised environment for handling patient information. The decentralised application offers a tamper-proof ledger meaning if data is recorded at a certain time, it cannot be altered or deleted. Blockchain makes it easily possible to share medical records with only the authorized personnel because the data is encrypted and protected through cryptographic keys that meet the POLs. (Hulsen, T (2024) Self-sovereign identity (SSI) in Blockchain helps patients manage their data with the ability to determine who gets access to it and for what reason. This also benefits the patients as well as enhances the confidence that patients have in the health sector. In addition, the openness of Blockchain guarantees that there will always be a record of who accesses the data, who changed it, and when the change was made. Smart contracts relate to the automation of data sharing arrangements which cuts costs related to compliance with privacy policies.

Figure 1. Managing Patient Data with Blockchain in Virtual Spaces

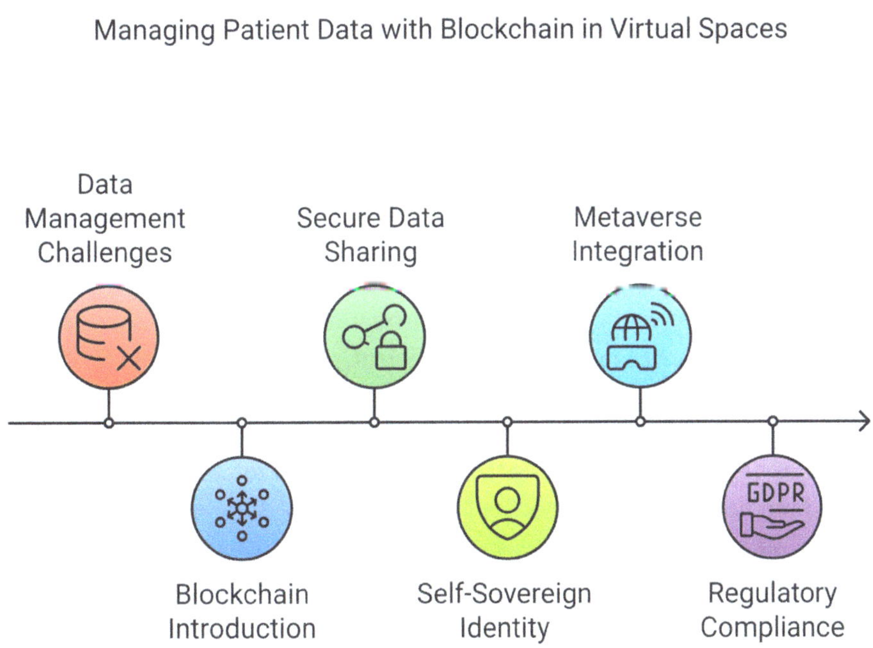

3.3 Virtual Spaces

The advent of the Metaverse means that there are increased possibilities for handling patient data in virtual space. In these environments, consultations, treatments and therapies are done virtually, and therefore, appropriate measures need to be provided to ensure privacy of sensitive health information. A major function of blockchain technology is to ensure that data exchanged in the Metaverse space is encrypted and can only be accessed by entitled parties. Blockchain also is essential for compliance with different regulations, since blockchain has an immutable record of data usage and access. This means that patients can place all their digital health records on the Blockchain and refer to them during interactions in the Metaverse. This de-centralized approach offsets the hazards of data fade that is related to central database systems. When linked with Blockchain's security functionality and the Metaverse's interactive features, healthcare providers can establish trust, safeguard the patient's identity and guarantee equal access to virtual health care. Both of these technologies provide a revolutionary approach to the problem of patient data handling in the context of increasing digitization.

4. VIRTUAL CARE DELIVERY AND TELEMEDICINE IN THE METAVERSE

4.1 Telemedicine Evolution

Telemedicine has been progressive especially over the last decade as a result of increased technology and health care needs. At first, restricted to only distant consultations, telemedicine has expanded its scope and covers diagnosis, distant patients' monitoring, and chronic diseases treatment. It got a boost during the COVID-19 pandemic because it provides efficient, scalable and remote-first models for healthcare. However, existing telemedicine models based on a traditional approach have certain problems, including data protection, patients' activity, and insufficient compatibility of platforms. Solving these problems calls for new technologies that improve both the use and quality of telehealth services.

4.2 Role of the Metaverse

Metaverse is the next generation of telemedicine solutions that provide highly engaging environments for healthcare delivery. In virtual Metaverse, doctors and clients can meet in three-dimensional avatars and work in 3D clinics, which will make the conversation more successful. This level of engagement improves the patient's comprehension of a disease or a treatment regime through illustrations and animations. (Musamih, 2022)

The Metaverse also makes it possible to use AR and VR in remote surgeries and perform real-time collaborations from different continents. Introducing the remote patient monitoring system into virtual settings means that patients and clinicians receive round-the-clock care with real-time data representation. For instance, smart wearable devices can feed health status data into the Metaverse where clinicians can use them to make decisions. These innovations employ geographic issues and enhance availability of quality services especially in the developing world.

Figure 2. Telemedicine Evolution

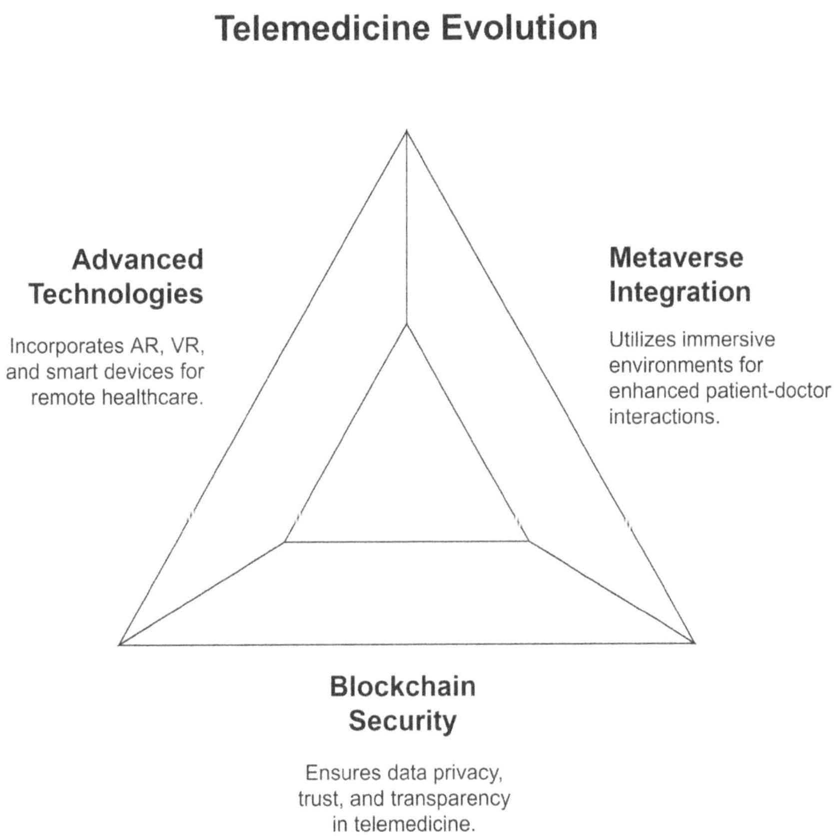

4.3 Blockchain in Telemedicine

Telemedicine services within the Metaverse require trust, privacy, and transparency, where blockchain technology provides or meets those requirements. Telehealth systems, thus, can use Blockchain to store and/or exchange patient's data as the access rights are granted only to the authorized persons/organizations. Medical records' data are fully protected under Blockchain thus eradicating the risks of having records altered or modified by unauthorized individuals.

Blockchain based smart contracts can take on repetitive activities including patient enrolment, obtaining their consent, and handling of payments so that further complexities do not hinder the process. Furthermore, Blockchain enhances the openness of interactions so that all the records can be audited hence improving the trust of the patient in virtual digital care delivery methods. (Ganapathy, K. 2022)

Combined, the Metaverse and Blockchain pave the way to the future of virtual healthcare with both highly engaging environments and safe and effective data solutions. These technologies have the potential to revolutionize the practice of telemedicine and bring ICTs to areas that have rarely or never seen them before.

5. THE SELF-SOVEREIGN IDENTITY (SSI) FOR HEALTHCARE USERS

5.1 SSI in Healthcare

Self-Sovereign Identity (SSI) is one of the new identity models that give the subject a full right of ownership over their data without any central authority regulating. In the context of healthcare, SSI allows the patient to control the health information, give or withdraw the access to it. Health care databases which are normally centralized to cater for the large number of patients storing patient records are vulnerable to data leakages and unauthorized access. SSI provides that control to patients through decentralization of their digital health identities thus privacy and security are guaranteed. It provided an opportunity to share the healthcare information on the basis of intelligent patient control, which increases the level of trust and patient's independence.

SSI can also be of help to the healthcare service providers too since it eliminates the time wasted to authenticate a patient and also offers a way for the provider to access the patient's health details. The model also increases patient involvement, which is the extent to which patients can customize their records, deciding who may access them, when, and why. It complies with the emerging concept of precision medicine, where patients can transmit concrete information to doctors but keep complete ownership of their profiles.

5.2 Blockchain Implementation

Blockchain technology is instrumental in the use of SSI to support healthcare services. Blockchain being decentralized and secure enables the development of digital identities that are both authentic and nonchangeable. Blockchain allows patient's identity details, including medical history, prescriptions, and vaccination certifications, to be stored safely and cannot be changed. This way if a patient wants to grant a healthcare provider access to his/her data, then he/she provides the key to the health information allowing only the relevant parties to read or write on the data.

As for blockchain's function in delivering SSI, it is to make a decentralised environment, which means that there is no need in checking the patient's identity and medical history by a central instance. However, the consensus mechanisms of the Blockchain guarantees the authenticity of all the information and therefore provides for the basis of accurate patient-credentialed provider interaction. (Vetrivel et al., 2024) Besides, Blockchain provides for the function of smart contracts that can handle consent management and protect patients' rights ensuring that only agreed parties will utilize patient's data and for how long.

SSI integrated with Blockchain provides a great solution to protect the patient's information and increase privacy. It means that a patient has an opportunity to manage his or her records, and, at the same time, a health care provider can be sure that he or she has corrected, verified information to make proper decisions. This way, Blockchain and SSI prevent the domination of the centralized authorities while maintaining the complete transparency and giving the power mostly to the patients and remove the obstacles in the healthcare field.

6. BLOCKCHAIN-ENABLED INTEROPERABILITY IN HEALTHCARE

6.1 Interoperability Challenges

Lack of interoperability has emerged as one of the most complicated problems that affect virtually every healthcare system around the world today. In the context of the traditional environment of healthcare organizations, medical records and data are commonly located in systems that are not integrated. Healthcare institutions such as hospitals, clinics, laboratories, insurance companies and others normally employ different applications from various vendors that have different structures and data formats. This fragmentation results to some of the delays on getting information from other care givers and ensures that patient's information is correct to avoid any mistake in the treatment that may result to harm of the patient.

Many view data silos as possibly being the most significant obstacle towards attaining perfect integration. Current systems have independently managed databases where a provider cannot easily share information or access a patient's record if this patient has been treated by other providers. (Ahmad, M et al., 2024) They also found that a lack of coordination can not only slow down diagnoses, treatment, and overall care but can also be a negative factor. Further, privacy and security become a major issue when data will be transferred between one organisation and another, and each organization has different levels of protection. Healthcare systems consequently have the double burden of dealing with scattered data while at the same time addressing data privacy and security of the patients.

6.2 Blockchain as a Solution

Blockchain addresses the main challenges in the exchange of health information more effectively compared to current existing solutions as it is a decentralized, secure, and standardized exchange of health information. Blockchain is different from the normal systems that work on the centralized data base, through the distributed ledger where data is stored at several nodes and cannot be manipulated without complete consensus. This decentralized characteristic ensures that data is safe and can only be accessed by the correct parties making healthcare organizations trust the system.

Figure 3. Blockchain-Enabled Interoperability in Healthcare

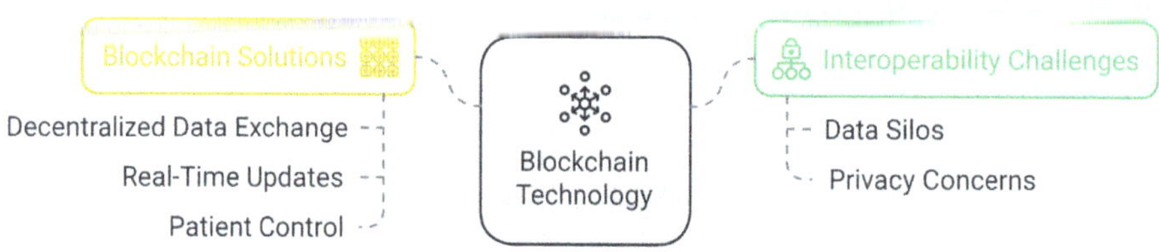

Blockchain can easily allow any kind of data sharing between different health care givers since it produces a distributed, immutable health record of all the interactions that the patient has had with the caregivers. With Blockchain, each healthcare provider gets all the verified information to make reasonable decisions taking into account the patient's complete and true medical history. Patients are able to allow providers to view some of their medical information, so they have control over their records and there is continued protection of the information.

Blockchain in healthcare can also help enhance real-time update and data validation within the systems among different party stakeholders. The smart contracts that will run on Blockchain platforms can execute data sharing protocols so that patient data can only be shared under certain protocols. This automation cuts on the many processes that are usually involved before one is attended by a health expert.

Blockchain thus removes the problem of having data silos, increases the reliability of medical records and consequently the quality of care to the patients. Blockchain technology has enormous potential for improving how different healthcare systems communicate and exchange data through secure, standard, and decentralized networks.

7. SMART CONTRACTS FOR HEALTH TRANSACTIONS AND INSURANCE

7.1 Smart Contracts Overview

Smart contracts are contracts that execute automatically where the terms and conditions of the contract are coded. These contracts have the function of automatically performing and fulfilling the provisions of an agreement where the conditions have been specified before. Smart contracts remove the middleman, including banks or legal counsellors, which lowers overhead expenses and disposal, mistakes, and time. In the healthcare sector, many activities such as patient transactions, medical records, insurance claims, as well as payments can all be automated with smart contracts, which execute the contracts based on set terms of agreement without outside interference.

Smart contracts run on blockchain that makes them secure, transparent and tamper proof. After being launched on the blockchain, the contract's provisions cannot be changed, which ensures everyone's trust. This makes it possible for all participants to have an insight of the execution process and provide guarantee to the effect that action is being taken as stated in the contact, and accountability is being uphold.

7.2 Blockchain Integration

Smart contracts integration into blockchain has great advantages for health transactions and insurance activities. Healthcare, main traditional forms of payment, and insurance claims are more often are difficult, elaborate procedures with many middlemen and high chances of mistakes or fake. Such operations, with the help of smart contracts, can be implemented through blockchain to maximise efficiency and minimise manual auditing and verifying.

In the health transactions, smart contracts can be employed to disburse of payments based on pre-defined conditions in a patient healthcare provider relation for instance, upon a medical procedure or delivery of healthcare services. For instance, in a surgery case a smart contract can state that the provider is paid after the surgery is conducted and the patient discharged. This cuts much on time and bureaucracy enabling the payments to be made on time so as to improve trust between the patients and the providers.

In insurance smart contract therefore benefits the insurance sector most especially in the area of claims section. In general, the evaluation of health insurance claims is conducted using a standard process, which may take a lot of time or contain some mistakes. (Wang, Y et al 2024) Smart contracts on blockchain technology can help to automatically check and pay the insurance claims whenever the set conditions are met, for instance where the insured persons produce their medical records or a doctor's recommendation. This automation helps to minimise fraud, speeds up the process of claim approval and improves overall performance.

Reducing intermediaries, increasing the transparency and reducing the cost of administration, smart contracts enhance the full cycle of health transactions and insurance claims. The incorporation of blockchain with smart contracts makes it even more efficient, less fraudulent but above all improves healthcare by making it safer, more transparent, and focused on patients. By means of these innovations, operation in the healthcare systems can be made much more efficient and better services can be provided to the patients and providers.

8. DIGITAL THERAPEUTICS AND VIRTUAL CARE IN THE METAVERSE

8.1 Digital Therapeutics(DT)

DT are defined as clinically endorsed therapeutic tools that are offered through and accessed by digital devices including mobile applications, software or programs. These interventions are meant to be used for the prevention, management or cure of diseases using individual patient data for treatment plans. DT can be used in chronic diseases such as diabetes, cardiovascular diseases, and mental health diseases. They provide patients an opportunity for the active participation in the treatment process, frequently including monitoring processes, behavioral changes and data analysis in the concept.

DT has several advantages such as increased access, decreased cost and the opportunity to deliver comprehensive care outside clinical environment. They can also allow for differential treatment plans, in which the patient is at liberty to embrace a specific disease or condition in the best possible way, all this as the patient complies with the practitioner prescribed intercessions. Digital therapeutics are moving to the forefront of the healthcare industry in terms of becoming an acceptable addition to traditional treatments for diseases and a potential solution to increasing the quality of patient's lives.

Figure 4. The Components and Benefits of Digital Therapeutics

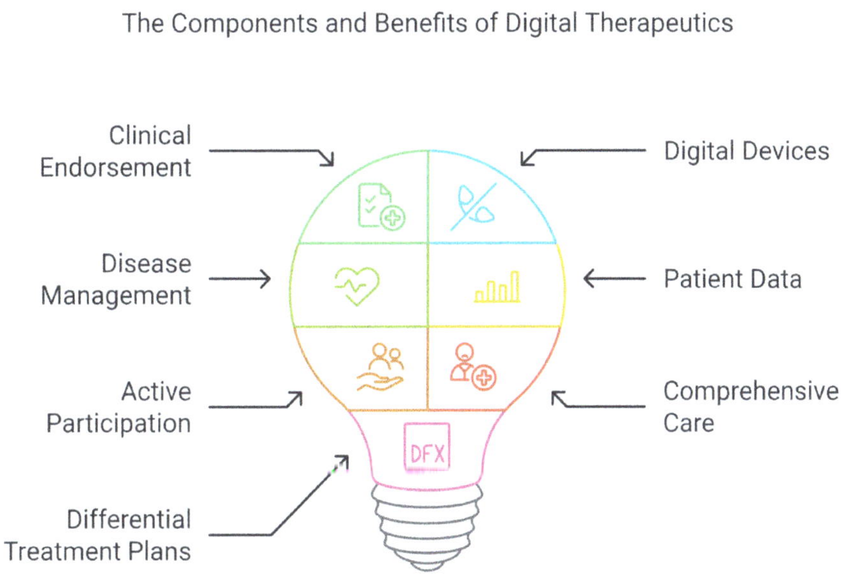

8.2 Metaverse Integration

The Metaverse, a virtual reality (VR) space consisting of digital spaces with interactive and immersive experience, can disrupt healthcare in digital therapeutics and virtual care. It is possible to perform virtual therapies, wellness programmes, and improve patient experiences and involvement through virtual 3D worlds where they can meet with healthcare providers, follow up with prescribed exercises and/or treatment regimes in a more physical way.

For example, in mental health, patient can practice CBT where through virtual reality, they face real life and learn to cope with anxiety or phobia. In the same way, concerning the physical therapy, patients can perform exercises independently and get elaborate instructions as well as have a feedback session in the Metaverse in order to make therapy enjoyable for patients. It can also give patients social support through interaction with patient support groups or other health care people in a virtual reality environment which is needed to change the location of chronic patients and mental health illness patients.

8.3 Blockchain for Digital Therapeutic

Blockchain is an important component of the proper functioning, security and transparency of digital therapeutics. Since, digital therapeutics frequently use patient data to deliver targeted treatment, protecting this information is of the essence. Blockchain allows the creation of an immutable register for patient management health records are highly secure, and only relevant parties may access them.

By integration of blockchain technology, digital therapeutics assure the patients that their information will only be shared securely with other healthcare providers, the researchers, and the patients themselves without compromising the information integrity. (Mozumder et al 2022) Further, there is also an opportunity to use smart contracts to automate the control over consent and therapeutic progress. For example, a smart contract might be used to monitor the completion of a digital therapeutics program and execute subsequent actions based on achieved objectives to minimize paper work and guarantee compliance with the treatment plan.

In conclusion, it is possible to state that the Metaverse along with a blockchain is a brand-new approach to digital therapeutics which give a chance to deliver the treatment and engage patients within immersive virtual environments. Blockchain also guarantees the safe, efficient, and transparent delivery of digital therapies to address efficiency and trust problems with such therapies.

9. SECURITY AND COMPLIANCE IN METAVERSE HEALTHCARE APPLICATIONS

9.1 Security Risks

When healthcare services move to the online platform like the Metaverse they raise massive security issues. The Metaverse refers to full-video virtual space through which healthcare services are provided and patients use avatars or interfaces to connect with their providers. This shift new exposes the healthcare industry to specific risks such as data leakage, cybercrimes, and unauthorized access to a patient's data. Since health information comprises of personal records, treatment history, and genetic information, it is important to secure health information.

Phishing, ransomware attacks, man in the middle can threaten patients' data or destabilize virtual healthcare. Further, virtual environments can also be exposed to identity theft whereby fake patients or fake healthcare professionals create an account and access patient's information. (Yang, Y et al 2023) Being based on different platforms and technologies, the Metaverse increases the attack surface almost uncontrollably to manage it effectively in terms of security threats and risks prevention. These challenges raise the question of sophisticated security solutions that can protect the patient information and privacy, as well as preserve the healthcare services credibility in the Metaverse(Priyadharshini et al., 2025; Shiny Irene et al., 2025).

9.2 Blockchain for Security

By using blockchain technology, it is possible to address a number of the security issues connected with the Metaverse when it comes to the storage of health information. Blockchain characteristic of decentralization prevents the data from being modified making it ideal to prevent alteration of patient records. This is because every transaction on the blockchain is agreed by so many nodes that hacking it in order to change data is virtually impossible.

The basic concept of blockchain, encryption, guarantees the protection of important patient information during storage and transfer. By means of cryptographic technologies, patient data can be encrypted, which means that only authorized individuals can access it. Moreover, blockchain offers protection of identity and patient's ownership of their data while also permitting certain access to healthcare providers. This approach addresses the issue of having third parties gain access into the data and guarantees that the patients' privacy is protected.

Moreover, blockchain opens up an opportunity for smart contracts in healthcare applications. These contracts include elements like patient consent that enable authorisation of use of data or participation in virtual health care services only under certain conditions. Similarly, telehealth payments can also be done automatically by the smart contract as soon as the conditions of the agreement are fulfilled so that the contract is highly secure and transparent.

10. ETHICAL AND REGULATORY CONSIDERATIONS IN THE METAVERSE

10.1Ethical Dilemmas

The incorporation of the Metaverse in the healthcare sector presents some legal challenges on privacy, consent, and AI. One of the main issues is the processing of patient data in virtual environments. In the Metaverse, healthcare providers and patients can communicate and share information in virtual environments creating new health risks for the patient's information. Preserving the patient data in these environments has to be secure and private. It is important that patient rights to privacy always be respected since health related information can be transferred from one virtual platform to another.

Several areas have also been identified, such as the concept of informed consent. The privacy of patient information received through virtual health services may not be well-understand by the patients themselves. The dilemma lies in the manner in which patients are to be educated on how the information about them will be utilized, safeguarded and even disseminated. Virtual platforms must have clear and easily understandable consent models so that the patients do not have to make the forced consent. Further, with the use of AI to make decisions for Metaverse currently it is unclear who will be accountable for bias and fairness of the decisions made. AI models being employed in virtual healthcare may recreate current bias and thus create similar inequalities in provision of care. This is the reason why steps must be taken in order to make sure that the usage of AI is ethical and the decision process is not a closed one.

Furthermore, the problems of digital divide and access should also be considered. The Metaverse uses sophisticated technology which may be unavailable or difficult to obtain for the patients especially those in the vulnerable groups, such as the elderly, low-income earners or those who have less experience working with technology gadgets. It is imperative to determine the ethical approaches to make a virtual healthcare service accessible to everyone irrespective of the issues of concerns, such as economic or technological differences.

10.2 Regulatory Frameworks

This is more so since virtual Healthcare services are likely to grow more and more as the use of Metaverse continues to grow. The existing legal requirements, while useful for conventional and physical systems of health care may not sufficiently capture the new challenges that come with virtual care. New rules have to be set in place because such technologies in healthcare environments are relatively new and have not been regulated to any extent. One of the major issues in the regulation of the Metaverse for healthcare is that these platforms must meet privacy as well as security requirements. Blockchain for example can offer a secure decentralized management of patient data but how such systems fit into current legal framework is something that may have to be determined by regulators. Further, virtual healthcare platforms need to be made to answer to the general standards of quality of care, patient safety, and non-discrimination. In addition, cross boundary regulation can be viewed as a factor that is another constraint. Since the Metaverse enables interaction across jurisdictions, healthcare givers and consumers across jurisdictions may engage in virtual health care. This complicates harmonisation of several national laws and policies over privacy, consent and data sharing. As a result, ethical and regulatory issues of virtual healthcare in the Metaverse are described in reference to privacy and consent of patients and fair use of AI. To this end, there is a need to design and formulate particular regulations that can adequately deal with these issues in the event of the use of the Metaverse in healthcare.

Figure 5. Regulatory Frameworks for Virtual Healthcare

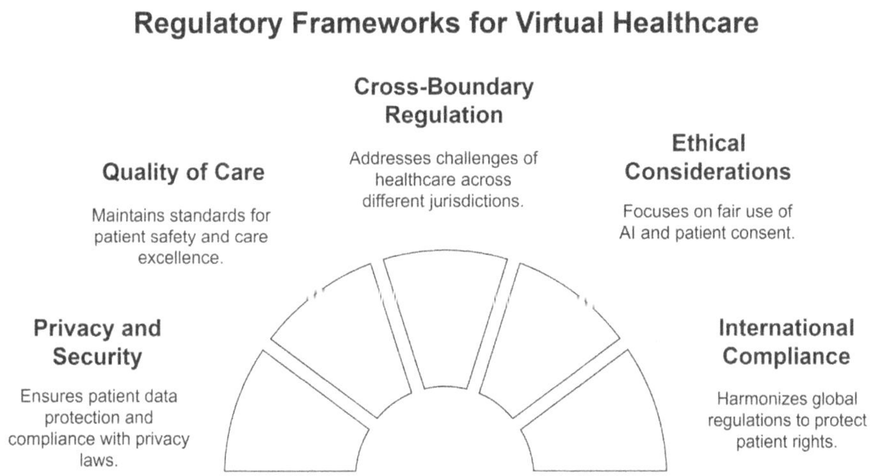

11. INNOVATIVE APPLICATION AND NEW TRENDING USAGE

11.1 Emerging Trends

When Blockchain and the Metaverse were introduced in the healthcare sector, it opened up various possibilities that are changing the current scenario. The most perspective trend is virtual clinical trials based on the use of Blockchain and Metaverse technologies to facilitate the process of trials. Some of the common issues associated with conventional clinical research include; restricted patients' accessibility, cases of compromised data credibility, and the relative difficulty of patients' anonymity. A virtual clinical trial means patients from all over the world can join a trial with a fully interactive digital environment where patients' data is recorded and transferred through the Blockchain. This saves on expenses, also expedites the recruitment process and safeguards the accuracy of trial data. Structurally, the blockchain has potentiality to preserve the data from participants in an unchallengeable manner, with clear record of consent and interactions.

Another one is artificial intelligence aided diagnosis. In virtual healthcare context, AI pattern recognition can be applied to read images or patient data for diagnosing illnesses, ranging from routine to exotic ones. In combination with the Metaverse it can be applied to virtual consultations where patient and the doctor and other diagnostic tools are in the 3D environment. Blockchain improves this process since it guarantees the safety of all the collected diagnostic information and enables free exchange of records between many different facilities.

Another major innovation is decentralised clinical research. Typically, clinical research is conducted in institutions or hospital basing it may not be diverse enough to incorporate data from different regions. Combined with the Metaverse, blockchain can facilitate organization of decentralized global research networks, that include researchers, doctors and patients. It is possible to share the data safely and receive only the necessary information at the same time; more people can get access to questionnaires and surveys, which is important for obtaining broader information and development of medical researches.

12. PRACTICAL IMPLEMENTATIONS OF BLOCKCHAIN IN HEALTHCARE

12.1 Current Implementations

The use of blockchain technology has been incorporated in many areas of healthcare to respond to problems relating to security, transparency, and efficiency.

Some of the most well-known includes patient record management as a clinical information system. Health care organizations and healthcare institutions are trying to implement blockchain for maintaining patients' electronic health records through a secure distributed network. Blockchain provide a single and immutable record for patient data that is secured and owned by the patient. Another important one is supply chain management. Some of the issues affecting the healthcare supply chain include; fraud, counterfeit and poor or even lack of traceability of the pharmaceuticals throughout the process from manufacturing to delivery. The major benefit of the Blockchain is that it offers an open ledger that can track every transaction made within the supply chain.

12.2 Challenges

However, the use of blockchain in healthcare has some challenges as explained below. Technological constraints include the issue of how Blockchain can be deployed in a clinical environment with the current structures already in place. Most healthcare facilities today still operate from their older infrastructures, which may not integrate well with Blockchain technologies hence requiring costly and extensive overhauls.

Other challenges that are likely to slow the industry's growth include regulatory problems. Inherent in blockchain technology is that it is decentralized, a model that can go against the grain of conventional legal systems that attempt to centralize data away from various publics. Current laws lack comprehensive guidelines on managing distributed data storage hence raises questions on compliance and protection of data.

One of the perpetual challenges of Blockchain in healthcare is scalability. As mentioned above, Blockchain applications manage massive data in healthcare organizations, and the ability to achieve that level of volume without affecting performance or security is a technical issue. Moreover, some of the implemented Blockchain systems can cause additional challenges in terms of scalability and sustainability when introduced to the large-scale healthcare systems at the same scale.

In conclusion, despite the success of applying Blockchain in patient record, supply chain tracking and prescription, there are several technological, regulatory and scaling issues. Eliminating these barriers shall be the critical success factor when it comes to harnessing Blockchain to its full potential in the healthcare sector.

13. AI AND MACHINE LEARNING INTEGRATION IN BLOCKCHAIN-BASED VIRTUAL HEALTHCARE IN THE METAVERSE

13.1 AI and ML in Healthcare

AI and ML are transforming the health sector through increased accuracy in diagnosis, better treatment plans and better patient solutions. AI systems can then use such raw data as medical images, patient records, and genomics data to detect the patterns and prognosis the health conditions[Sudha et al 2024]. For instance, AI's can help make diagnoses in such areas as cancer, detect features in medical images or estimate the likelihood of heart diseases from patients' information (Yamini et al 2024).

There are the following, AI leads to the automation of these processes of data analysis and Machine learning that is a part of it makes these systems learn from new data on their own (Maithili et al., 2024). ML models make predictions of the efficacy of treatments, offer advice on patients' care, and enhance patient satisfaction. Both AI and ML have been found to be most essential in the area of precision medicine since it is a medical condition that seeks to deliver treatment to a patient depending on the patient genotype. They also can perform a number of clerical procedures, manage the work of a hospital, and even improve the interaction with individuals by utilizing AI-based applications such as chatbots and assistants (Sreelakshmi et al., 2024 ;Lakumarapu et al., 2024).

13.2 Blockchain Integration

However, it is crucial to concentrate on the fact that both AI and ML contribute greatly to the improvement of healthcare, however, the key success factor for such technologies greatly depends on the availability of accurate, secure, and comprehensive data. This is where Blockchain integration comes to the rescue. Blockchain is relevant to AI and ML to improve the security of the data used in models by storing and sharing health data via a decentralized, tamper-proof ledger. The use of Blockchain in the context of AI-driven systems in healthcare guarantees that the information used to create the models is not only accurate but also secure and trustworthy since all the data fed to the AI models is transparent, and its traceability is unerring.

Moreover, Blockchain facilitates data compatibility in the sharing of patient records and information by different healthcare facilities by adhering to provisions on the protection of data. This guarantees that the models of AI and ML get to work with large and versatile datasets thus improving their performance of the predictions and the recommendations. Blockchain Also, due to its capabilities of verifying and auditing data transactions, blockchain helps avoid the use of the faulty or biased data for machine learning models, thus, making AI decision making more accurate (Subha et al., 2024 ;Ambhika et al., 2024).

13.3 Metaverse Application

The Metaverse is possibly one of the best opportunities to bolster developments in the domain of AI/ML for healthcare since it will create an environment in which patients can be accommodated virtually. Patients can encounter virtual doctors and Medical AI agents, get individualised treatment and participate in virtual health promotion activities including virtual therapy and virtual physiotherapy.

The use of AI/ML in the Metaverse will also improve virtual care services by feeding the AI/ML system with patients' real-time information drawn from their interactions in the metaverse (Selvi et al., 2024). For instance, the AI can change the environment for mental health therapy since it had shown that blue light was effective in making patients less anxious; or change the difficulty level of an exercise in physical therapy depending on the patient's improvement pattern. Blockchain guarantees the integrity and privacy of the patient data created in such environments and creates an environment in which AI models and virtual caregivers can easily and efficiently interact with each other due to privacy preservation.

Finally, it may be stated that the utilization of AI and ML in combination with Blockchain in the Metaverse will cause a transition in the healthcare industry through providing enhanced diagnostic and treatment services, as well as the protection of personal data of patients. Blockchain does more than improve the accuracy of AI decisions it also allows for the safe transfer of healthcare data through multiple systems. Metaverse enhances these possibilities with immersive and individualised care solutions based on technologies (Sudha et al., 2024).

14. USER EXPERIENCE AND ACCESSIBILITY IN BLOCKCHAIN-ENABLED HEALTHCARE SYSTEMS

14.1 UX Challenges

Optimizing the user experience in healthcare systems, especially those that are built on Blockchain and the Metaverse technologies are crucial to increasing patient and healthcare provider satisfaction. Currently, conventional health care systems have many challenges such as they are complex, integrated system are not well co-ordinated, and lack of proper access hence they are slow, lengthy, and less engaging to patients. Specifically, UX issues experienced in virtual healthcare settings relate to system interfaces, speed of access and lack of focus on the user. People requiring telecare, patients, and healthcare workers require simple, easy to operate and interpret interfaces when it comes to telehealth, records, and appointments.

There are also issues concerning data entry, how the data will fit into the existing work flow, and issues of compatibility. Such barriers may lower efficiency and impose stress on the healthcare workers, thus compromising on the quality of services to the patients. This is what makes enhancing the UX all about creating functional systems, which are easy to navigate and efficient for both users and the providers as well as aesthetically pleasant to the eyes while at it all this while at the same time ensuring that the providers do not experience undue operational difficulties in implementing the reviewed systems enough to make them wish they never embarked on the process in the first place.

14.2 Blockchain Solutions

Blockchain has potential to reduce time and enhance experience for patients in healthcare sector through providing the transparency, security and data integrity. For example, by leveraging blockchain in managing electronic health record (EHR) in healthcare enables health care providers to decrease the instances of manual data entry of information, increase automation of the processes and make sure that data is readily retrievable across various health care providers yet secure and private. Blockchain provides a shared ledger that patients and healthcare providers can use where data is immediate, transparent, and unchangeable, this removes hurdles that may hinder users from getting key health information.

14.3 Ensuring Inclusivity

Reducing the digital divide is important for making virtual healthcare services available to everyone, irrespective of ethnic background, age or physical disability or lack of funds to acquire hardware and software for home use. The use of blockchain in the healthcare sector can enhance the delivery of health care services through secure means like telemedicine, digital health, and remote health care. But there are still barriers, which include; access to high-speed internet connection, the ability to afford the devices and knowledge on how to use them.

To be inclusive for as many patients as possible, healthcare systems need to address the issue of languages and cultures, as well as to introduce user-friendly interfaces to the platform for those doctors and patients who do not have experience with the usage of the modern technology. These efforts remain crucial for changing the context of monolithic healthcare delivery, and making integrated virtual environments for everyone, who might not know much about technology or could be located far away from facilities in the developed countries.

15. FUTURE RESEARCH DIRECTIONS FOR BLOCKCHAIN IN METAVERSE HEALTHCARE

15.1 Key Research Areas

As Blockchain and the Metaverse develop, a number of specific research directions are discernible that should be explored in detail. Another imperative area of Blockchain research is the issue of Blockchain scalability. While Blockchain brings secure decentralized solutions, it provides constrained scalability to accommodate extensive healthcare data in different healthcare settings across the globe. Further study needs to be conducted to make consensus mechanisms more efficient, storage more effective, and transactions occur faster so that Blockchain technology can accommodate the demand of the healthcare industry especially in a metaverse setting where real time processing is significant and there is need for large scale integration.

A second important area that needs to be addressed specifically for Blockchain-based healthcare systems is user trust. Trust is an essential component in healthcare and Blockchain while being decentralized presents issues to do with openness, responsibility and ease to use. Research should be directed towards the following topics, User authentication, identity verification, and privacy in decentralized environments. Furthermore, trust in automated processes, like smart contracts or artificial intelligent computerized healthcare assistants, will need innovation through interdisciplinary collaboration with methods on how to secure data, especially in the field of sensitive health data.

There is also a need to address the growth of Blockchain in the Metaverse application as well as explore more potentials to apply Blockchain. Blockchain has been applied in such areas as patient data, telemedicine, and drugs traceability; however, other areas of healthcare may also benefit from blockchain as well. Further studies can evaluate new uses of Blockchain in virtual clinical trials, medical data sharing, and patient-led health projects as well as consider using Blockchain with other advanced technologies including IoT, 5G, and wearable health- related devices to foster an interrelated, efficient health system (Subramanian et al., 2025).

15.2 Vision for the Future

That is why the synthesis of the Blockchain and Metaverse trends may bring global changes in the field of healthcare in the future. More than ever, as Blockchain scales up, gets more secure, and efficient, or when the Metaverse grows to be a more real environment, virtual healthcare could become more normalized, mainstream, and even more personalized. As mentioned, through decentralised healthcare networks, the Metaverse can offer virtual doctor's appointments and virtual surgeries, country-to-country cooperations, and overall, an opportunity for people worldwide to receive proper treatment.

The future vision of this case could be that patients could own all their health data through SSI and share it securely with the healthcare providers using Blockchain. Physicians and other healthcare practitioners and students could leverage the Metaverse for actual and simulation-based clinical practice while patients could also rely on virtual health and wellness programs, digital medicine, and constant remote real-time tracking by Internet of Things devices. These would all be supported by blockchain technology to provide the authenticity, privacy, and security, as well as removing waste in the health care system.

In conclusion, Blockchain and Metaverse integration might unlock the best of possible healthcare systems and revolutionize medicine for the better worldwide provision of better patient data privacy and the ability to offer unique patient-centered care to a level that the world has never seen before. This vision will also need to be constantly investigated, cannot be achieved in isolation of other disciplines and is ahead of its time because of the issues that have to do with regulations, security, and ethical considerations.

16.CONCLUSION

In this chapter, we sought to find out how Blockchain and the Metaverse are set to transform the healthcare sector. Major conclusions show that Blockchain characteristics, namely decentralization and security, can solve the healthcare problems including data ownership, privacy, and integration. The Metaverse with its virtual reality environments is a great potential for increasing the level of patient's involvement, using virtual consultations, surgeries, and precise care. Altogether, these technologies can build a new, efficient, open, and accessible healthcare system. The prospects of Blockchain and the Metaverse when it comes to health care are enormous. Blockchain can bring patients' control over their data through Self-Sovereign Identities (SSI) while making the data secure and private. Healthcare may be delivered and enhanced in the Metaverse through impacting patient and health care consumer engagement; and through the delivery of wellness programs and real-time monitoring. These will enhance efficiency, mitigate fraud and enhance data quality particularly in telemedicine and digital therapeutics.

However, there are still certain issues arising from the application of Blockchain and Metaverse technology in health care. Several technical challenges that come with implementing the system including scalability, compatibility with existing systems, and legal requirements come into question. In addition, the legal issues related to patient's consent, patients' privacy and the security of virtual environments are worth noting. However, the prospects offered by these technologies are vast despite the challenges described herein. The future of care in virtual space will strengthen the general and patient-oriented access to healthcare and medical services for patients of different parts of the world. Through continuous research, Blockchain and the Metaverse offer better frameworks for enhancing the healthcare delivery system to become more secure and efficient in the future years.

REFERENCES

Ahmad, M., Bangash, S. A., Shah, S. S., Chemingui, H., & Abubakar, M. (2024). Revolutionizing Healthcare in the Metaverse: The Power of Blockchain. In *Examining the Metaverse in Healthcare: Opportunities, Challenges, and Future Directions* (pp. 51-76). IGI Global.

Ali, S., Abdullah, Armand, T. P. T., Athar, A., Hussain, A., Ali, M., ... & Kim, H. C. (2023). Metaverse in healthcare integrated with explainable AI and blockchain: Enabling immersiveness, ensuring trust, and providing patient data security. *Sensors (Basel)*, *23*(2), 565.

Ambhika, C., Gayathri, S., & Sheena, B. G. (2024, August). Enhancing predictive modeling in high dimensional data using hybrid feature selection. In *2024 5th International Conference on Electronics and Sustainable Communication Systems (ICESC)* (pp. 873-879). IEEE.

Bansal, G., Rajgopal, K., Chamola, V., Xiong, Z., & Niyato, D. (2022). Healthcare in metaverse: A survey on current metaverse applications in healthcare. *IEEE Access : Practical Innovations, Open Solutions*, *10*, 119914–119946.

Dhinakaran, D., Kumar, N. J., & Ponnuviji, N. P. (2025). Safeguarding confidentiality and privacy in cloud-enabled healthcare systems with spectrasafe encryption and dynamic k-anonymity algorithm. *Expert Systems with Applications*, *279*, 127584.

Ganapathy, K. (2022). Metaverse and healthcare: A clinician's perspective. *Apollo Medicine*, *19*(4), 256–261.

Hulsen, T. (2024). Applications of the metaverse in medicine and healthcare. *Advances in Laboratory Medicine/Avances en Medicina De Laboratorio, 5*(2), 159-165.

Lakumarapu, S., Nithyanandhan, R., Bhargavi, V. S., & TP, A. (2024, August). Machine Learning Approaches for Liver Disease Prediction: A Comparative Analysis. In *2024 5th International Conference on Electronics and Sustainable Communication Systems (ICESC)* (pp. 159-164). IEEE.

Maithili, K., Ponmalar, A., Yamini, B., Karthikeyan, M., Anish, T. P., Maheswari, B., & Subramanian, R. S. (2024). Advances in AI and Machine Learning for Healthcare Informatics. In *Machine Learning and Generative AI in Smart Healthcare* (pp. 1–22). IGI Global.

Mozumder, M. A. I., Sheeraz, M. M., Athar, A., Aich, S., & Kim, H. C. (2022, February). Overview: Technology roadmap of the future trend of metaverse based on IoT, blockchain, AI technique, and medical domain metaverse activity. In *2022 24th International Conference on Advanced Communication Technology (ICACT)* (pp. 256-261). IEEE.

Musamih, A., Yaqoob, I., Salah, K., Jayaraman, R., Al-Hammadi, Y., Omar, M., & Ellahham, S. (2022). Metaverse in healthcare: Applications, challenges, and future directions. *IEEE Consumer Electronics Magazine*, *12*(4), 33–46.

Ponnuviji, N. P., Elangovan, G., Sujatha, K., Jambulingam, U., Ganesan, I., & Lalitha, S. D. (2024). IoT-Enabled Assistive Technologies Approach for Personalized Geriatric Health Monitoring and Safety. In *Future of AI in Biomedicine and Biotechnology* (pp. 125–146). IGI Global.

Priyadharshini, S. I., Irene, D. S., Beulah, J. R., & Ponnuviji, N. P. (2025). Enhancing real-time health monitoring with hybrid recurrent long short-term tyrannosaurus search for menstrual cups. *Biomedical Signal Processing and Control*, *100*, 107065.

Rosaline, R. A. A., & Ponnuviji, N. P., TC, S. L., & Manisha, G. (2023). Enhancing lifestyle and health monitoring of elderly populations using CSA-TkELM classifier. *Knowledge-Based Systems*, *276*, 110758.

Selvi, D. K., Aswini, J., Balakrishnan, C., Suganya, K., & Sheena, B. G. (2024, May). Revolutionizing cardiovascular care: The role of AI, ML, and DL in early heart disease prediction and treatment. In *2024 International Conference on Electronics, Computing, Communication and Control Technology (ICECCC)* (pp. 1-6). IEEE.

Shiny Irene, D., Ponnuviji, N. P., & Kalaivani, A. (2025). EHECA-HSWS: A Holistic Method for Improving Menstrual Health App User Experience. *Journal of the Institution of Electronics and Telecommunication Engineers*, •••, 1–12.

Sreelakshmi, S., Babu, A. A., Lakshmipriya, C., Gracious, L. A., Nalini, M., & Subramanian, R. S. (2024, October). Enhancing Intrusion Detection Systems with Machine Learning. In 2024 2nd International Conference on Self Sustainable Artificial Intelligence Systems (ICSSAS) (pp. 557-564). IEEE.

Subha, S., Balakrishnan, C., & Anish, T. P. (2024, August). Optimizing Machine Learning Algorithms for Heart Disease Prediction in Healthcare: A Comparative Study. In *2024 5th International Conference on Electronics and Sustainable Communication Systems (ICESC)* (pp. 866-872). IEEE.

Subramanian, R. S., Ramana, T. V., Ramana, K. V., Prabha, S., & Nivaskumar, V. (2025). Converging Horizons: Synergies of 6G Wireless Communication, Machine Learning, and Embedded Systems for Intelligent Connectivity. *The Intersection of 6G, AI/Machine Learning, and Embedded Systems*, 67-93.

Sudha, K., Lakshmipriya, C., Pajila, P. B., Venitha, E., & Anita, M. (2024, January). Enhancing Diabetes Prediction and Management through Machine Learning: A Comparative Study. In *2024 Fourth International Conference on Advances in Electrical, Computing, Communication and Sustainable Technologies (ICAECT)* (pp. 1-6). IEEE.

Sudha, K., Nithyanandhan, R., Girija, P., & Nalini, M. (2024, July). Enhancing Healthcare Data Security in the Cloud: Integrating ML-Based Intrusion Detection Systems. In *2024 2nd World Conference on Communication & Computing (WCONF)* (pp. 1-7). IEEE.

Vetrivel, S. C., & Mohanasundaram, T. (2024). Blockchain-empowered metaverse healthcare systems and applications. *Digital Transformation in Healthcare 5.0: Volume 2: Metaverse, Nanorobots and Machine Learning*, 61.

Wang, Y., Zhu, M., Chen, X., Liu, R., Ge, J., Song, Y., & Yu, G. (2024). The application of metaverse in healthcare. *Frontiers in Public Health*, *12*, 1420367.

Yamini, B., Saraswathi, T., Radhakrishnan, P., Nalini, M., Shanmuganathan, M., & Siva, S. R. (2024). Machine learning algorithms for predicting of chronic kidney disease and its significance in healthcare. *International Journal of Advanced Technology and Engineering Exploration*, *11*(112), 388.

Yang, Y., Zhou, Z., Li, X., Xue, X., Hung, P. C., & Yangui, S. (2023). Metaverse for healthcare: Technologies, challenges, and vision. *International Journal of Crowd Science*, *7*(4), 190–199.

Chapter 2

Blockchain Technology in Healthcare: Transforming Data Management and Security

Priya Tanwar
https://orcid.org/0000-0002-8361-247X
Manav Rachna International Institute of Research and Studies, India

Neha Gupta
https://orcid.org/0000-0003-0905-5457
Manav Rachna International Institute of Research and Studies, India

ABSTRACT

As one of the most disruptive forces across industries, blockchain technology holds immense promise for the healthcare sector. In this chapter, we will discuss the advantages, applications, and challenges of integrating blockchain into healthcare systems. The chapter opens by outlining the key features of blockchain technology, highlighting its decentralization, immutability, and transparency. It then looks at individual use cases in health care, such as patient data management, drug traceability, and supply chain logistics. The ethical and legal implications of using blockchain in healthcare with a particular emphasis on patient confidentiality and consent. Case studies from real life and existing efforts are utilized to show the potential of blockchain-based solutions in healthcare. This chapter aims to provide researchers, medical professionals, and policymakers with a comprehensive understanding of blockchain's potential to improve the management of healthcare information and security, as well as insights into the challenges and concerns associated with its implementation.

DOI: 10.4018/979-8-3373-1225-5.ch002

1.1. INTRODUCTION

Blockchain technology is emerging as a transformative force in a variety of industries, maybe most notably healthcare. Blockchain may be classified into three types, as illustrated in Figure 1: public, private, and consortium, each having distinct characteristics suitable for diverse healthcare applications.

Figure 1. Types of Blockchain Architectures in Healthcare

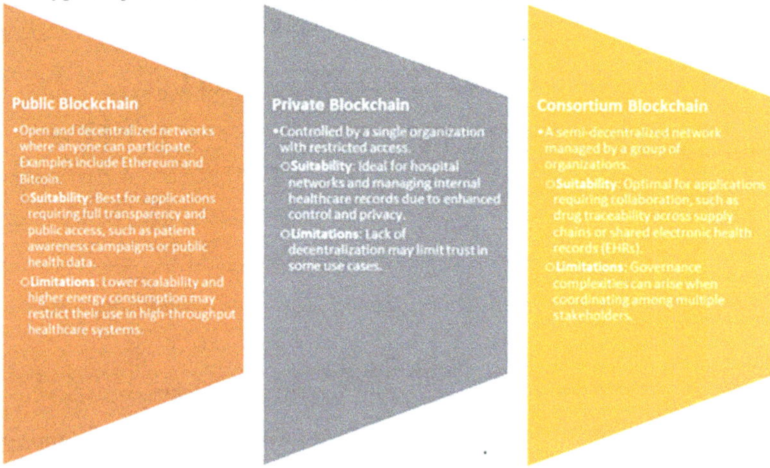

The healthcare industry has long grappled with issues of data security, interoperability, and patient privacy. In this era of digital transformation. The need for innovative solutions to address challenges has never been more pressing. Blockchain, originally developed as the basic technology driving cryptocurrency, has proven to be a formidable contender in redefining the way healthcare data is maintained and kept safe.

The healthcare industry is known for its complexities and intricacies, with vast amounts of sensitive patient data generated and exchanged among numerous Stakeholders, including patients, healthcare professionals, insurance, and pharmaceutical corporations. Protecting this data from unauthorized access, ensuring its accuracy, and enabling seamless, secure data sharing have been formidable challenges. Blockchain technology, with its decentralized (No single authority controls the system), immutable cannot be changed once added to the blockchain). and transparent (All stakeholders can view and verify the transaction history) ledger, holds the promise of transforming the healthcare landscape in profound ways.

This chapter strives to offer a detailed analysis of the impact of blockchain on health care data management and security. It also references blockchain features (e.g., immutability; smart contract) that hold promise for enabling secure and efficient data security support for healthcare processes. Then it gets further into the critical issues around patient privacy and consent management, and how blockchain here is delivering powerful solutions.

The chapter also considers the challenges of healthcare data interoperability, which has traditionally been a challenge in that specific area. The capacity of blockchain to serve as a single shared source of truth and enable secure data sharing between multiple healthcare systems is noteworthy.

In the first part of this ride from blockchain and health, usages, projects in progress, and the legal and regulatory environment that enables and slows down the blockchain integration as a disruption. As this chapter's readers may have grasped the revolutionary contributions of blockchain in health care, a way forward for a secure, scalable, patient-centric health care environment is provided.

The following discussion should be helpful for researchers, doctors, politicians, and IT professionals discovering the world of blockchain in healthcare. As we examine the potential for blockchain in healthcare, the opportunities for revolutionising an industry reach new levels of possibility. Figure 2: Integrity and interoperability between diverse distributed systems with the help of blockchain technology and its decentralized, tamper-resistant, and transparent ledger structure.

Figure 2. Components for Ensuring Data Integrity

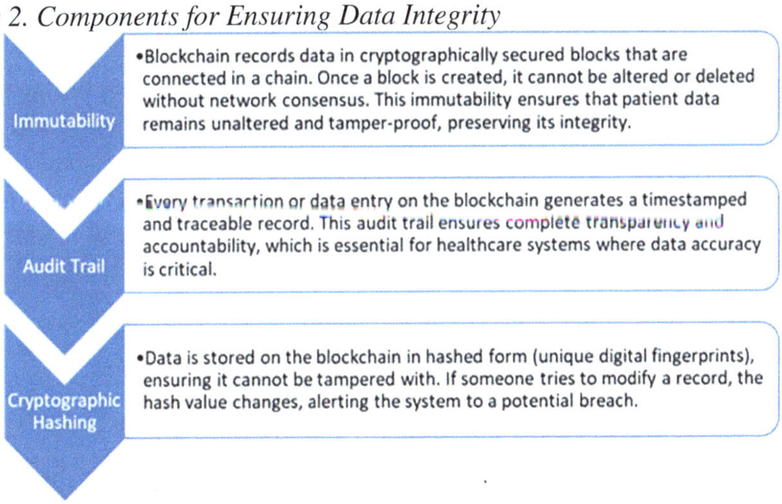

Example: Healthcare providers can store patient records on a blockchain to preserve the accuracy of data. And should a hospital try to rewrite a person's history, the blockchain ledger will red flag the change because it doesn't correspond with the cryptographic hash of the original data. Blockchain facilitates the free connection of systems by providing a single registry for secure data exchange among various healthcare systems (as in Figure 3: which can be of incompatible formatting and databases. Example: A patient from a private clinic can keep his clinical record safe

Figure 3. Key Benefits of Blockchain in Healthcare Data Management

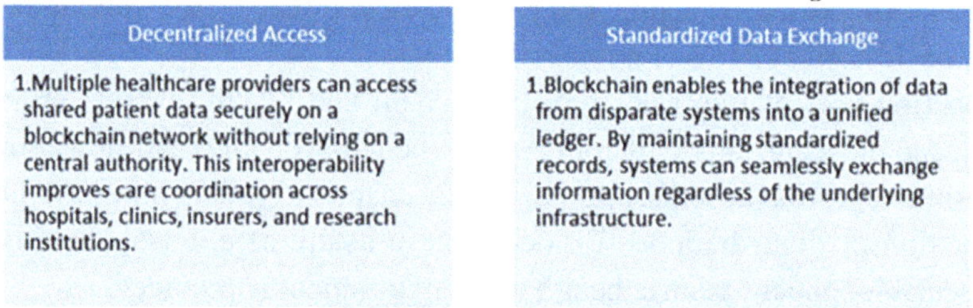

Example: A patient receiving therapy at a private clinic can share their medical records with a government hospital in a secure, permissioned manner through a blockchain network such that the continuity of care is maintained and yet with privacy.

1.2 SMART CONTRACTS

Smart contracts are self-executing contracts where the terms of the agreement is implemented automatically in the event that specified terms are met and are recorded on a blockchain. To mention also a healthcare application, in smart contracts are used for controlling patient consent and access to confidential medical data, as illustrated in Figure 4.

Figure 4. Blockchain-Based Patient Consent Management and Access Control

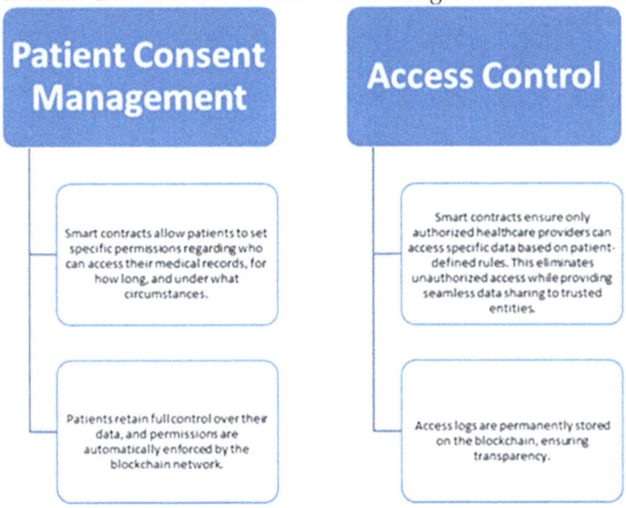

Example: A research organization is given authorization by a patient to use the patient's deidentified medical history for a 6-month study. Historic consent storage. After 6 months of expiry, the access is withdrawn automatically by the smart contract, and then it comes under Patient Consent Management. And when a specialist requests to review a patient's diagnostic data. Smart contract verifies the authenticity of the specialist and the permission of the patient and grants access. If the specialist exceeds their authorization, access is removed right away. This is equivalent to Access Control.

It's the blockchain that supplies us with the integrity of our data (which comes from such things as immutability, hashing, and auditable transactions) and interoperability (which is derived from a shared, peer-to-peer platform). Smart contracts facilitate the optimal handling of patient consent and access by making them secure and transparent, which in turn gives patients secure and transparent control over their data. That respect (disruptive tech) re-revolutionizes trust and cooperation within health care ecosystems.

1.3 PATIENT PRIVACY CONCERNS AND BLOCKCHAIN

The greater use of blockchain in healthcare is anticipated to help address some of the key challenges, such as data integrity, interoperability, and secure patient records. However, despite blockchain operating in terms of transparency and trust, there is a great need to ensure the patient's privacy. It can be seen that the perfect point of transparency and privacy is difficult to achieve in the healthcare blockchain (as depicted in Figure 5).

Figure 5. Central Issues of Patient Privacy in Blockchain-Enabled Healthcare

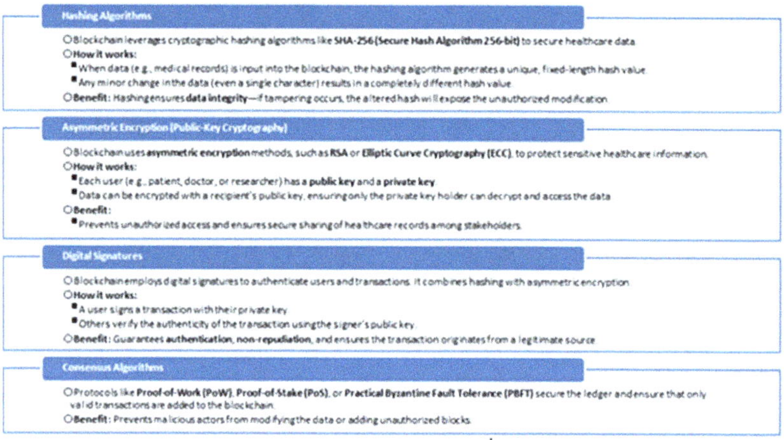
Hashing Algorithms
Blockchain leverages cryptographic hashing algorithms like SHA-256 (Secure Hash Algorithm 256-bit) to secure healthcare data
How it works:
When data (e.g., medical records) is input into the blockchain, the hashing algorithm generates a unique, fixed-length hash value
Any minor change in the data (even a single character) results in a completely different hash value
Benefit: Hashing ensures data integrity—if tampering occurs, the altered hash will expose the unauthorized modification
Asymmetric Encryption (Public-Key Cryptography)
Blockchain uses asymmetric encryption methods, such as RSA or Elliptic Curve Cryptography (ECC), to protect sensitive healthcare information
How it works:
Each user (e.g., patient, doctor, or researcher) has a public key and a private key
Data can be encrypted with a recipient's public key, ensuring only the private key holder can decrypt and access the data
Benefit:
Prevents unauthorized access and ensures secure sharing of healthcare records among stakeholders
Digital Signatures
Blockchain employs digital signatures to authenticate users and transactions. It combines hashing with asymmetric encryption
How it works:
A user signs a transaction with their private key
Others verify the authenticity of the transaction using the signer's public key
Benefit: Guarantees authentication, non-repudiation, and ensures the transaction originates from a legitimate source
Consensus Algorithms
Protocols like Proof-of-Work (PoW), Proof-of-Stake (PoS), or Practical Byzantine Fault Tolerance (PBFT) secure the ledger and ensure that only valid transactions are added to the blockchain
Benefit: Prevents malicious actors from modifying the data or adding unauthorized blocks

Transparency vs. Confidentiality in Blockchain

The issue of transparency vs. confidentiality is evident in Blockchain Centralization, Security, and Privacy. One of the main pitfalls of traditional healthcare systems is the centralization of data, resulting in security problems, including unauthorized access and single failure points.

Blockchain disintermediates data, in the process removing these issues of centralization. That way, no one person can take control over a single source of truth, and there is more visibility and trust. But the transparency of blockchain — when all nodes on the network verify transactions and see the ledger — is problematic with health care data. For instance, when it comes to patient records, they must comply with HIPAA (Health Insurance Portability and Accountability Act) and GDPR (General Data Protection Regulation). To mitigate this, blockchain-based systems utilize cryptographic techniques such as:

- **Zero-Knowledge Proofs (ZKP):** Allow verification of a transaction without revealing underlying data.
- **Encryption (e.g., asymmetric encryption):** Ensures that only authorized parties with private keys can access patient data.

- **Off-Chain:** Off-Chain Storage Sensitive data, such as detailed patient medical records, can be stored off-chain, and only secure metadata or hash value will be placed on chain for validation.

These are the solutions that enable blockchain to stay transparent, ensuring the validation and integrity of the data while securing the confidence of the patient.

Challenges in Patient Consent in Decentralized Environments

Another strong requirement is to obtain and manage patients' consent in healthcare systems based on blockchain. Centralized approaches take the first approach, simplifying the process by having the healthcare providers obtain consent directly from the patients. In a distributed setting, the control of consents is made even more complex by a heterogeneous topology of the network. Key challenges include:

Fine-grained Consent Control: A patient might want to approve access every time data is used (eg, research project, doctor visit) rather than providing blanket permission. Consent management might be automated with the help of smart contracts, although steering more fine-grained policies is challenging.

No revocability of consents: Even if a patient wants to withdraw consent, the immutability of a blockchain is in conflict with the revocation of consent by the patient. Proposed solutions were on-time, limited smart contracts, and off-chain references, though it is not a general practice.

1.4 LITERATURE REVIEW

Recent advances towards the introduction of blockchain-based technologies into health IT systems have brought more focus on potential solutions to patients' privacy, interoperability, and security, with which healthcare has historically faced. The decentralized nature of blockchain has received much attention as it is considered a candidate solution to profile heterogeneity and redundant traditional data management. But, as digital health records and telemedicine have taken off, so have fears of data breaches and illicit access, leading experts to consider how blockchain could be used to boost trust, transparency, and control. In this context, a growing corpus of research has been conducted to investigate the manner in which blockchain-based solutions have been developed, implemented, and evaluated in a variety of healthcare contexts, as shown in Table 1.

Table 1. Literature Review

Author(s) and Year	Summary	Research Findings	Research Gaps
Jayabalan & Jeyanthi (2022)	A scalable blockchain model using IPFS storage was proposed for better privacy and data security in healthcare.	Better privacy and scalability were achieved using off-chain IPFS storage.	Real-world implementation and cost-effectiveness were not tested.
Kumar et al. (2022)	A decentralized blockchain design was developed to protect healthcare data from cyberattacks.	High resistance to cyberattacks and better privacy were ensured.	Scalability and regulatory concerns were not deeply explored.
Siyal et al. (2019)	Challenges and future uses of blockchain in medicine were explored in detail.	Practical barriers and adoption challenges were pointed out.	Empirical validation and user adoption studies were missing.
Zaabar et al. (2021)	A secure blockchain-based system named HealthBlock was introduced for managing healthcare data.	Secure and efficient healthcare data exchange was enabled.	Limited discussion on integration with legacy systems was found.
Prybutok & Sauser (2022)	Both theoretical ideas and real-world uses of blockchain in healthcare information systems were reviewed.	Both academic and industrial implications of blockchain were clarified.	Real-time implementation outcomes were not shown.
Dimitrov (2019)	Various blockchain applications for handling healthcare data were described.	Improved data control and integrity were demonstrated.	User-centric design and large-scale case studies were not provided.
Attaran (2022)	Opportunities and difficulties in using blockchain in healthcare were examined.	Adoption challenges in real-world healthcare were emphasized.	Policy and ethical concerns were not fully addressed.
Rajawat et al. (2022)	The use of AI and blockchain together for healthcare security in smart cities was studied.	Enhanced data security through AI-blockchain integration was shown.	Practical deployment challenges in diverse cities were not examined.
Farouk et al. (2020)	A vision for blockchain use in industrial healthcare systems was presented.	A futuristic vision for blockchain in healthcare was proposed.	Technical feasibility under varied conditions was not assessed.
Yaqoob et al. (2021)	Opportunities, issues, and suggestions for blockchain in healthcare data were discussed.	Clear benefits with integration challenges were identified.	Standardization and regulatory frameworks were not detailed.
Alhadhrami et al. (2017)	The idea of using blockchain in healthcare settings was introduced.	Basic blockchain concepts for healthcare were introduced.	Practical deployment steps were not discussed.
Linn & Koo (2016)	Early views on how blockchain could help health IT and research were shared.	Potential uses in research and IT management were explained.	Comprehensive data on implementation effects was missing.
Angraal et al. (2017)	Applications of blockchain in various areas of healthcare were highlighted.	Various real-time healthcare applications were mentioned.	Security limitations and data standard challenges remained unexplored.

continued on following page

Table 1. Continued

Author(s) and Year	Summary	Research Findings	Research Gaps
Ahram et al. (2017)	New ideas in blockchain technology and their healthcare impact were explored.	Conceptual innovations with healthcare relevance were discussed.	Scalability and healthcare compliance standards were not evaluated.
Chen et al. (2019)	A patient-centered blockchain model was proposed for improving data access.	Patient ownership and secure access to data were supported.	Wide-scale testing and adoption readiness were not reviewed.
Ben Fekih & Lahami (2020)	A detailed study of blockchain uses in healthcare was performed.	Different use cases and advantages were categorized.	Impact on healthcare equity and access was not addressed.
Pandey & Litoriya (2020)	Problems in large-scale healthcare service delivery and blockchain-based solutions were discussed.	Barriers to scaling blockchain in healthcare were noted.	Performance under stress or emergency situations was not studied.
Sharma et al. (2021)	A distributed healthcare application using blockchain called Healthify was presented.	Improved patient data sharing was demonstrated.	Real-time privacy risks and usability issues were overlooked.
Qiu et al. (2018)	A blockchain-based secure and smart healthcare system for smart cities was designed.	Smart healthcare system features using blockchain were designed.	Adoption across different healthcare systems was not studied.
Tandon et al. (2020)	A full review and future roadmap for blockchain in healthcare were created.	A synthesized framework and future roadmap were developed.	Dynamic patient needs and stakeholder feedback were underexplored.

1.5 TOWARD A BALANCED APPROACH

To effectively balance transparency and confidentiality while addressing consent management challenges, blockchain healthcare systems must adopt hybrid approaches:

- **Permissioned Blockchains:** Unlike public blockchains, permissioned systems restrict access to validated participants, providing enhanced privacy.
- **Privacy-Preserving Protocols:** Techniques like homomorphic encryption and secure multi-party computation (SMPC) allow computations on encrypted data without revealing sensitive information.
- **Dynamic Consent Models:** Combining smart contracts with user-friendly interfaces can enable patients to grant, monitor, and revoke consent dynamically.

By employing the said means in parallel, blockchain can meet both ends of having patient data privacy and data integrity/security. While Blockchain holds great potential for successfully managing health data, striking a balance between transparency and data privacy is currently problematic. Powerful consent, protection of patients' data, and user-orientation are the keys to success. The balance can be struck with cryptological advances, hybrid models that allow for secure, transparent, patient-oriented health solutions. Cryptographic techniques in the blockchain for securing the patients' health information, emphasizing on its private ledger mechanism.

1.6 CRYPTOGRAPHIC METHODS

Blockchain combines hashing, asymmetric encryption, and consensus for the security of healthcare data, as in Figure 6. The decentralized, non-mutable data value storage in the source data based on blockchain and secured access to the data without unauthorized tampering allows for a system for sharing confidential healthcare information.

Figure 6. Core Cryptographic Techniques Enabling Blockchain Security in Healthcare

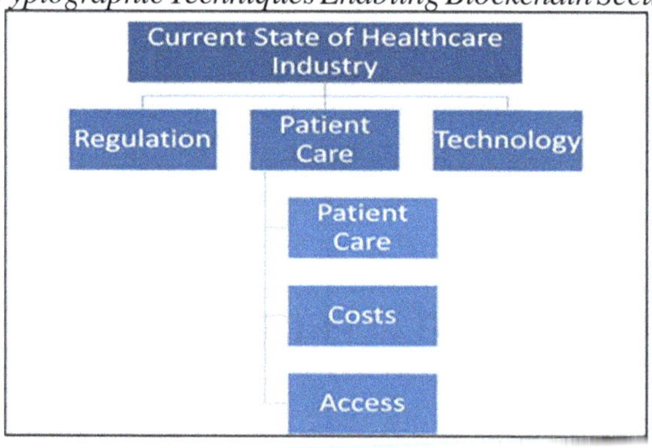

1.7 HOW BLOCKCHAIN'S LEDGER SYSTEM MITIGATES RISKS

It also offers insight into four major functionalities of blockchain in healthcare, viz, Data Tampering Prevention, Decentralization, Access Control, and Auditability with Transparency (Figure 7). The two sections are "designed to demonstrate how blockchain technology enhances the security and trust of data."

Figure 7. Blockchain Safeguards

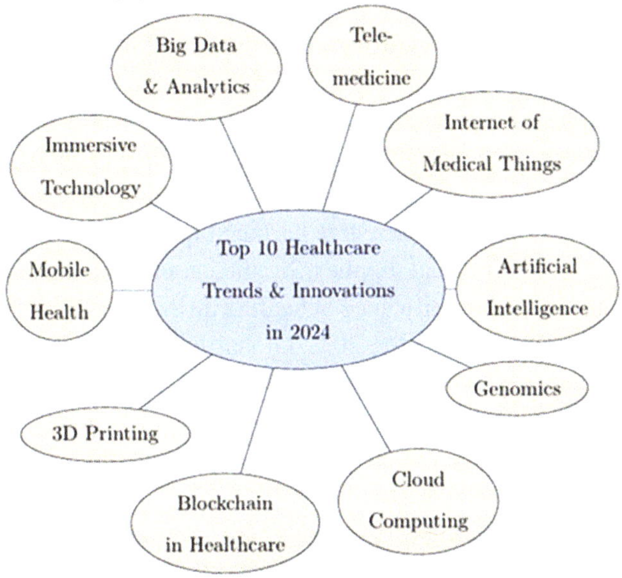

Data tampering protection: Blockchain is constructed on a decentralized and immutable ledger, where any transaction (e.g., healthcare data updates) is stored in a cryptographically protected block. The connecting thread between each block and its predecessor is the hash, binding them all together in a "chain". An attempt to edit a block will produce another hash, breaking the chain, and on it will go, destroying the network.

Appropriate use of Decentralization: Typical centralized databases can be easily hacked, and they are a single point of failure. In blockchains, there does not exist any central ledger; rather, each node keeps a ledger, and ledgers are broken (block initialization) and dispersed across all nodes.

Access Control: Health data can be accessed without permission using smart contracts and encryption. No one else, except for the holder of the appropriate cryptographic keys, can read or write data.

Auditability and Transparency: Blockchain maintains a transparent, chronological record of all transactions, making it easy to audit healthcare data while ensuring privacy through encryption.

1.8 CURRENT STATE OF THE HEALTHCARE INDUSTRY

The worldwide healthcare industry is persistently confronting the challenges posed by the ongoing pandemic, which demands constant attention and allocation of resources from healthcare systems. These organizations are diligently working to enhance the health of their staff, redefining the nature, methods, and locations of work, and rapidly expanding virtual healthcare services for patients. Also, they are focusing on establishing collaborative partnerships to manufacture and procure essential vaccines, treatments, and supplies. Simultaneously, healthcare organizations are addressing the growing significance of healthcare disparities, sustainability, and environmental concerns. As per the 2022 Global Healthcare Outlook report, the current status of the global healthcare sector has been assessed and focused on six critical sector issues, outlining actionable strategies to enhance resilience and strive for enhanced healthcare results in the years after the pandemic. Key parameters of the healthcare industry are illustrated in Figure 8.

The COVID-19 pandemic has expedited the advancement of various pre-existing or emerging trends in the healthcare sector. Notably, these trends encompass issues related to health equity, environmental sustainability, and the integration of life sciences into healthcare. Furthermore, healthcare executives worldwide remain focused on addressing shifting consumer preferences and behaviours, the swift evolution of digital health technologies, the introduction of new talent and care delivery models, as well as ongoing clinical innovations. Managing these challenges while concurrently addressing the ongoing pandemic will be of paramount significance in the year 2022. Figure 8 shows the main parameters that play a major role in the healthcare industry, including regulation, patient care, and technology.

Figure 8. An illustration of key parameters of the healthcare industry

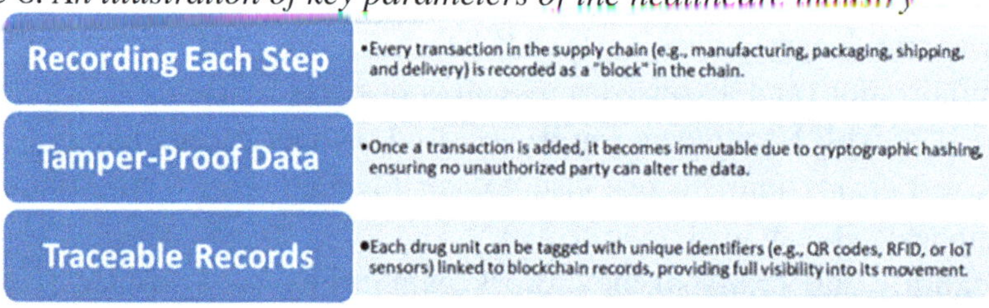

1.8.1. What is one current industry trend in healthcare?

Innovations in healthcare encompass a wide spectrum, including electronic consultations, telemedicine, instant diagnostics, and the availability of digital therapeutics through immersive technology tools. Progress in healthcare technology, such as genetic analysis and the utilization of big data and analytics, has paved the way for precision medicine.

These solutions are being developed very quickly in response to the novel coronavirus Covid-19 pandemic and span disinfection, transmission control, disease detection, treatment, patient engagement, and immunity." These innovative healthcare technologies are e-consultations, m-telemedicine, real-time diagnostics, and marrying digital therapeutics with immersive technology-based interventions.

There have been tremendous technological developments in health care, particularly in genetics, clinical data archiving, and big data analytics, on which precision medicine is built. Enterprising startups have leveraged these advances to tailor care to the patient, thanks to the use of real-time remote monitoring devices.

This convergence of AI, the IoT, and enhanced data management is helping to transform hospitals into more intelligent health facilities. As well as facilitating best workflows and staffing, the solutions also link infrastructure, devices, and systems, which deployment agencies and SEND providers also have oversight of, so that the right services can be delivered as quickly as possible, which supports this.

1.8.2. Top 10 Healthcare Trends & Innovations in 2024

In healthcare, it is imperative to stay at the forefront of emerging trends and innovations. In this section, the top 10 transformative trends that are projected to shape the healthcare industry in 2024 are discussed. Figure 9 shows the current trends and areas for the healthcare industry that will offer valuable insights for healthcare professionals, policymakers, and stakeholders.

Figure 9. Top 10 healthcare advancements and developments predicted for 2024

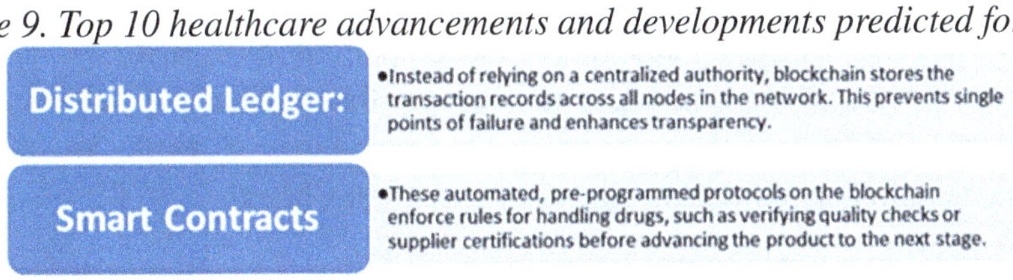
Distributed Ledger:
•Instead of relying on a centralized authority, blockchain stores the transaction records across all nodes in the network. This prevents single points of failure and enhances transparency.
Smart Contracts
•These automated, pre-programmed protocols on the blockchain enforce rules for handling drugs, such as verifying quality checks or supplier certifications before advancing the product to the next stage.

1.9. BLOCKCHAIN IN HEALTHCARE

For the secure storing, sharing, and restoration of Electronic Health Records (EHR), blockchain technology, a disruptive technology with a dependable decentralized structure, can be utilised to address issues with standard healthcare architecture. In this study, a blockchain-based framework for EHR in healthcare administration that is integrated with IPFS is suggested. By implementing Blockchain, healthcare institutions can establish decentralized, fail-safe, and highly secure healthcare ledgers. Patients' nodes may vary in complexity, ranging from full nodes to lightweight nodes, whereas hospitals and physicians typically function as lightweight nodes. To thwart potential fraudulent node activities, the model recommends the adoption of both two-factor and multi-factor authentication. Em-bracing a patient-centric access approach empowers individuals to digitally manage their health data, allowing healthcare providers access as needed and the ability to revoke permissions after a designated period. The content is encrypted via symmetric encryption (AES-128), and the keys to the information are supplied in a digital envelope sealed with asymmetrical encryption (RSA-4096) to the recipients while uploading to IPFS. Authentication of a transaction and verification of the other nodes' members' authenticity are carried out with the help of digital signatures (RSA-1024); the data are hashed by the SHA-256 for an encrypted data object.

The stack of models utilized for security prevents any exploiter from getting anything about the IPFS data. Moreover, if they did gain access, the data would be worthless because it's encrypted. The proposed off-chain storage method with IPFS can be scaled out and fits the blockchain structure. Leveraging the blockchain and IPFS, the healthcare system can enjoy better security, scalability, availability, and patient privacy.

Data Exchange is a safe and secure data sharing; the blockchain is making a mark in the healthcare industry for that. This is revolutionizing age-old health care into something safe to go for an accurate diagnosis and successful treatment. The blockchain technology is so exciting: pairing up current clinical data related to an individual's health status and plugging it into a secure health ecosystem. This chapter reviews the healthcare industry and future industry patterns by using the metaphor of blockchain to underpin the challenges and changes that the industry is facing. This chapter aims to understand the potential of blockchain in creating the key pillar of the next-generation personalized, smart, and secure healthcare.

1.9.1 Blockchain in Drug Traceability

The blockchain enhances the ability to track drugs, solutions against fake drugs, and is compliant with the current supply chain:

1. Mechanisms of Blockchain for Drug Traceability

Blockchain technology is a distributed, decentralized ledger that safely logs transactions at several supply chain nodes. For drug traceability, it creates a tamper-proof, transparent, and auditable record of each step, from manufacturing to final delivery. The key mechanisms include: Transaction Recording, Secure Verification, End-to-End Visibility, as shown in Figure 10, and decentralization for secure verification, Figure 11.

Figure 10. Steps of Immutable Ledger for Transaction Recording

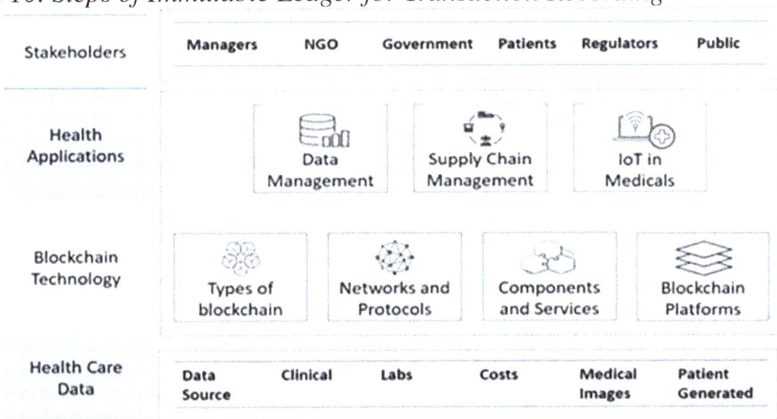

Figure 11. Decentralization for Secure Verification

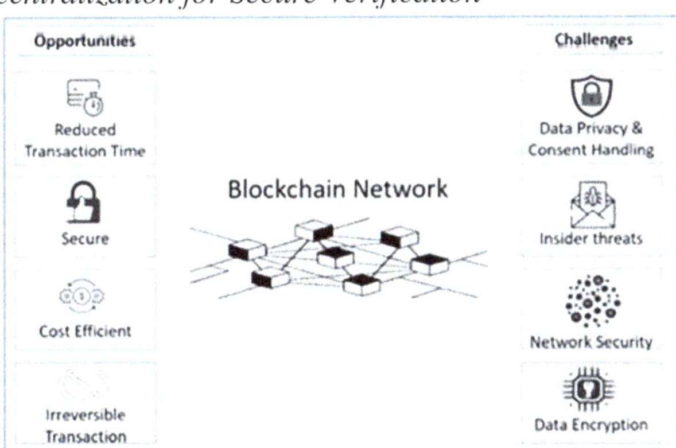

End-to-End Visibility

- Stakeholders (manufacturers, distributors, pharmacists, and regulators) can access real-time data to verify the origin, authenticity, and handling of drugs.
- At each checkpoint, data is updated and linked, creating a chain of custody that reduces the likelihood of tampering.

1.9.2. Preventing Counterfeit Drugs

Counterfeit drugs are a major global issue, and blockchain addresses this problem through:

Authentication of Drug Origins

- By linking blockchain data to **unique serial numbers, barcodes, or digital certificates**, every drug package can be traced back to its exact origin.
- Patients, pharmacists, and healthcare providers can scan QR codes or RFID tags to verify whether the drugs are genuine.

Eliminating Gaps in the Supply Chain

- Blockchain ensures that all participants (e.g., manufacturers, logistics providers, warehouses) are verified and compliant.
- Counterfeit drugs often enter the system through unmonitored or unauthorized intermediaries. Blockchain reduces such vulnerabilities by creating a transparent and tamper-proof ecosystem.

Enhanced Real-Time Monitoring

- IoT sensors integrated with blockchain provide real-time data on drug temperature, humidity, and handling during shipment. This ensures compliance with storage standards and prevents tampering that often accompanies counterfeit distribution.

Regulatory Compliance

- Regulators can access blockchain data to ensure compliance with drug safety laws, such as the FDA's **Drug Supply Chain Security Act (DSCSA)**. Non-compliant transactions are flagged, preventing counterfeit products from infiltrating the supply chain.

1.9.3. Integration with Current Supply Chain Frameworks

Integrating blockchain with the current supply chain infrastructure involves the following steps:

Data Standardization

- Existing systems (ERP (Enterprise Resource Planning) and WMS (Warehouse Management Systems)) can be integrated with blockchain via standardized Application Programming Interfaces (APIs).
- Data formats (e.g., GS1 standards for barcodes and serialization) allow for smooth communication between blockchain and legacy systems.

Use of IoT and RFID Tags

- Sensors, RFID chips, and barcodes linked to blockchain records enable automated updates at various checkpoints. Existing tracking systems can be augmented with blockchain to ensure transparency and tamper detection.

Scalability with Permissioned Blockchains

- Supply chains can use **permissioned blockchain networks** where only verified stakeholders have access to data.
- This ensures privacy, scalability, and efficient integration without overhauling existing systems entirely.

Smart Contracts for Automation

- Existing logistics and inventory systems can use smart contracts to automate routine processes like shipment verification, invoicing, and payments.
- For example, once a drug batch passes all checkpoints (verified on the blockchain), smart contracts trigger the next action, such as releasing the batch for distribution.

Blockchain enhances drug traceability by creating a secure, transparent, and tamper-proof record of every step in the supply chain. It combats counterfeit drugs through authentication, real-time monitoring, and the elimination of weak points in the distribution process. By integrating seamlessly with existing systems through APIs, IoT devices, and standardized protocols, blockchain ensures a scalable and efficient solution for modern pharmaceutical supply chains. This approach not only improves drug safety and regulatory compliance but also builds trust among manufacturers, distributors, healthcare providers, and patients.

1.10 BENEFITS OF ADOPTING BLOCKCHAIN IN HEALTHCARE

The blockchain system's main advantages are:

- Quicker credentialing throughout the employment process for healthcare organizations.
- A chance for healthcare providers, insurers, and medical institutions to profit from their current credential data on current and former employees.
- Openness and certainty for partners, such as subcontracting organizations

Figure 12. Schematic Representation of the Blockchain-Enabled Healthcare System

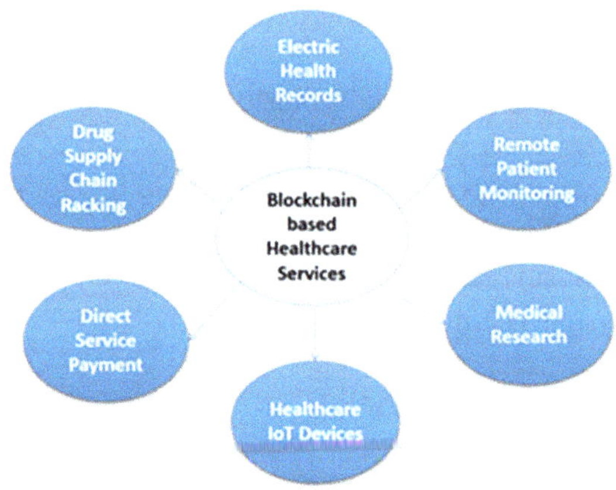

In Figure 12, the Integration of Healthcare Raw Data, Blockchain Technology, Healthcare

Applications, and Stakeholder Engagement illustrating the architecture of a blockchain-based healthcare system. At the top, a header row lists various stakeholders involved in the system, including managers, NGOs, government entities, patients, regulators, and the public. Below this, a section labelled "Health Applications" contains three boxes representing key functionalities: Data Management (icon of a database), Supply Chain Management (icon of supply chain-like elements), and IoT in Medicals (icon of a medical device connected to a network). The next layer is labelled "Blockchain Technology". It includes sections detailing types of blockchain, networks and protocols, components and services, and blockchain platforms. Each of these subsections also features a corresponding icon. At the very bottom, the section labelled "Health Care Data" lists different sources of data: Data Source, Clinical, Labs, Costs, Medical Images, and Patient Generated. That's providing a framework and a systematic way to enter into blockchain for healthcare.

1.11. WHY BLOCKCHAINS IN HEALTHCARE -REASONS TO USE BLOCKCHAIN FOR HEALTHCARE

When it comes to disrupting the healthcare sector, blockchain continues to chew off a big mouthful, one problem at a time. Blockchain application in medicine is driven by several factors, such as the requirement of improved data protection, interoperability, and patient-centred care.

This chapter is the first to investigate the prominent factors of blockchain applications in the trends of healthcare development.

Improved Security of Data: The craving for more secure data has become one of the leading reasons for the adoption of blockchain in the healthcare scene. Health care organizations handle vast amounts of sensitive patient information, such as medical records, insurance information and personal identifying information. Aggregated solutions are also subject to data breaches and hacking. With the cryptographic algorithms in place and a decentralized network that no one person controls, this is a protocol that is safe and secure, greatly reducing risks and keeping your personal information safe from theft or prying eyes.

Data Interoperability: Heterogeneous health systems are old sore barriers to reach interoperability. 3 Decentralizing blockchain Decentralized ledger offered by blockchain can facilitate the building of a comprehensive, immutable patient ledger Not only does the data become more integrated and shareable between the different health institutions, but data quality and validity is also preserved, improving the coordination of patient care.

Transparency and Traceability: Two of blockchain's most critical attributes for health care are transparency and traceability. Every time something is done against a block chain network it is recorded, with a timestamp, providing an unchangeable historical record. This traceability is invaluable for tracking sources of medical records, medications, and clinical trial data, and can limit cases of fraud, counterfeiting, and ensure adherence to regulatory standards.

Patient-Centred Care: Blockchain puts the patients in control of their medical data. Blockchain health records would grant users access and control over their health records, while maintaining data privacy, enabling user-centred care. This movement towards patient empowerment and data ownership is consistent with the direction of medicine in a world of patient-centred, personalized medicine and the next era of shared decision-making.

Research and Innovation:

Both healthcare providers and academic institutions have seen enough potential in leveraging blockchain to do joint research projects. The blockchain accelerates the development of medical research and enhancements in diagnostics, drug treatment, and development.

1.12. BLOCKCHAIN CHALLENGES IN HEALTHCARE

Various challenges are going to be settled in the healthcare sector by means of blockchain.

However, the application has its own difficulties, shown in Figure 13.

Figure 13. Conceptual summary of the complex problems and challenges in blockchain technology incorporation into the healthcare industry.

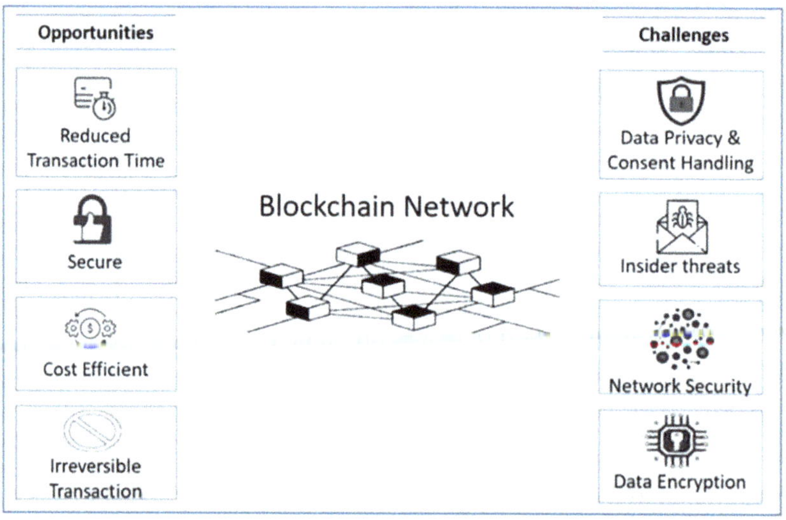

This Figure itself captures the challenges, such as privacy, data sharing, security, and compliance, that must be overcome for the healthcare sector to fully utilize blockchain technology.

1.13. SECURITY CHALLENGES

Healthcare blockchain also brings some security concerns that need to be have to be addressed to ensure the security of medical sensitive information, as well as system integrity. The following are a few of the distinct security challenges related to blockchain in healthcare:

- **Data Privacy and Consent Management:** Since healthcare data is very private, with patient consent as a major concern. It is an issue how to ensure that the balance between them, data sharing with only the authorized people, and having data control on the blockchain for patients.
- **Identity Management:** It is a crucial aspect of security in blockchain. Stronger identity proofing is needed to protect blockchain from unauthorized access by only allowing access to approved entities.
- **Secure smart contracts:** In healthcare, it is possible that smart contracts can be applied to monitor essential processes, for instance, settlements of insurance or cases of treatment. And we need to ensure the security of these contracts and that there will be no vulnerability or exploit of this sort from now on.
- **Data entry-security and Oracles:** preserving the validity of data entry to blockchains is essential. The blockchain, if not correctly protected, may become a target of security risks while receiving external data sources (oracles) to the blockchain.
- **Network Consensus Security:** The consensus security, e.g., PoW or PoS, of the base(blockchain) network, such as 51% attack resistance, double-spending resistance, etc.
- **Encrypted Data:** While the data is stored permanently on the blockchain, having assets encrypted before being placed onto the chain will make it secure. But these approaches make querying and analyzing the data more complicated.
- **Legal and regulatory adherence:** Compliance with healthcare regulations such as HIPAA is essential. Also, making sure your implementation complies with these laws while keeping the transparency of the blockchain can get tricky.
- **Insider Threats:** Although it acts as a distributed ledger, Insider threats from malicious insiders within the organization could be dangerous for the security of the blockchain and its information.
- **End-User Security:** It is further desirable for the end user (e.g., patient, health-care worker) to be aware of best practices to secure their own blockchain technology investment and avoid falling victim to phishing or scams.

- o **Long-term protection:** Blockchain systems should not be undermined by disguised new attacks or defence technologies, so they should be maintained, updated, and evaluated for reasonable new subtle attack systems or defence strategies constantly throughout their life.
- o **Data Recovery and Erasure**: Immutability of data remains a core benefit of blockchain, but there are times when data must be deleted due to regulation or patient request. It is difficult to reconcile immutability with the right to be forgotten.

This security model is viewed from all these vantage points: the technical solution space, the regulatory compliance model, and general awareness across all the stakeholders. A collaboration between blockchain craftsmen, cybersecurity leaders, healthcare providers, and legal experts is required to create a secure and compliant blockchain industry.

1.14. RISKS ASSOCIATED

Using blockchain in healthcare presents some security issues, but the security is strong enough to ensure that the private information of the patient will not be leaked, and the system cannot be compromised. The following are just some of the security challenges specific to the healthcare blockchain:

- o **Data Privacy and Consent Management:** Healthcare is personal. Patient consent is sacred, unlike many other things. Control of patients' data on the blockchain and with whom it is shared is complicated.
- o **Identity:** It's incredibly important to be able to access and secure identities stored on a blockchain. A wrong ID verification system needs to be implemented to ensure access is controlled to avoid unwanted access, such as only the rightful users should be able to make transactions on the blockchain.
- o **Reliable Smart Contract:** In healthcare, it is necessary to rationalize the use of smart contracts (e.g., drug and dispute agreements, insurance claims, validation processes). These contracts need to be audited to prevent hearing exposure and take-down.
- o **Data Ingress and Oracles to be secure:** All data coming into the blockchain must be secure, including all of the data that gets entered into the blockchain. The access to oracles (external data feeds), which supply information for the blockchain, involves security aspects that the protocol needs to defend itself against.

- **Network Consensus Security: The** security of the consensus (PoW/ PoS in the blockchain network) must be robust against 51% attacks and double-spending.
- **Coexistence with the current system:** Care must be taken when coexisting with the blockchain with the old systems so as not to make the healthcare system vulnerable to threats. A secure way of communication must exist between traditional systems and blockchain.
- **Encrypt data:** one could argue that encoding is not a necessity, while with blockchain, as it provides its own data integrity, but then again, encoding sensitive information before recording it into the blockchain is more tactical. The final component of the Solution Architecture that allows the SME to take control of their SCRM strategy is the Data Dashboard. But that adds some complication for querying, for processing the data.
- **Compliance:** Adherence to health regulations like HIPAA is mandatory. Yet it is challenging to ensure compliance with this model while preserving blockchain's transparency benefits.
- **Insider Threats:** Insider attacks by internal malicious entities (an employee who has access to the blockchain itself may pose a threat to an organization's blockchain as well as its data).
- **End-User Security:** To avert end-users, including patients and healthcare providers, from getting entangled in phishing-related scams, it is important that they are informed about blockchain and also educated on how best to protect it.
- **Lasting Security:** Maintenance perspective, update, and ongoing oversight of vulnerabilities for Blockchain systems are needed to handle the attacks/ threats of today and tomorrow.
- **Data Recovery and Deletion:** While immutability is one of the strong aspects of blockchain, there may be some instances when data needs to be scrubbed, by rule, or as required by the patient. There could well be tensions between immutability and the right to be forgotten.

Interdisciplinary teamwork between developers, cybersecurity professionals, doctors, and lawyers is key to building safe and regulatory-compliant blockchain applications for healthcare.

1.15. DATA PROTECTION CHALLENGE

Privacy One of the biggest concerns about adopting the use of the blockchain in the healthcare industry is Privacy. Some of the typical privacy concerns of using blockchains in healthcare include:

- o **Immovability:** The immovability of blockchain is perfect for security and trust, but not great for putting in wrong or outdated data. Health data may have to be changed or corrected but not so much on blockchain.
- o **Privacy and Confidentiality of Patient Information:** Healthcare data are private and confidential. If a hacker were able to intercept the blockchain, they would also be able to intercept a patient's file — if that were to be broadcast, even worse privacy is gone because everyone would know a patient's private history (AuthorBlock Transaction History) with full confidence. Even more crucial is to strike a balance between the transparent sharing of data and the privacy of patients.
- o **Right to Be Forgotten:** Legislation like the GDPR grants individuals the power to have their past forgotten. And interfere with the trust and unchangeability of blockchain on the way in attempts to do the same to the blockchain.
- o **Consent management** (consent for the patient's health information to be included in the blockchain — an intricate issue.) Consent is also not static, but on top of sharing, when having received consent (at the correct level!), the picture becomes even more entangled.
- o **Data protection / Encryption** - encryption can be used to protect data but also can block transparency and interoperability. It's neutral to find an encryption scheme which will retain the security of the data while allow some other party to decrypt the data and verify it.
- o **Access Control:** Access control of data in a decentralized blockchain is daunting and fine-grained. It is desirable that certain healthcare information be accessible only to authorized users and/or entities.
- o **Interoperability:** Health systems' landscapes often consist of multiple stakeholders/systems. Integration and security: Working with blockchain and traditional systems in healthcare and securing data can be complex.
- o **Data validity & Integrity:** Making sure that only valid data is submitted to the blockchain. Inaccurate information may disturb patient care and decision making if appropriate precautions are not taken.
- o **Regulatory Compliance:** Complying with a heathcare regulations (e.g., HIPAA, GDPR) with its unique properties is challenging on the blockchain. Getting blockchain implementations compatible with these sort of laws isn't easy.

- o **Big Data Off-Chain:** Storing vast amounts of data on the blockchain would be much too expensive and impractical. The challenge of what needs to be off-chain and how to secure it and keep the off-chain/on-chain linkage is a difficult problem.
- o **Identity Management:** Retaining patient identities and genuine records are important with health. The actual problem is that it is really difficult to ensure that those who should be able to see a certain piece of data have access to it, without undermining the security of the network.
- o **Smart Contract Security of Healthcare:** Healthcare applications might need to manage critical task smart contracts. It is critical to secure and make these contracts free of weakness to protect from unauthenticated access.

These data privacy issues demand a good blend of technology, legislation, and the involvement of all stakeholders and need to be redressed. As we continue to see blockchain with health systems, a holistic approach that respects both patient privacy and data protection — and complies with regulations — is necessary.

a workaround to respond to your query regarding scalability/compliance:

1.16. SCALABILITY PROBLEM: OVERVIEW AND SOLUTION APPROACHES OF THE BLOCKCHAIN

The scalability issue is still one of the biggest hurdles for the adoption of blockchain-based systems, such as those in the health sector, because by nature, transactions need to be instant, private, and legally compliant. There are two main scaling problems (i) transaction throughput and (ii) energy consumption.

- o **Throughput of Transactions:** Transactions are the vital fluid in a blockchain system and the pace of transactions in the blockchain network is called `transaction throughput. Traditional blockchains like Bitcoin and Ethereum have extremely low throughput, due to:
- o **Consensus algorithms:** PoW is time-consuming and expensive in terms of resource usage. Bitcoin can handle, at best, 7 transactions per second (TPS), and Ethereum can manage ~15 TPS.
- o **Block Size Limits:** There is a maximum size for blocks to prevent too many transactions from being included.
- o **Network cloggy:** More and more users use networks to get caught up in a backlog of transactions, so that a transaction takes longer to handle, and the fees will be higher.

Solutions for Transaction Throughput:

- o **Layer 2 Protocols:** Second-layer solutions like the Lightning Network (Bitcoin) and Optimistic Rollups (Ethereum) help offload the main chain. That is, off-gained on-chain security through on-L1 batching of transactions that the L2 system has transacted.
- o **Sharding**: It cuts the blockchain into pieces (of data) called shards that can process transactions in isolation. Sharding is a key improvement in Ethereum 2.0 that will scale the number of transactions that it can process.
- o **Energy Consumption:** PoW consensus mechanism is very energy-consuming, and this is a problem when the health sector is increasingly focused on sustainability. And bitcoin alone gobbles up at least 100 terawatt-hours of power annually — about as much as a small country.

Solutions for Energy Efficiency:

- o **PoS:** PoS dramatically reduces power consumption as validators must stake tokens and cannot spend energy solving cryptographic puzzles.
- o **Mixed consensus mechanisms:** Integrating PoS and DPoS can stimulate decentralization.
- o **Green Blockchain Networks:** Next-generation blockchains like Algorand and Cardano are designed to be energy lean while maintaining security.

1.17. COMPLIANCE WITH HEALTHCARE REGULATIONS

Compliance: Compliance with HIPAA, GDPR, and country-specific regulations is a must in blockchain-based healthcare solutions.

1. HIPAA (U.S. Healthcare Regulation)

In a logical world, Personal Health Information (PHI) should be safeguarded by statute under the Health Insurance Portability and Accountability Act (HIPAA). Blockchain apps will need to secure patient data in motion and at rest. HIPAA Role Based limitations should follow and allow access only to those users who have been explicitly granted permission, user access to PHI Role based where the hashes are stored on the blockchain, can sit off-chain also secure, encrypted.

2. GDPR (General Data Protection Regulation)

In the EU, GDPR regulates privacy and data protection. The right to be forgotten, which gives people the ability to ask for their data to be deleted under GDPR, is one of the main compliance issues. But

The immutability of blockchain goes against this idea.

Solution:

- Store only **pseudonymous data** or **encrypted hashes** on-chain. Actual data can be stored in off-chain databases where it can be deleted upon request.
- Implement **Zero-Knowledge Proofs (ZKPs)** to validate transactions without revealing sensitive data.

3. Country-Specific Regulations

Each country may have unique requirements for healthcare data storage and access. Blockchain developers must:

- Collaborate with legal and compliance experts to tailor solutions for jurisdictional needs.
- Integrate **smart contracts** with regulatory logic to automate compliance.

1.18. BLOCKCHAIN BASED HEALTHCARE SERVICES

Blockchain technology has emerged as a promising innovation within the healthcare sector, offering the potential to introduce a transformative era by effectively tackling critical issues such as data security, interoperability, and the promotion of patient-centric care, as shown in Figure 14. There are some examples of how blockchain can be applied to healthcare services:

- Electronic Health Records (EHRs): In the realm of Electronic Health Records (EHRs), blockchain technology emerges as a promising solution, offering a robust and interoperable framework for the storage and dissemination of electronic health records. This innovative approach empowers patients with the ability to exercise control over their sensitive health information and selectively authorize healthcare providers to access it when required McGhin et al. 2019.

Figure 14. Illustration of the Innovative Integration of Blockchain Technology in Healthcare

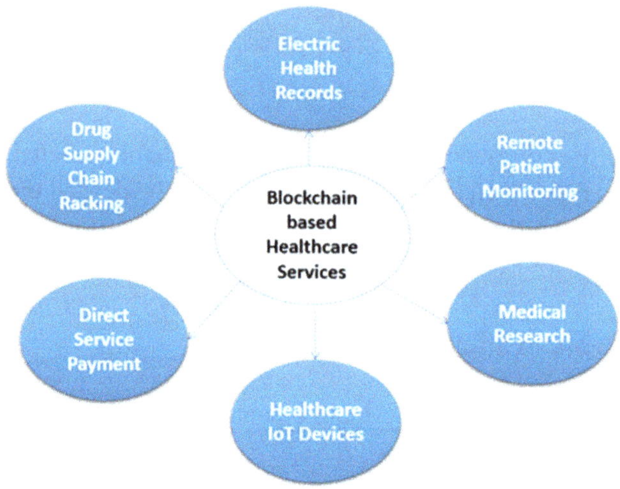

- Data transmission and interoperability: Blockchain has the potential to enable efficient and secure data sharing among various healthcare providers and institutions, ensuring the preservation of data integrity and safeguarding patient confidentiality.
- Medical Supply Chain Management: Blockchain can track the entire journey of medical supplies, drugs, and equipment, ensuring authenticity, reducing counterfeits, and enhancing the transparency of the supply chain.
- Clinical Trials & Research: Blockchain also plays a role in enhancing transparency and traceability in clinical trials, where a secure record for the trial data (in a hack-proof and immutable way) can be safely maintained. This minimizes data fabrication and promotes spread of facts.
- Health Billings and Claims – Bringing health billings and insurance claims to blockchain will lead to reduced fraud, better transparency and can also make claims process more streamlined.
- Telemedicine and Remote Monitoring: Blockchain technology allows secure sharing of healthcare data with decentralized access and data sharing—such as sharing of patient history summary, drug summary without revealing patient's identity and securely share only the required patients data (like patient history or drug list) with the consulting doctor so that the required medication (not more) is provided to the patients, thus maintaining patient privacy.

- Drug Prescription: Blockchain can assure and offer an auditable means to confirm a drug prescription, it could reduce the possibility of Drug Prescriptions, and give control back to patients over their Drugs.
- Consent Management: Patients can manage their consent for health data sharing across their healthcare providers through blockchain ensuring that their data is not used without their prior consent.
- Healthcare IoT sensor devices: Blockchain could protect data and privacy; that is, any data being generated by a healthcare-related internet-of-things (IoT) device, such as a wearable health tracker and monitoring device.
- Medical Credentials Verification: Secured and tamper-proof verification of credentials for medical using blockchain ensuring qualified skills of health professionals.
- Medical Research and Sharing: Patients can manage of their privacy and consent by giving and revoking access, in a secure way, to facilitate the doctor sharing information among the researchers in a secure data sharing platform of blockchain technology.
- Patient-Inputted Data: Patients may input their own health data — such as wellness and fitness data — into blockchain networks so that they feel secure about who can access that data and guarantee privacy.

Implementing blockchain-based healthcare services requires collaboration among healthcare providers, technology experts, regulatory bodies, and patients.

While the potential benefits are substantial, addressing challenges such as data privacy, interoperability, and regulatory compliance is essential to realizing the full potential of blockchain in healthcare services.

1.19. CURRENT MARKET DYNAMICS

Blockchain technology's application in healthcare has gained significant attention due to its potential to address various challenges in the industry.

Some key dynamics observed in the blockchain in healthcare market:

- Pilot Projects and Proof of Concepts: Many organizations, including healthcare providers, pharmaceutical companies, and startups, were conducting pilot projects and proof of concepts to explore how blockchain could be integrated into various aspects of healthcare, from data sharing to supply chain management.
- Data Interoperability: With large numbers of disaggregated systems and data stores, interoperability has been a major problem in the healthcare sector. The

potential of such blockchain technologies to develop secure information settings in which this 'data exchange' seems to be maintained without concern of patient care was of concern. There has been an increased usage of blockchain in order to expand access to pharmaceuticals and to track each one throughout the distribution chain. This seems to be essential for validating the medicinal products' originality and reducing the number of imitations.

- Stability and Privacy of Data: The health sector suffered many data crimes and cyber-attacks. The cryptographic security and decentralization of the Blockchain make patient information secure and prevent unauthorized access.
- Health Data Exchange: Blockchain could be utilized by clients for managing their medical records and transferring them even more confidentially to health suppliers and researchers, allowing more information liquidity without compromising on patient secrecy.
- Identity and Credentials: Attention was concentrated on keeping close relations with companies in the healthcare field; however, this became a major source of concern for enforcing the identities of each of the healthcare experts. Blockchain allowed for the authentication of skills and professional qualifications for experts in fitness care, essentially facilitating precision and removing scammers. Critical reflection was provided.
- Regulation: Since the healthcare sector works on a rule-based platform, there have been talks on how blockchain implementations could affect HIPAA in the US and GDPR in the European Union.
- Partnerships and Collaborations: A large number of contracted partnerships between different blockchain solutions providers and healthcare companies emerged to achieve and offer blockchain results that fit their needs.
- Implementation Challenges: Despite all its advantages, blockchain also had some drawbacks when it came to its adoption, such as integrating current systems, raising the bar for developers and establishing guidelines and benchmarks.
- Public VERSUS Private Blockchains: Public or private? The case of health care was addressed, highlighting several factors, such as the privacy of data, active patients in using their data and consensus mechanisms
- Research and Innovation: Research institutions were studying the technical, economic, and ethical implications of blockchain in healthcare to better understand its potential impact on patient care, data security, and the overall healthcare ecosystem.

1.20. SUCCESSFUL BLOCKCHAIN IMPLEMENTATIONS IN HEALTHCARE

Blockchain technology has demonstrated significant potential in healthcare, offering solutions to enhance data security, interoperability, and operational efficiency. Examples are followed by their outcomes and inherent lessons:

MediLedger: MediLedger, developed by Chronicled, is built on blockchain and helps with DSCSA compliance. It is capable of enhancing the traceability of drugs along the value-added chain.

- Enhanced drug verification and reduced counterfeit drug exposure. An enhanced network in which manufacturers, distributors, and dispensers are a part, without the need for the sharing of proprietary business information.
- In highly regulated industries, such as pharmaceuticals, compliance can be mitigated through blockchain.

Creating consensus and stimulating cooperation among various factions is the premise for the industry-wide application of new technologies.

Patientory: Patient's Data Access and Management System providing a secure environment for patients' data access and management using blockchain technology.

- Patient access and control of healthcare information was facilitated securely. Fostered interoperability by linking providers and facilitating patient care.
- Decentralized data storage can empower patients, but practitioners and patients must be educated on the use of the technology.
- Scalability and compatibility with existing healthcare infrastructure are concerns.

Estonia National Health System: The country implemented blockchain technology to secure medical records under its e-Health project.

- Number of people without an ID card, since over 1.3 million citizens have tamper-proofed.
- Lower costs and increased transparency of access to data through greater efficiency.
- Pro-blockchain regulation and a dedicated government are key for the proliferation of blockchain technology.

My Health My Data (MHMD): MHMD is a European Union-funded project that focuses on the use of blockchain for consent management and sharing health data for research.

- Have patients control over and the ability to profit from their own data.
- Ethical and secure data access: Lightning-fast science.
- The Information: Blockchain is opening up ethical data sharing, but can it combat privacy risk too?
- Ease of use. Ease of use is another important aspect to be adopted by non-technical users.

1.21. HOW INDIAN HEALTHCARE FIRMS ARE GAINING FROM BLOCKCHAIN

The blockchain is gaining ground at a steady pace in various sectors in the country, and healthcare is no different. This section offers a look at how blockchain has been reshaping Indian health firms until now:

- Data transmission and interoperability: Blockchain was studied to improve the sharing of patient information between healthcare providers, where health data was securely shared between various entities/organizations, which still maintained data privacy and integrity.
- EHRs – with EHR are spread throughout India, blockchain may be used to secure EHR and make more available. (As a patient, you would have control over your EHRs, which you could make available to doctors or hospitals as needed.)
- Drug Supply Chain Traceability: In a country like India with a widespread pharmaceutical industry, blockchain was being pilot tested to trace the entire drug supply chain so as to stop the distribution of spurious and NSQ drugs and ensure patient safety.
- Clinical Trials: As blockchain is an immutable distributed ledger technology, it can bring transparency and data integrity within clinical trials and aid in minimizing fraud and ensuring the authenticity of data in clinical trials. The data was of particular significance since India was undertaking medical research.
- Telemedicine and Remote Patient Monitoring: There are possibilities that blockchain could facilitate the secure and private sharing of patient data for telemedicine, while enabling remote patient monitoring or consultation in a secure manner.

- Health insurance: The visibility and security of blockchain would make claims less susceptible to tampering, resulting in decreased insurance fraud involving health insurance claims.
- Identity Credentials Verification: With blockchain, identity credentials of healthcare workers can be verified, which can reduce the number of fake claims to a credential, which will provide more confidence to patients.
- Health Data Marketplace (Proof of Concept): Loosely coupled, centralized Health Data marketplace blockchain test beds where pecifically, we envision the development of Proof of Concept blockchain test beds for patients to Powerful actors in the health domain, including researchers and research organizations (including pharmaceuticals, universities, and National Institute of Health institutes), hospitals, life insurance companies, and other options grantee's discretion, to be transferred to the Assistant Secretary for Planning and Evaluation at upon of the Secretary, waive such options in whole or in part to expeditiously achieve the endgame (which is still illusory).
- Regulatory Assent and secure as well as regulatory compliance: The decentralization and transparency inherent to blockchain technology would allow Indian healthcare organizations to not only comply with data protection laws but also to maintain secure and compliant data usage.
- Startups And Innovation: There were already a few Startups in India who were working on blockchain applications for the healthcare sector, And were trying to come out with new-age solutions to age-old problems of healthcare.

However, it should be noted that the adoption of blockchain is still in a formative state for Indian healthcare organisations and faces issues such as technology unification, compliance, and awareness. In the last few years, regulatory and technical evolutions, Regulations, and Technology have evolved.

1.22. TECHNICAL AND INFRASTRUCTURAL REQUIREMENTS FOR INTEGRATING BLOCKCHAIN INTO HEALTHCARE SYSTEMS

1.22.1. Technical Requirements

a) Data Security and Privacy

Blockchain must comply with healthcare regulations such as HIPAA (in the U.S.) and GDPR (in Europe) to ensure patient data privacy and security. This involves implementing:

- End-to-end encryption to protect information while it's being transmitted and stored.
- Permissioned blockchain systems to restrict access to authorized participants.
- Smart contracts to automate compliance and access controls.

b) Interoperability

Healthcare systems often use varied Electronic Health Record (EHR) platforms. Blockchain must:

- Integrate with existing EHR systems using standard APIs.
- Support cross-platform data exchange using interoperable protocols such as HL7 or FHIR.

c) Scalability

Every day, healthcare systems produce enormous volumes of data. Blockchain solutions need:

- Layer 2 solutions (e.g., sidechains) or sharding to process large transaction volumes efficiently.
- Storage off-chain for bulky medical records, with only essential metadata stored on-chain.

d) Consensus Mechanisms

Consensus algorithms should balance security, energy efficiency, and speed:

- Proof-of-Authority (PoA) or Proof-of-Stake (PoS) are more suitable than energy-intensive Proof-of-Work (PoW) for healthcare use cases.

e) Smart Contracts

Smart contracts automate healthcare processes such as insurance claims or consent management. These require:

- Rigorous auditing to eliminate vulnerabilities.
- User-friendly interfaces for medical staff and patients.

1.22.2. Infrastructural Requirements

a) Network Infrastructure

- **Hardware:** Decentralized nodes distributed across healthcare organizations for redundancy and fault tolerance.
- **Connectivity:** High-speed internet and low-latency networks to ensure smooth data sharing.
- **Cloud Integration:** Cloud platforms can host blockchain nodes to reduce initial infrastructure costs.

b) Identity and Authentication Systems

- Blockchain must integrate with existing identity systems like biometrics or government-issued IDs.
- Decentralized identifiers (DIDs) can provide patients control over their healthcare data.

c) Regulatory Compliance Infrastructure

- Real-time monitoring systems to ensure that blockchain operations adhere to local and international laws.
- Auditable trails to simplify compliance reporting and legal investigations.

1.23. NEED FOR CROSS-INDUSTRY COLLABORATION AND STANDARDS DEVELOPMENT

Successful implementation of blockchain in healthcare requires stakeholders across industries to align on various fronts:

1. Development of Standards

a) Data Standards

- Uniform data formats (e.g., HL7, FHIR) for seamless interoperability.
- Standardized metadata for blockchain entries, ensuring consistency.

b) Smart Contract Standards

- Common templates for smart contracts to facilitate trust and scalability.
- Legal recognition of smart contracts to enforce agreements in healthcare contexts.

2. Cross-Industry Collaboration

a) Stakeholder Involvement

- **Healthcare Providers:** Hospitals and clinics need to collaborate to define use cases and share infrastructure.
- **Technology Companies:** Blockchain developers and cloud providers must tailor solutions to healthcare needs.
- **Insurance Firms:** Integration is necessary for claims automation and fraud detection.

b) Public-Private Partnerships

Governments, tech companies, and healthcare providers should work together to fund pilot projects and establish proof-of-concept models.

c) Global Consortia

Organizations like WHO and IEEE can lead efforts in:

- Establishing global blockchain standards for healthcare.
- Sharing best practices and lessons learned from pilot implementations.

3. Education and Awareness

- Educating IT personnel and medical experts on blockchain applications.
- Raising patient awareness about the benefits and risks of blockchain systems.

Implementation of blockchain technologies in health institutions requires careful planning, technical and infrastructure aspects, and collaboration strategies. On the other hand, technical and policy readiness and maturity in security, scalability, interoperability, infrastructure development, and the like make room for decentralized networks, such as identity systems. Furthermore, industry-to-industry cooperation needs to be established to implement rules and gain the confidence of all stakeholders. By concentrating its efforts in these three areas, blockchain stands to revolutionize healthcare and improve data security, operational efficiency and patient empowerment.

1.24 FUTURE RESEARCH DIRECTIONS

- Healthcare and the use of IoT and blockchain: Secure Management of Patient Data, which examines the secure storage of patient data on blockchain and whether IoT devices can send out their health-related data securely and privately.
- Decentralized Healthcare Systems - Find out how the blockchain can decentralize patient records that are transferable between devices and doctors while maintaining privacy and adhering to HIPAA.
- Smart Contract Use Case-This white paper looks at how smart contracts can be applied to automate healthcare-related transactions such as invoicing, prescriptions, and insurance requests.
- AI-Powered Blockchain Data Analytics: Predictive Analytics - AI models that analyse blockchain transaction patterns to spot anomalies, fraud, and market predictions.
- Blockchain Data Mining: Experiment with advanced AI algorithms for blockchain data mining and unearth hidden patterns that can be used for business intelligence or security.
- AI Empowered Consensus Algorithms: Investigate AI techniques to make the blockchain consensus mechanisms smarter, such as for energy efficiency or to improve scalability and performance.
- Blockchain Based Cross-Border Data Sharing Mechanism:
- Global Privacy Laws: Discuss how blockchain can solve cross-border data sharing and still comply with varying national privacy rules (GDPR, CCPA, etc.)
- Decentralised ID Verification – Learn how blockchain can enable cross-border ID verification and authentication, sharing of private data on a secure basis across global business networks.
- End-to-End Encrypted Blockchains for Safe Information Sharing: Adaptable on-chain protocols that allow for secure and transparent data sharing between countries or organizations with additional placement of data integrity, auditability, and tampering prevention to reduce risk for information tampering or loss.

REFERENCES

Ahram, T., Sargolzaei, A., Sargolzaei, S., Daniels, J., & Amaba, B. (2017, June). Blockchain technology innovations. In *2017 IEEE technology & engineering management conference (TEMSCON)* (pp. 137-141). IEEE.

Alhadhrami, Z., Alghfeli, S., Alghfeli, M., Abedlla, J. A., & Shuaib, K. (2017, November). Introducing blockchains for healthcare. In *2017 international conference on electrical and computing technologies and applications (ICECTA)* (pp. 1-4). IEEE.

Angraal, S., Krumholz, H. M., & Schulz, W. L. (2017). Blockchain technology: Applications in health care. *Circulation: Cardiovascular Quality and Outcomes, 10*(9), e003800. PMID: 28912202

Attaran, M. (2022). Blockchain technology in healthcare: Challenges and opportunities. *International Journal of Healthcare Management, 15*(1), 70–83.

Ben Fekih, R., & Lahami, M. (2020). Application of blockchain technology in healthcare: a comprehensive study. In *The Impact of Digital Technologies on Public Health in Developed and Developing Countries: 18th International Conference, ICOST 2020, Hammamet, Tunisia, June 24–26, 2020* [Springer International Publishing.]. *Proceedings, 18*, 268–276.

Chen, H. S., Jarrell, J. T., Carpenter, K. A., Cohen, D. S., & Huang, X. (2019). Blockchain in healthcare: A patient-centered model. *Biomedical Journal of Scientific & Technical Research, 20*(3), 15017. PMID: 31565696

Dimitrov, D. V. (2019). Blockchain applications for healthcare data management. *Healthcare Informatics Research, 25*(1), 51–56. PMID: 30788182

Farouk, A., Alahmadi, A., Ghose, S., & Mashatan, A. (2020). Blockchain platform for industrial healthcare: Vision and future opportunities. *Computer Communications, 154*, 223–235.

Jayabalan, J., & Jeyanthi, N. (2022). Scalable blockchain model using off-chain IPFS storage for healthcare data security and privacy. *Journal of Parallel and Distributed Computing, 164*, 152–167.

Kumar, A., Singh, A. K., Ahmad, I., & Kumar Singh, P., Anushree, Verma, P. K., ... & Tag-Eldin, E. (2022). A novel decentralized blockchain architecture for the preservation of privacy and data security against cyberattacks in healthcare. *Sensors (Basel), 22*(15), 5921. PMID: 35957478

Linn, L. A., & Koo, M. B. (2016, September). Blockchain for health data and its potential use in health it and health care related research. In *ONC/NIST Use of Blockchain for Healthcare and Research Workshop. Gaithersburg, Maryland, United States: ONC/NIST* (pp. 1-10).

Pandey, P., & Litoriya, R. (2020). Implementing healthcare services on a large scale: Challenges and remedies based on blockchain technology. *Health Policy and Technology*, *9*(1), 69–78.

Prybutok, V. R., & Sauser, B. (2022). Theoretical and practical applications of blockchain in healthcare information management. *Information & Management*, *59*(6), 103649.

Qiu, J., Liang, X., Shetty, S., & Bowden, D. (2018, September). *Towards secure and smart healthcare in smart cities using blockchain. In 2018 IEEE international smart cities conference (ISC2)*. IEEE.

Rajawat, A. S., Bedi, P., Goyal, S. B., Shaw, R. N., Ghosh, A., & Aggarwal, S. (2022). Ai and blockchain for healthcare data security in smart cities. *AI and IoT for Smart City Applications*, 185-198.

Sharma, P., Jindal, R., & Borah, M. D. (2021). Healthify: a blockchain-based distributed application for health care. *Applications of blockchain in healthcare*, 171-198.

Siyal, A. A., Junejo, A. Z., Zawish, M., Ahmed, K., Khalil, A., & Soursou, G. (2019). Applications of blockchain technology in medicine and healthcare: Challenges and future perspectives. *Cryptography*, *3*(1), 3.

Tandon, A., Dhir, A., Islam, A. N., & Mäntymäki, M. (2020). Blockchain in healthcare: A systematic literature review, synthesizing framework and future research agenda. *Computers in Industry*, *122*, 103290.

Yaqoob, I., Salah, K., Jayaraman, R., & Al-Hammadi, Y. (2021). Blockchain for healthcare data management: Opportunities, challenges, and future recommendations. *Neural Computing & Applications*, 1–16.

Zaabar, B., Cheikhrouhou, O., Jamil, F., Ammi, M., & Abid, M. (2021). HealthBlock: A secure blockchain-based healthcare data management system. *Computer Networks*, *200*, 108500.

Chapter 3
Blockchain Technology for Smart Healthcare

Ahmad Tasnim Siddiqui
https://orcid.org/0000-0002-1884-9331
Horizon University College, UAE

Mehedi Masud
https://orcid.org/0000-0001-6019-7245
Taif University, Saudi Arabia

ABSTRACT

Blockchain technology, renowned for its decentralized and immutable nature, is poised to revolutionize the landscape of smart healthcare. In this transformative paradigm, patient data becomes securely stored and efficiently managed, fostering unprecedented levels of trust, transparency, and interoperability among healthcare stakeholders. By leveraging blockchain, institutions can ensure the integrity and confidentiality of medical records, mitigating the risk of data breaches. Smart contracts embedded within the blockchain facilitate automated execution of agreements, streamlining processes such as insurance claims, medication adherence monitoring, and patient consent management. Moreover, it enables the creation of comprehensive patient-centric networks, facilitating seamless data sharing across disparate healthcare systems while maintaining patient privacy. This technology holds immense promise for reforming smart healthcare, fostering a future where data is securely shared, patient outcomes are optimized, and the delivery of healthcare services is truly patient-centric.

DOI: 10.4018/979-8-3373-1225-5.ch003

INTRODUCTION

A blockchain functions as a public, decentralized record-keeping system, storing transaction data across many computers so that past records cannot be retroactively changed. In fact, Blockchain is the record's name, because it is validated and attached to the preceding block. Blockchain provides a high level of accountability because each transaction is recorded and verified publicly. In addition to public record-keeping and verification of transactions, Blockchain ensures a high level of responsibility. It is impossible to modify every entry saved on the Blockchain once it has been written. It verifies that the information remains up-to-date, actual and unaltered. Blockchain enhances stability and shows the vulnerability of central databases by keeping data on networks instead of a single database. It provides a fantastic platform for developing innovative business models to compete with those of traditional models of business (Khezr et al., 2019; Kumar et al., 2018; Moona et al., 2019;). Blockchain networks are distributed ledger networks that add records to the database and never modify them without a consensus for doing so. Blockchain hashes are calculated by connecting newly added records with each added data block using a cryptographic hash.

Blockchain technology ensures patient records remain confidential, as well as store and prevent the modification of medical records. All commonly available hardware in the hospital is connected to this decentralized network. Utilizing the resources stored by these devices, researchers can generate estimates for therapies, medicines, and remedies for a range of health conditions and ailments (Kassab et al., 2019 & Shen et al., 2019). Blockchain ledger architecture prevents data from being processed centrally, allowing all network participants to access and access it. By decreasing clinical practice and monitoring by twice as much, this decentralized system strengthens and secures health records. By reducing medical interventions and supervision, it improves patient care while minimizing the time and effort required from both patients and healthcare providers. Health records will be stored on a blockchain, allowing patients to keep track of where their information is going (Chelladurai & Pandian, 2021; Zhang et al., 2018).

Figure 1. Working procedure of Blockchain Technology (Haleem et al., 2021)

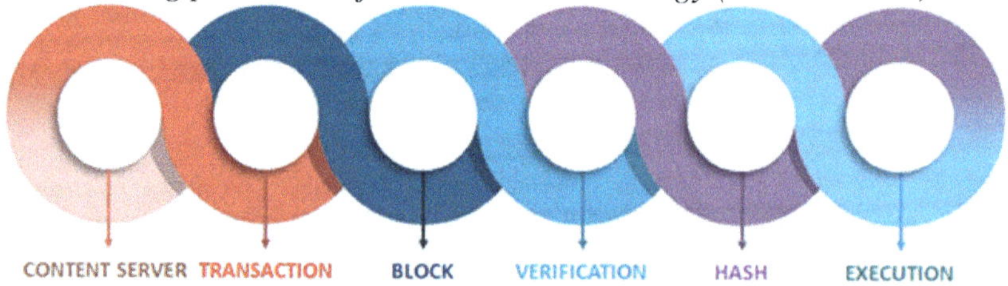

Blockchain technology runs atop internet infrastructure, using peer-to-peer interconnected computing devices running the same protocol and keeping an identical copy of the ledger, facilitating P2P value exchange without the need for an intermediary. Blockchain technology comes in many forms, incorporating public, private, hybrid, and consortium categories. Each blockchain network comes with its own advantages and disadvantages that will ultimately determine how well it performs for its intended application (Haleem et al., 2021).

Bitcoin and other cryptocurrencies were conceptualized on the public Blockchain, which represents the first type of blockchain system. Distributed ledger technology (DLT) was started on the public Blockchain. As a result, the system eliminates the security and transparency drawbacks of centralization. Rather than storing data in one place, DLT distributes it across a network of peers. It requires some form of data authentication due to its decentralized nature.

- The term "private Blockchain" refers to a Blockchain network that is restricted to a specific context, like a closed network. It means an entity controls or operates a private Blockchain network, such as a closed network or a private network. The network functions in much the same way as a public blockchain network concerning P2P connectivity and decentralization, but it is considerably smaller. When a blockchain network is private, the network's creator is aware of the participants before the network is established. A public web can't be used to develop permission-based applications, and users are completely anonymous (Haleem et al., 2021).
- Sometimes, organizations that aim for the best of both worlds use hybrid Blockchains, which include both private and public Blockchain features. Using Blockchain technology, businesses can create both private and public permission-less systems, allowing them to control access to specific data and what data becomes public.

BLOCKCHAIN IN HEALTHCARE

In healthcare, development is moving faster and faster than ever before. In today's world, it is necessary to have high-quality health facilities with cutting-edge technology. Blockchain can play a critical role here, and the health system is becoming more patient centered. Moreover, the healthcare sector is transitioning to a patient-centered model based on two key factors: service accessibility and the availability of healthcare resources around the clock. With the blockchain system within healthcare organizations can provide patients with high-quality care and facilities that are of adequate quality. By using this technology, we can quickly solve time-consuming and repetitive health data exchange processes that are costing the health industry a lot of money. Citizens will be able to participate in health study programs using Blockchain technology, and there will be better research and the sharing of data on the wellbeing of the public will enhance treatment for a wide range of communities. Management of the healthcare system and organizations is carried out using a centralized database (Hölbl et al., 2018; Farouk et al., 2020; Ekblaw et al., 2016).

A blockchain architecture, which uses intelligent contracts and immutable bookkeeping, can be used to facilitate the transfer of medical information (Dubovitskaya et al., 2017). As shown in Figs 2, 3, and 4, BCT plays a crucial role in sharing health information and enabling IoT-based remote care, security & confidentiality as well as supply chain management.

Figure 2. a) BCT has been used in Security and Privacy (Dubovitskaya et al., 2017).

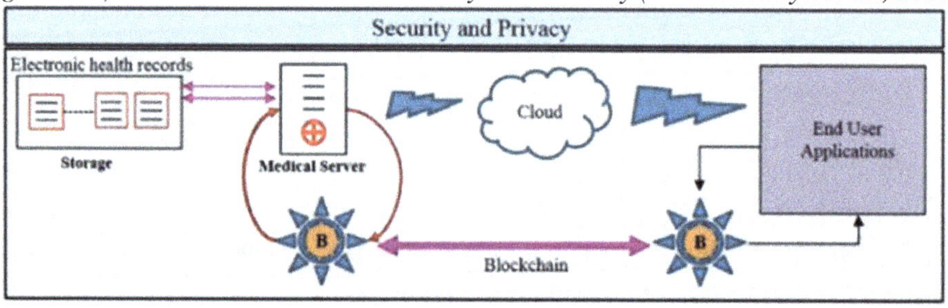

Security and privacy play an important role everywhere. Figure 2(a) shows how BCT has been used to security and privacy.

Figure 3. b) BCT has been used in Sharing Health Information (Dubovitskaya et al., 2017).

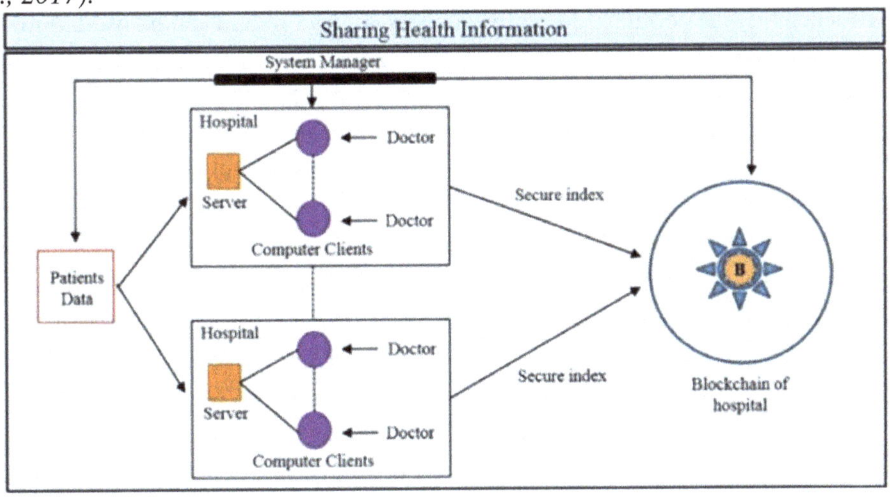

BCT has been also used for sharing health information among the managers, medical professionals, and other people involved in the system.

Figure 4. c) BCT has been used in Remote Care with IOT (Dubovitskaya et al., 2017).

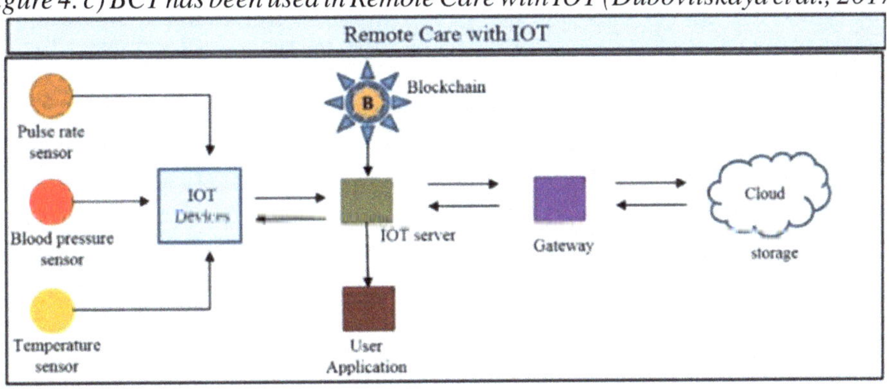

Figure 2(c) explains that BCT is being used for remote care with combination of IOT devices in cloud environment.

BLOCKCHAIN APPLICATIONS FOR HEALTHCARE

Blockchain was popularized by the success of Bitcoin and can be used to make secure and reliable transactions on an unknown network without the help of any third party (Taherdoost, 2023). The expansion of electronic health data, cloud storage of healthcare data, and patient privacy protection creates new options for health data administration, patient data sharing, and quick access to patient data. For every data-driven firm, but especially for the healthcare industry, protecting data, storing it, and managing its smooth integration are essential. Blockchain technology has the potential to effectively address these issues (Mijwil et al., 2025).

Blockchain is an emerging innovative technology that has been effectively utilized within healthcare through innovative applications. By sharing data efficiently and efficiently across the prominent healthcare providers and network members, many diseases can be treated at a lower cost and with more sophisticated treatments. This will quicken the growth in healthcare soon. Recently, Blockchain technology has been revealed to offer opportunities to the logistics industry, which can be useful in the healthcare industry. Digital transformation improves and innovates life quality directly in this area, as it directly affects quality of life. As blockchain technology becomes more prevalent, especially in the financial sector, it is becoming increasingly common. From scientific research and logistics to interactions between medical practitioners and patients, it provides numerous valuable opportunities for the healthcare industry (Griggs et al., 2018; Fu et al., 2020; Satamraju, 2020). Blockchain is being used in healthcare in several significant ways, as illustrated in Table 1 below:

Table 1. Major uses of blockchain in the healthcare sector

S. No	Applications	Description	References
1	Maintain patient-specific information	A large volume of patient health records and related data are generated before and after the various phases of clinical study. Health assessments, health polls, and quality assessments are available to many people. A document or record can be found in this way. By matching the data with the original records stored and maintained using blockchain technology, healthcare providers can determine whether the stored data is valid. To facilitate data sharing, Blockchain is built upon existing cryptography methods. Patient details, including name, date of birth, diagnoses, treatments, and ambulatory history, are recorded by healthcare providers in electronic health records. A cloud computing system or current database stores this information.	(Ejaz et al., 2021; De Aguiar et al., 2020; Aggarwal et al., 2021; Mackey et al., 2019)
2	Examine the impact of a specific procedure	With authorized access to patient data, researchers can effectively analyze any procedure. Consequently, these groups of patients respond better to this mode of management. Pharma firms will be able to deliver precise prescription drugs and services to patients in real time thanks to the Blockchain infrastructure. Since blockchain contains all the data, pharmacists have an easier time operating. With these results, they can give patients efficient instructions on how to take their medication. With real-time information collected from wearable devices, clinicians will get an update on the patient's status and be alerted to any emergencies.	(Khatoon, 2020; Abu-Elezz et al., 2020; Vaishya et al., 2021; Hussien et al., 2021)
3	Validation	The Blockchain validates transactions Until they join the chain by using algorithms. A digital signature and encryption seal the authenticity of a piece of material. Technology innovators, healthcare companies, and industry are looking for ways to create safer and cheaper healthcare in the future. If healthcare management can validate blockchain results adequately, it can revolutionize the health ecosystem.	(Bhuvana et al., 2020; Onik et al., 2019; Agbo et al., 2019; Engelhardt, 2017; Tanwar et al., 2020)
4	Transparency and safety	It facilitates patient safety and transparency while allowing doctors to spend more time treating them. Moreover, it would permit the development of clinical trials for rare diseases and the implementation of treatments for them. A healthcare ecosystem can be cost effective if patient data is exchanged smoothly among the medical solution providers. Blockchain promotes greater safety and transparency in healthcare by allowing organizations to remain linked and exchange data via a shared ledger. This system enables users to exchange information and monitor actions while ensuring confidentiality and integrity, without the need for additional tools.	(Wang et al., 2018; Jiang et al., 2018; Zhang et al., 2017; Hathaliya et al., 2019)

continued on following page

Table 1. Continued

S. No	Applications	Description	References
5	Maintaining health record	Record-keeping in the medical field can be made easier by blockchain technology. Health care data can be shared, electronic records can be maintained, insurance can be managed, and administrative operations can be performed on the system. An app that connects to a Blockchain network can allow patients to send their health information. By connecting all data in the same place, blockchain will consolidate all information and provide patients with access to their complete medical history. Therefore, Blockchain would safeguard the users' privacy and ensure the information was legitimate and authentic.	(Berdik et al.,2021; Du et al., 2021; Peterson et al., 2016; Celesti et al., 2020; Zhang & Boulos, 2020)
6	Clinical Test	Implementing blockchain in clinical trials addresses issues such as false results and data breakdown that don't correspond to the research's objectives and purposes. By examining the evolving market dynamics, the business analysis platform will increase transparency and trust in clinical trials. This information will help the healthcare sector make informed decisions. Blockchain enables the creation and monitoring of the medicine supply chain, ensuring traceability from the manufacturer to the customer.	(Gökalp et al., 2018; Leeming et al., 2019; Javaid & Haleem, 2019; Bhattacharya et al., 2021)
7	Presenting information	To secure superior quality and accurate supply of the medication, the system will display origin-related information through blockchain. With appropriate use of blockchain, sensitive data is better protected than ever before. The blockchain app trend has been adopted by many sectors, such as finance, retail, and immobilization, achieving several benefits for displaying information. However, healthcare can be challenging and nuanced. Because of its complexity, fundamental changes have occurred across the market, affecting medicines, vaccines, clinical trials, and cloud computing.	(Al Omar et al., 2019; Zarour et al., 2020; Ribitzky et al., 2018; Khujamatov et al., 2020)
8	Fake content detection	Clinical studies involving participants and clients should be readily verifiable thanks to blockchain, which provides more clarity and identifies false content. In an intelligent agreement, protocol documents along with their findings are transparent and publicly verifiable, Which facilitates obtaining approval and keeping public transparency. Using this technology, patients can have real-time access to their health and insurance records in a safe and secure manner.	(Agbo & Mahmoud, 2019; Sun et al., 2018; Zheng et al., 2018; Pham et al., 2018; Ismail et al., 2019)

continued on following page

Table 1. Continued

S. No	Applications	Description	References
9	Eliminates unnecessary overhead expenses	By using blockchain technology, unnecessary overhead expenses are reduced, and health records can be used appropriately. Additionally, this technology will facilitate the efficient sharing of critical health information by reducing the need for multiple intermediaries. Therefore, healthcare providers are tasked with providing their patients with efficient, timely, and adequate care. Several problems plaguing the healthcare system can be fixed, such as challenges with interoperability, report processing, theft, and critical data failure.	(Tandon et al., 2020; Agbo & Mahmoud, 2020; Curbera et al., 2019; Srivastava et al., 2019)
10	Patient monitoring	When medical professionals need medical equipment, they can rely on Blockchain's trust. Watching patients and reacting to health-related events from a distance may be time consuming for doctors. Blockchain technology can be applied to improve the oversight of patient room conditions, bed utilization, and the management of supplies. Healthcare institutions and providers can establish stable digital identities with a Blockchain healthcare network. Improves healthcare logistics transparency by integrating Blockchain and leveraging IoT to improve supply chain tracking and reaction times.	(Ray et al., 2020; Mamoshina et al., 2018; Munoz et al., 2019; Soltanisehat et al., 2020)
11	Initiate research efforts	The blockchain can serve as a reliable source of information. Disputes and membership claims can be handled via blockchain, which can transform the manual process. Blockchains enable the exchange of patient data more broadly, which opens new and innovative research opportunities. In addition to controlling patient referrals, this technology can also help prevent fraud.	(Cyran, 2018; Chen et al., 2019; Mazlan et al., 2020; Vaishya et al., 2020)
12	Keep hospital financial statements up to date	The bookkeeping process relies on accurate records of financial statements. It is possible to conduct and assess the clinical trials smoothly. The process of accounting and reporting has been streamlined using Blockchain technology by companies. As a result of this application, everyone can prepare for their visit to the health care provider by completing documentation ahead of schedule. Also, they won't need to queue. because the paperwork is already done in advance.	(Syed et al., 2019; Al Omar et al., 2017; Ahmad et al., 2021; Ramani et al., 2018)

continued on following page

Table 1. Continued

S. No	Applications	Description	References
13	Improves safety	Interoperability and medication validity problems can be addressed with blockchain, and blockchain increases overall patient safety in health care. A supply chain management scheme can only replace the existing one if it prevents counterfeit drug manufacturers from entering the market with their illegal drugs. A centralized location for storing all data would be possible with blockchains. Kudos to blockchain's interoperability, doctors can easily access detailed patient information, helping them make more accurate diagnoses and develop better treatment plans.	(Nguyen et al., 2021; Gul et al., 2021; Islam & Shin, 2020; Dhagarra et al., 2019; Islam et al., 2019)
14	Lower the cost and duration of data conversion	Blockchain networks help lower the time and cost associated with data conversion. Blockchain holds the potential to solve the problem of fast and efficient verification of medical evidence. Blockchain secures patient data while enabling innovative, privacy-preserving health information sharing. As a decentralized, time-stamped ledger, it ensures transparent, trustworthy transactions and paves the way for transformative advances in global healthcare. Each node in the network can independently process and store every input.	(Angraal et al., 2017; Saha et al., 2019; Pandey & Litoria, 2020; Koshechkin et al., 2018; Ashima et al., 2021)
15	Tracking of medications and medical supplies	Blockchain allows for the tracking of medications and medical supplies from production to ultimate delivery.	(Smolenskas, 2024)
16	Claims and Billing	Insurance claims can entail intricate procedures that need to be verified and approved in several levels. Blockchains can simplify this by establishing a single, safe source of truth for data related to claims. A blockchain-based immutable ledger tracks all stages of the claims process, facilitating automatic verification.	(Smolenskas, 2024)

SECURITY AND PRIVACY IN HEALTHCARE

Healthcare professionals continue to manage and update personal health records using digital technology. Experts in the field recognize digital platforms like the UK's Health Navigator that handle ordering and payment processes for medical devices and supplies. Blockchain technology, which provides computational intelligence, auditability, robustness, and security, can help manage sensitive personal data by converting existing models to clean data exchange models (Stone, 2018). There are numerous blockchain-based platforms for medical record management. MedRec (Ekblaw et al., 2016), MedBlock (Fan et al., 2018), and BlockHIE (Jiang et al., 2018) all propose distributed management of health-related data. Blockchain technology can work alongside other technologies, including IoT. Research by Ichikawa et al. (2017) and Griggs et al. (2018) illustrated how smart contracts can automate medical interventions by capturing data from mobile devices.

Data is maintained and transferred in the smart healthcare store so that quality care can be provided. Organizations face numerous challenges when it comes to securing and protecting massive amounts of health data. There are several methods for ensuring protection of healthcare information. This problem has been addressed in several studies through a combination of administrative, physical, and technological strategies. To ensure the secure handling of patient data in digital health systems, healthcare providers implement multiple security strategies. To protect against unauthorized access, patient data is restricted using security protocols. This could be accomplished using operational controls within a covered entity. Blockchain technology, which securely stores and exchanges sensitive patient data, has the potential to transform the healthcare industry. Ensuring data security in healthcare is vital to protect sensitive patient information, such as medical histories, medications, and test results. Blockchain enables secure, decentralized storage and seamless sharing of data, functioning as a tamper-proof digital ledger. The information is stored in blocks, with each block connected to the one before it in a chain, hence the term "blockchain" (Taherdoost, 2023; Mohanasundaram et al., 2022; Sriram, 2022).

Since these records include a wealth of personal data, including names, residences, Social Security numbers, and comprehensive medical histories, cybercriminals can profit greatly from them. The frequency and expense of healthcare data breaches are startlingly high. According to IBM Security research, healthcare experiences the highest cost per data breach, averaging $9.23 million. Ransomware, insider threats, and phishing attempts are all potential sources of breaches. Significant consequences result, such as monetary losses, fines, harm to one's reputation, and a decline in patient confidence. Strict rules are placed on healthcare providers under the Health Insurance Portability and Accountability Act (HIPAA) in the U.S., which obliges the safeguarding of patient data. To guarantee compliance, a complex and continuous task, a great deal of resources and unwavering attention are needed. (Chowdary et al., 2024).

Blockchain technology can address several problems facing the healthcare sector, but there are some things to keep in mind. This may influence how well technology is implemented. Regulatory and compliance concerns are an important factor that healthcare providers need to consider when implementing blockchain health solutions. Strict regulations pertaining to clinical safety, patient privacy, and data protection apply to the healthcare industry, making compliance a major obstacle when deploying a medical blockchain. Healthcare institutions must follow data privacy laws, including the General Data Protection Regulation (GDPR) in Europe and HIPAA in the United States. Fifty-one percentage (51%) of attacks, in which a group takes over more than half of a blockchain's processing power and manipulates data, are one of the main security issues. This attack may affect clinical trial data, insurance claims, or patient records, raising questions about the accuracy of the information (Smolenskas, 2024).

Validation Issues in blockchain-based transaction

Environmental and health concerns about blockchain are directly linked to how its algorithms work (Schinckus, 2022). Blockchain technology employs cryptographic protocols to ensure that information is unalterable and traceable. In this context, creating or changing a record in the distributed ledger triggers a cryptographic problem that must be solved by updating the records. To validate a new record, there are several computational options available. A widely used method for solving such cryptographic puzzles is called the 'proof-of-work' (POW) consensus. This involves sending the puzzle to all nodes in the network, which then competes to solve the algorithmic challenge. Regarding this procedure, Schinckus (2021); " Each time a new block is created, containing transactions or activities, all network nodes attempt to solve its associated cryptographic puzzle. Once one node finds the solution, the block is validated and appended to the blockchain". Schinckus (2020) wrote that, even though there are several computation consensuses, most blockchain platforms rely on POW to guarantee that data remains intact and secure. "Proof-of-stake" (POS) is another popular algorithm that operates differently since it randomly selects a miner to validate the transaction and receive the reward, based on the wealth or age of the network participants.

With the POS, the reward is chosen based on a random selection among the computers rather than competition between them. As a result, proof-of-stake consumes less energy since only the selected computer validates the algorithmic enigma that is associated with the new block. In the first instance, the proof-of-stake protocol seems like a good alternative to the POW, but everything is not as it appears since it requires a specific authority to govern the mining process, meaning that any application working with it requires a supercomputer. When targeted hacking is attempted, such configurations may compromise data integrity. As a result, these applications' integrity and security cannot be algorithmically guaranteed, like those of the POW (Andoni et al., 2019), which relies on a distributed/decentralized validation of the data. In many health care and financial applications, the POW consensus is often used as a validation method for blockchain-based transactions due to this disadvantage. By utilizing POW led applications, applications are completely decentralized, so no critical node is susceptible to hacking. The algorithmic strength of POW is evident in its economic significance and its role in cryptocurrencies like

Ether and Bitcoin, which have market capitalizations of USD 137 billion and USD 386 billion, respectively.

In this environment, it is imperative that healthcare data remain secure, and the adoption of POW-based blockchain technology for secure validation and recording of all operations makes intuitive sense for the algorithmic reasons explained above.

It is worth acknowledging, however, that the POW algorithm also has a serious drawback related to its energy consumption, despite its technical advantages regarding security. POW validation involves all computer nodes racing to solve a generated puzzle, which validates the transaction and determines the reward. Consequently, the fees are awarded solely to the node that solves the enigma, which leads to the others consuming significant amounts of electricity without receiving anything in return.

Blockchain technology is well-suited for handling secure health data due to the following features:

Decentralized storage: The data stored in conventional data storage is centralized, making it vulnerable to hackers. With blockchain technology, information is spread across the web and stored decentralized, reducing its susceptibility to hacking.

Immutability: Data added to the blockchain cannot be altered or removed. This ensures its integrity and protects it from tampering.

Encryption: Data is protected by the most advanced encryption methods of blockchain technology, which ensures access only to authorized parties.

Smart contracts: Data exchange and access control processes can be automated using these self-executing legal agreements. This feature improves security by ensuring data is accessible only by authorized personnel.

Transparency: Blockchain technology improves transparency by allowing all network participants to access data easily. This can boost accountability and help reduce fraud.

Blockchain has the potential to transform the healthcare industry by providing a secure and decentralized way to store and exchange sensitive medical data. There are still issues that must be addressed before widespread acceptance can occur. They encompass statutory and regulatory requirements, issues with interoperability, and the necessity for standardized protocols (Zheng et al., 2018).

It is possible to enhance patient privacy with blockchain technology, but there are some problems that need to be addressed. One of the biggest subjects is the interoperability of various blockchain platforms since healthcare providers may use different systems that are not compatible. In addition, implementing blockchain technology in healthcare is complex, requiring resources and technology that may not be available to everyone. Data access rights and consent management are automated under blockchain technology, bringing increased transparency and accountability to healthcare data management. In addition to ensuring regulatory compliance, it also provides an auditable record of the data treatment process. Therefore, a decentralized and secure approach to exchanging and storing patient data is offered by blockchain technology.

DISCUSSION

Clinical trials are made credible and more reliable by blockchain technology. The digital thumbprint can be used to store those records as blockchain-based intelligent contracts. Blockchain Technologies in Healthcare offer an array of benefits, including Enhanced network security, verified authentication, identities, and standardized access to electronic health records. Blockchain technology is used to track and monitor medication responsibilities in the pharmaceutical supply chain. Using this technology, the effects of a particular procedure can be analyzed and validated for any individual patient. In addition to providing health records, clinical trials, and patient monitoring, blockchain has also been used to improve safety, display information, and foster transparency in healthcare. By using this technology, hospitals can maintain their financial statements and minimize the time and cost of data transformation.

This system solves several problems in the data-centered environment, such as generating hashes for blocks of patient health records. Patients would also feel more comfortable sharing their data with third parties while still maintaining their anonymity. Large number of data sets are required to conduct a clinical trial. To analyze, estimate, and determine the efficiency ratios under various conditions, researchers focus on these data sets and conduct routine experiments. Nevertheless, some scientists and researchers may manipulate the collected data and evidence to change the results.

The pharmaceutical industry is also eager to capture the findings that will allow them to benefit their business in such a way. To make clinical trials more straightforward and fairer, researchers use Blockchain technology. A secure, uneven, and straightforward clinical trial can be recorded with this tool. It is possible to use the collected knowledge to improve medical treatment and optimize efficiency benefits after market launch by providing post-market analysis. Consequently, these standards focus on key aspects of blockchain technology, such as open governance, transparent audit trails, data transparency, robustness, and enhanced privacy and security. As a result, healthcare providers can comply with contemporary healthcare standards, including safety standards for medications and related supplies. By easing the secure and decentralized exchange of sensitive medical data, blockchain could revolutionize the healthcare industry.

ISSUES WITH BLOCKCHAIN

Despite blockchain's potential advantages for managing medical data, there are still problems that need to be resolved. For instance, the blockchain's decentralized structure allows all network users to access the data it stores. Encryption techniques are used to protect this data, however maintaining data secrecy and privacy is hard. Blockchain systems' immutability may also provide problems in the case of data breaches or errors because it may be hard to change or remove erroneous data once it has been uploaded to the blockchain. The development of strong blockchain-based health record management systems that can satisfy the intricate requirements of the healthcare sector would require more investigation to overcome these obstacles. The Ethereum public network was used to construct most of the healthcare applications. Thus, this network flaw has an impact on applications in healthcare. The problems that are emerging in blockchain healthcare are covered here (Kasyapa & Vanmathi, 2024).

Technical Difficulties

One major obstacle to the adoption of blockchain is the integration of blockchain with current legacy systems. Traditional IT approaches that are incompatible with blockchain technology are still used by many healthcare organizations. Because switching to a decentralized approach requires large investments in infrastructure and technology, smaller suppliers may be put off. Additionally, healthcare practitioners who might lack the necessary technical competence may find the intricacy of blockchain technology to be a hurdle. Overcoming industrial resistance requires proper training on blockchain platforms. Initiatives for education will become increasingly important as the healthcare sector develops to guarantee a smooth transition to blockchain-enhanced systems. A carefully thought out, staged strategy might help lessen the difficulties; first, efforts should be directed at integrating blockchain with the most important systems before moving on to more general uses (Kasyapa & Vanmathi, 2024).

Maintenance of storage

The purpose of blockchain technology is to compile a list of transaction details and attach them to a block, which necessitates little storage capacity. MRI and X-ray images, test results, medical records, and other graphical data are just a few of the enormous volumes of data in the healthcare industry that require routine processing. The complexity of maintaining and replicating the entire blockchain across all network nodes increases with blockchain size, which leads to rising storage requirements and declining speed (Kasyapa & Vanmathi, 2024).

Security

Blockchain technology has eliminated one of the main risks to data security and privacy in conventional systems by prohibiting transactions from being completed by third parties. BT's decentralized structure, however, presents further security issues. Although every node on the network can see every piece of information, permissions are still needed to access data. Patients might have to designate multiple agents who have access to their medical records if external management is not in place. It can be challenging to assign permits during patient emergencies (Kasyapa & Vanmathi, 2024).

Scalability

As blockchain networks expand, scalability remains a significant issue, resulting in longer transaction processing times and higher storage requirements, which practically impacts the use and adoption of the blockchain across multiple industries (Morar & Popescu, 2024). Large data storage on blockchain can make it sluggish and ineffective. Given that EHR systems often hold a lot of patient data, this could be an issue. It became apparent that it was a major obstacle to the use of BT in medical settings. One of the main issues with blockchain networks' scalability is their low transaction throughput. Blockchain systems' increasing storage needs are another factor affecting scalability. Additionally, blockchain consensus techniques like proof-of-stake or proof-of-work may make scaling problems worse. The validation and verification process is time-consuming and resource-intensive since these solutions require network participants to engage in computationally costly operations or stake substantial amounts of money. As the network grows, the computational demands and energy usage related to attaining consensus can become unsustainable. Implementing off-chain computing can help address scalability difficulties in healthcare models (Kasyapa & Vanmathi, 2024).

Social Issues

Blockchain is evolving and dealing with societal challenges such as technological problems and social transformation. Technology that deviates from standard research techniques could be challenging to implement. Though the obstacle to fully implementing the technology, particularly blockchain, has not yet been identified, the healthcare sector is moving closer to digital data. It is challenging to persuade medical professionals to switch from research data to blockchain at the appropriate moment due to the medical industry's sluggish adoption of policy and technology. For example, established methods of data collecting and processing are accustomed to being used by medical researchers. They eventually come to trust these strategies. Because blockchain technology is thought to be complicated, there may be resistance to its use for safe and transparent data sharing and cooperation. Blockchain-based data management may encounter resistance from researchers because of social backlash. To persuade people to utilize blockchain, you must highlight its advantages, deal with data security concerns, and provide intuitive tools and interfaces (Kasyapa & Vanmathi, 2024).

Absence of Standards and Regulations

There is currently no standard for the application of blockchain technology to EHR management. Because of this, collaboration between multiple healthcare organizations may be difficult. Teamwork, careful consideration, and adherence to all relevant regulations are required for this process (Alexis, 2025). For example, two healthcare institutions are implementing blockchain-based electronic health records on their own. Both medical facilities select their own encryption and data format. It is challenging to share and integrate medical records among hospitals due to a lack of common data formats and interoperability methods. Doctors may have trouble getting important information, and patients may need many tests. It is because of these requirements that healthcare institutions find it difficult to exchange medical data (Kasyapa & Vanmathi, 2024).

LIMITATIONS AND FUTURE SCOPE

There are specific challenges associated with integrating blockchain technology into the healthcare industry. There are technical challenges, security issues, scalability problems, societal problems, and absence of any standard regulations. Apart from all this, lack of expertise is one of the major obstacles for medical facilities utilizing this advanced technology. As blockchain technologies are still in their infancy, more work needs to be done to explore them and research them. As a result, it is applicable to the obligations of medical associations and regulators. It's time for the healthcare industry to embrace innovation.

Blockchain in healthcare is expected to grow significantly in the future. With this technological innovation, it can be used more effectively in healthcare to explain the results of treatment and progress. Blockchain plays a key role in transaction validation and the exchange of information. Soon, by using blockchain, transactions can be authenticated and documented, subject to the approval of network members. Blockchain, as the foundation of next-generation health information exchange, provides security using public and private key encryption. Among the benefits this technology enables proper handling of medical records, prevents infringements, enhances interoperability, and streamlines procedure, medication and prescription control will be improved, and medical and supply chains will be monitored. Blockchain in healthcare is expected to perform spectacularly in the future (Kassab et al., 2019).

One of the main issues with blockchain technology is security since anything can happen, from little flaws to massive attacks that might damage the entire network. Standardized frameworks, thorough testing, and staying abreast of evolving cyberthreats are essential for preserving the blockchain's high level of security (Morar & Popescu, 2024).

The regulatory and compliance trouble involve the navigation of exceedingly complex, nontechnical policy environments. Simplified research into these frameworks is necessary to guarantee that blockchain operations will comply with strict regulations. Because of this, educational initiatives are very important. To effectively increase awareness of blockchain technology and encourage wider adoption, specialized programs and public outreach initiatives must be developed with strong support from government and academic institutions (Morar & Popescu, 2024).

Blockchain and AI together can improve predictive healthcare and data analytics. By having total control over their medical records, patients can lessen their reliance on centralized systems. Blockchain-based healthcare solutions are attracting the interest of governments and businesses. Tokenized rewards for patients taking part in wellness and research initiatives can be made possible via blockchain technology (Blockchain Consultant, 2025).

CONCLUSIONS

Since Blockchain is decentralized and encrypted, it can be applied to healthcare in innovative ways. It improves the interoperability between healthcare organizations, strengthens the security of patient health records, and helps fight counterfeit drugs. Blockchain technology may bring significant changes to a range of healthcare sectors; for example, digital contracts, which can facilitate intelligent agreements, can have a significant impact on healthcare. The cost of cash transfers will be minimized with intelligent contracts since intermediaries will be removed from the process. For Blockchain to be of significant value in healthcare, it depends heavily on the implementation of supporting advanced technologies. Clinical trials, healthcare insurance, and system tracking are among the areas that are covered. With the help of blockchain, hospital services can be tracked throughout their entire lifecycle, including patient monitoring. In addition to improving patient history management, blockchain technology can also improve insurance mediation, allowing clinical actions to be completed more quickly with optimized data management. Ultimately, this technology would improve the quality of healthcare services for both patients and physicians by improving how clinical records are treated and used (Haleem et al., 2021).

REFERENCES

Abu-Elezz I, Hassan A, Nazeemudeen A., Househ M., Abd-Alrazaq A. (2020). The benefits and threats of blockchain technology in healthcare: a scoping review Int. J. Med. Inf. (2020 Aug 14), p. 104246

Agbo, C. C., & Mahmoud, Q. H. (2019, September). Comparison of blockchain frameworks for healthcare applications. *Internet Technology Letters*, *2*(5), e122.

Agbo, C. C., & Mahmoud, Q. H. (2020, July 1). Blockchain in healthcare: Opportunities, challenges, and possible solutions Int. *J. Healthc. Inf. Syst. Inf.*, *15*(3), 82–97.

Agbo, C. C., Mahmoud, Q. H., & Eklund, J. M. (2019). Blockchain technology in healthcare: a systematic review Healthcare, vol. 7, Multidisciplinary Digital Publishing Institute (2019 Jun), p. 562

Aggarwal, S., Kumar, N., Alhussein, M., & Muhammad, G. (2021, February 16). Blockchain-based UAV path planning for healthcare 4.0: Current challenges and the way ahead. *IEEE Network*, *35*(1), 20–29.

Ahmad R. W., Salah K., Jayaraman R., Yaqoob I., Ellahham S., Omar M. (2021). The role of blockchain technology in telehealth and telemedicine Int. J. Med. Inf. (2021 Jan 28), p. 104399

Al Omar, A., Bhuiyan, M. Z., Basu, A., Kiyomoto, S., & Rahman, M. S. (2019, June 1). Privacy-friendly platform for healthcare data in cloud-based on blockchain environment Future Generat. *Comput. Syst.*, *95*, 511–521.

Al Omar, A., Rahman, M. S., Basu, A., & Kiyomoto, S. (2017). Medibchain: a Blockchain-based privacy-preserving platform for healthcare data International Conference on Security, Privacy and Anonymity in Computation, Communication and Storage, Springer, Cham (2017 Dec 12), pp. 534-543

Alexis. (2025). Blockchain in Healthcare: Benefits, Challenges, and Future Potential. HealthPoint; healthpoint.com. https://healthpoint.com/technology/blockchain-in-healthcare-benefits-challenges-and-future-potential/ Accessed on: 29/04/2025

Andoni, M., Robu, V., Flynn, D., Abram, S., Geach, D., Jenkins, D., McCallum, P., & Peacok, A. (2019). Blockchain technology in the energy sector: A systematic review of challenges and opportunities. *Renewable & Sustainable Energy Reviews*, *100*, 143–174.

Angraal, S., Krumholz, H. M., & Schulz, W. L. (2017, September). Blockchain technology: Applications in health care. *Circulation: Cardiovascular Quality and Outcomes*, *10*(9), e003800. PMID: 28912202

Ashima, R., Haleem, A., Bahl, S., Javaid, M., Mahla, S. K., & Singh, S. (2021). Automation and manufacturing of smart materials in Additive Manufacturing technologies using Internet of Things towards the adoption of Industry 4.0. *Materials Today: Proceedings*. Advance online publication. DOI: 10.1016/j.matpr.2021.01.583

Berdik, D., Otoum, S., Schmidt, N., Porter, D., & Jararweh, Y. (2021, January 1). A survey on Blockchain for information systems management and security. *Information Processing & Management*, *58*(1), 102397.

Bhattacharya, P., Tanwar, S., Bodke, U., Tyagi, S., & Kumar, N. (2021). Bindaas: Blockchain-based deep-learning as-a-service in healthcare 4.0 applications. *IEEE Transactions on Network Science and Engineering*, *8*(2), 1242–1255.

Bhuvana R., Madhushree L.M., & Aithal P.S. (2020). Blockchain as a disruptive technology in healthcare and financial services-A review-based analysis on current implementations International Journal of Applied Engineering and Management Letters (IJAEML), 4 (1) (2020), pp. 142-155

Blockchain Consultant. (2025). The Role of Blockchain in Healthcare: Use Cases & Challenges - Chain Consult. https://www.chainconsult.io/the-role-of-blockchain-in-healthcare-use-cases-challenges/ Accessed on: 29/04/2025

Celesti, A., Ruggeri, A., Fazio, M., Galletta, A., Villari, M., & Romano, A. (2020, January). Blockchain-based healthcare workflow for telemedical laboratory in federated hospital IoT clouds. *Sensors (Basel)*, *20*(9), 2590. PMID: 32370129

Chelladurai U., Pandian S. (2021). A novel blockchain based electronic health record automation system for healthcare. J. Ambient Intell. Humanized Comput.

Chen, H. S., Jarrell, J. T., Carpenter, K. A., Cohen, D. S., & Huang, X. (2019). Blockchain in healthcare: A patient-centred model. *Biomedical Journal of Scientific & Technical Research*, *20*(3), 15017. PMID: 31565696

Chowdary, C. D., Chigurupati, S., Surapaneni, P., & Maguluri, L. P. (2024). Blockchain for healthcare management: Enhancing data security and transparency. In community practitioner (Vol. 21, Number 07, pp. 651–665). *Zenodo*. https://doi.org/DOI: 10.5281/zenodo.12704770

Curbera, F., Dias, D. M., Simonyan, V., Yoon, W. A., & Casella, A. (2019, April 26). Blockchain: An enabler for healthcare and life sciences transformation. *IBM Journal of Research and Development*, *63*(2/3), 8–1.

Cyran, M. A. (2018, March 23). Blockchain as a foundation for sharing healthcare data. *Blockchain in Healthcare Today*, *1*, 1–6.

De Aguiar, E. J., Faiçal, B. S., Krishnamachari, B., & Ueyama, J. (2020, March 13). A survey of blockchain-based strategies for healthcare. *ACM Computing Surveys*, *53*(2), 1–27.

Dhagarra D., Goswami M., Sarma P. R., & Choudhury A. (2019). Big Data and blockchain supported conceptual model for enhanced healthcare coverage Bus. Process Manag. J. (2019)

Du, X., Chen, B., Ma, M., & Zhang, Y. (2021, January 12). Research on the application of blockchain in smart healthcare: Constructing a hierarchical framework. *Journal of Healthcare Engineering*, •••, 2021. PMID: 33505644

Dubovitskaya, A., Xu, Z., Ryu, S., Schumacher, M., & Wang, F. (2017). Secure and trustable electronic medical records sharing using blockchain. [). American Medical Informatics Association.]. *AMIA ... Annual Symposium Proceedings - AMIA Symposium. AMIA Symposium*, *2017*, 650. PMID: 29854130

Ejaz, M., Kumar, T., Kovacevic, I., Ylianttila, M., & Harjula, E. (2021, January). Health-BlockEdge: Blockchain-edge framework for reliable low-latency digital healthcare applications. *Sensors (Basel)*, *21*(7), 2502. PMID: 33916700

Ekblaw, A., Azaria, A., Halamka, J. D., & Lippman, A. (2016). A Case Study for Blockchain in Healthcare: "MedRec" prototype for electronic health records and medical research data In *Proceedings of IEEE Open & Big Data Conference*, vol. 13, p. 13

Ekblaw, A., Azaria, A., Halamka, J. D., & Lippman, A. (2016). A case study for blockchain in healthcare: "MedRec" prototype for electronic health records and medical research data. *Proceedings of IEEE Open & Big Data Conference*, *13*, 13.

Engelhardt, M. A. (2017). Hitching healthcare to the chain: An introduction to blockchain technology in the healthcare sector. *Technology Innovation Management Review*, *7*(10).

Fan, K., Wang, S., Ren, Y., Li, H., & Yang, Y. (2018). Medblock: Efficient and secure medical data sharing via blockchain. *Journal of Medical Systems*, *42*(8), 136. PMID: 29931655

Farouk, A., Alahmadi, A., Ghose, S., & Mashatan, A. (2020, March 15). Blockchain platform for industrial healthcare: Vision and future opportunities. *Computer Communications*, *154*, 223–235.

Fu, J., Wang, N., & Cai, Y. (2020, January). Privacy-preserving in healthcare blockchain systems based on lightweight message sharing. *Sensors (Basel)*, *20*(7), 1898. PMID: 32235389

Gökalp, E., Gökalp, M. O., Çoban, S., & Eren, P. E. (2018). Analysing opportunities and challenges of integrated blockchain technologies in healthcare InEurosymposium on Systems Analysis and Design, Springer, Cham (2018 Sep 20), pp. 174-183

Griggs, K. N., Ossipova, O., Kohlios, C. P., Baccarini, A. N., Howson, E. A., & Hayajneh, T. (2018, July). Healthcare blockchain system using smart contracts for secure automated remote patient monitoring. *Journal of Medical Systems*, *42*(7), 1–7. PMID: 29876661

Gul, M. J., Subramanian, B., Paul, A., & Kim, J. (2021, February 1). Blockchain for public health care in smart society. *Microprocessors and Microsystems*, *80*, 103524.

Haleem, A., Javaid, M., Singh, R. P., Suman, R., & Rab, S. (2021). Blockchain technology applications in healthcare: An overview, International Journal of Intelligent Networks, Volume 2, Pages 130-139, ISSN 2666-6030, https://doi.org/DOI: 10.1016/j.ijin.2021.09.005

Hathaliya, J., Sharma, P., Tanwar, S., & Gupta, R. (2019). Blockchain-based remote patient monitoring in healthcare 4.0 In2019 IEEE 9th International Conference on Advanced Computing (IACC), IEEE (2019 Dec 13), pp. 87-91

Hölbl, M., Kompara, M., Kamišalić, A., & Zlatolas, L. N. (2018). A systematic review of the use of Blockchain in healthcare. *Symmetry*, *10*(10), 470.

Hussien, H. M., Yasin, S. M., Udzir, N. I., Ninggal, M. I., & Salman, S. (2021, June 1). Blockchain technology in the healthcare industry: Trends and opportunities. *Journal of Industrial Information Integration*, *22*, 100217.

Ichikawa D., Kashiyama M., Ueno T. (2017). Tamper-resistant mobile health using blockchain technology, Journal of Medical Internet Research, mHealth uHealth 5 (7) (2017) e111.

Islam, A., & Shin, S. Y. (2020, June 1). A blockchain-based secure healthcare scheme with the assistance of unmanned aerial vehicles in the Internet of Things Comput. *Electrical Engineering*, *84*, 106627.

Islam, N., Faheem, Y., Din, I. U., Talha, M., Guizani, M., & Khalil, M. (2019, November 1). A blockchain-based fog computing framework for activity recognition as an application to e-Healthcare services Future Generat. *Comput. Syst.*, *100*, 569–578.

Ismail, L., Material, H., & Zeadally, S. (2019, October 15). Lightweight blockchain for healthcare. *IEEE Access : Practical Innovations, Open Solutions*, *7*, 149935–149951.

Javaid, M., & Haleem, A. (2019, May 1). Industry 4.0 applications in medical field: A brief review. *Current Medicine Research and Practice*, *9*(3), 102–109.

Jiang, S., Cao, J., Wu, H., Yang, Y., Ma, M., & He, J. (2018). Blochie: a blockchain-based platform for healthcare information exchange 2018 IEEE International Conference on Smart Computing (Smart Comp), IEEE (2018 Jun 18), pp. 49-56

Jiang, S., Cao, J., Wu, H., Yang, Y., Ma, M., & He, J. (2018). BlocHIE: a blockchain-based platform for healthcare information exchange, in: IEEE International Conference on Smart Computing (SMARTCOMP), IEEE, 2018, pp. 49–56.

Kassab, M.H., DeFranco j., Malas T., Laplante G.D., & Neto V.V. (2019). Exploring research in Blockchain for healthcare and a roadmap for the future. *IEEE Transactions on Emerging Topics in Computing*.

Kasyapa, M. S. B., & Vanmathi, C. (2024). Blockchain integration in healthcare: A comprehensive investigation of use cases, performance issues, and mitigation strategies. *Frontiers in Digital Health*, *6*, 1359858. DOI: 10.3389/fdgth.2024.1359858 PMID: 38736708

Khatoon, A. (2020, January). A blockchain-based innovative contract system for healthcare management. *Electronics (Basel)*, *9*(1), 94.

Khezr, S., Moniruzzaman, M., Yassine, A., & Benlamri, R. (2019). Blockchain technology in healthcare: A comprehensive review and directions for future research. *Applied Sciences (Basel, Switzerland)*, *9*(9), 1736.

Khujamatov, K., Reypnazarov, E., Akhmedov, N., & Khasanov, D. (2020). Blockchain for 5G healthcare architecture In2020 International Conference on Information Science and Communications Technologies (ICISCT), IEEE (2020 Nov 4), pp. 1-5

Koshechkin, K. A., Klimenko, G. S., Ryabkov, I. V., & Kozhin, P. B. (2018, January 1). Scope for the application of blockchain in the public healthcare of the Russian federation. *Procedia Computer Science*, *126*, 1323–1328.

Kumar, T., Ramani, V., Ahmad, I., Braeken, A., Harjula, E., & Ylianttila, M. (2018). Blockchain utilisation in healthcare: key requirements and challenges. In2018 IEEE 20th International Conference on E-Health Networking, Applications and Services (Healthcom), IEEE (2018 Sep 17), pp. 1-7

Leeming, G., Cunningham, J., & Ainsworth, J. (2019, July 24). A ledger of me: Personalising healthcare using blockchain technology. *Frontiers of Medicine*, *6*, 171. PMID: 31396516

Mackey, T. K., Kuo, T. T., Gummadi, B., Clauson, K. A., Church, G., Grishin, D., Obbad, K., Barkovich, R., & Palombini, M. (2019, December). 'Fit-for-purpose?'– challenges and opportunities for applications of blockchain technology in the future of healthcare. *BMC Medicine*, *17*(1), 1–7. PMID: 30914045

Mamoshina, P., Ojomoko, L., Yanovich, Y., Ostrovski, A., Botezatu, A., Prikhodko, P., Izumchenko, E., Aliper, A., Romantsov, K., Zhebrak, A., & Ogu, I. O. (2018, January 19). Converging Blockchain and next-generation artificial intelligence technologies to decentralise and accelerate biomedical research and healthcare. *Oncotarget*, *9*(5), 5665. PMID: 29464026

Mazlan, A. A., Daud, S. M., Sam, S. M., Abas, H., Rasid, S. Z., & Yusof, M. F. (2020, January 24). Scalability challenges in healthcare blockchain system—A systematic review. *IEEE Access : Practical Innovations, Open Solutions*, *8*, 23663–23673.

Mijwil, M. M., Aljanabi, M., Abotaleb, M., Shukur, B. S., Al Sailawi, A. S. A., Bala, I., Hiran, K. K., Doshi, R., & Dhoska, K. (2025). *Exploring the Impact of Blockchain Revolution on the Healthcare Ecosystem: A Critical Review*. Mesopotamian Journal of CyberSecurity., DOI: 10.58496/MJCS/2025/006

Mohanasundaram, S., Ramirez-Asis, E., Quispe-Talla, A., Bhatt, M. W., & Shabaz, M. (2022). Experimental replacement of hops by mango in beer: Production and comparison of total phenolics, flavonoids, minerals, carbohydrates, proteins and toxic substances. *International Journal of System Assurance Engineering and Management*, *2022*(13), 132–145.

Moona G., Jewariya M., Sharma R. (2019). Relevance of dimensional metrology in manufacturing industries MAPAN, 34, pp. 97-104, DOI: 10.1007/s12647-018-0291-3

Morar, C. D., & Popescu, D. E. (2024). A Survey of Blockchain Applicability, Challenges, and Key Threats. *Computers*, *13*(9), 223. DOI: 10.3390/computers13090223

Munoz, D. J., Constantinescu, D. A., Asenjo, R., & Fuentes, L. (2019). Clinicappchain: a low-cost blockchain hyperledger solution for healthcare International Congress on Blockchain and Applications, Springer, Cham (2019 Jun 26), pp. 36-44

Nguyen, D. C., Pathirana, P. N., Ding, M., & Seneviratne, A. (2021). BEdgeHealth: A decentralised architecture for edge-based IoMT networks using blockchain. *IEEE Internet of Things Journal*, *8*(14), 11743–11757.

Onik, M. M., Aich, S., Yang, J., Kim, C. S., & Kim, H. C. (2019). Blockchain in healthcare: challenges and solutions Big Data Analytics for Intelligent Healthcare Management, Academic Press (2019 Jan 1), pp. 197-226

Pandey, P., & Litoriya, R. (2020, March 1). Implementing healthcare services on a large scale: Challenges and remedies based on blockchain technology. *Health Policy and Technology*, *9*(1), 69–78.

Peterson, K., Deeduvanu, R., Kanjamala, P., & Boles, K. (2016). A blockchain-based approach to health information exchange networks InProc. NIST Workshop Blockchain Healthcare, 1 (No. 1) (2016 Sep), pp. 1-10

Pham, H. L., Tran, T. H., & Nakashima, Y. (2018). A secure remote healthcare system for hospital using blockchain smart contract In2018 IEEE Globecom Workshops (GC Wkshps), IEEE (2018 Dec 9), pp. 1-6

Ramani, V., Kumar, T., Bracken, A., Liyanage, M., & Ylianttila, M. (2018). Secure and efficient data accessibility in Blockchain-based healthcare systems In2018 IEEE Global Communications Conference (GLOBECOM), IEEE (2018 Dec 9), pp. 206-212

Ray, P. P., Dash, D., Salah, K., & Kumar, N. (2020, January 21). Blockchain for IoT-based healthcare: Background, consensus, platforms, and use cases. *IEEE Systems Journal*, *15*(1), 85–94.

Ribitzky, R., Clair, J. S., Houlding, D. I., McFarlane, C. T., Ahier, B., Gould, M., Flannery, H. L., Pupo, E., & Clauson, K. A. (2018, March 23). Pragmatic, interdisciplinary perspectives on Blockchain and distributed ledger technology: Paving the future for healthcare. *Blockchain in Healthcare Today*, *1*, 24.

Saha, A., Amin, R., Kunal, S., Vollala, S., & Dwivedi, S. K. (2019, September). Review on "Blockchain technology-based medical healthcare system with privacy issues. *Security and Privacy*, *2*(5), e83.

Satamraju, K. P. (2020, January). Proof of concept of scalable integration of internet of things and Blockchain in healthcare. *Sensors (Basel)*, *20*(5), 1389. PMID: 32138380

Schinckus, C. (2020). The good, the bad and the ugly: An overview of the sustainability of blockchain technology. *Energy Research & Social Science*, *69*(1), 101614.

Schinckus, C. (2021). Proof-of-work based blockchain technology and Anthropocene: An undermined situation? *Renewable & Sustainable Energy Reviews*, *152*, 111682.

Schinckus, C. (2022). A Nuanced perspective on blockchain technology and healthcare. Technology in Society, Vol 71, (2022), ISSN 0160-791X, https://doi.org/DOI: 10.1016/j.techsoc.2022.102082

Shen, B., Guo, J., & Yang, Y. (2019). Med Chain: Efficient healthcare data sharing via Blockchain. *Applied Sciences (Basel, Switzerland)*, *9*(6), 1207.

Smolenskas, A. (2024). Blockchain in healthcare: Benefits, use cases, & challenges. BitDegree. Retrieved from https://www.bitdegree.org/crypto/tutorials/blockchain-in-healthcare#challenges-and-considerations Accessed on 22/04/2025

Soltanisehat, L., Alizadeh, R., Hao, H., & Choo, K. K. (2020). Technical, temporal, and spatial research challenges and opportunities in blockchain-based healthcare: A systematic literature review. *IEEE Transactions on Engineering Management*, •••, 1–16.

Sriram, G. (2022). Edge computing vs. Cloud computing: An overview of big data challenges and opportunities for large enterprises. *International Research Journal of Modernization in Engineering Technology and Science*, *2022*(4), 1331–1337.

Srivastava, G., Crichigno, J., & Dhar, S. (2019). A light and secure healthcare blockchain for IoT medical devices In2019 IEEE Canadian Conference of Electrical and Computer Engineering (CCECE), IEEE (2019 May 5), pp. 1-5

Stone, D. (2018). Blockchain: The challenges and opportunities in healthcare. *Divurgent*, *1*, 1–14.

Sun, Y., Zhang, R., Wang, X., Gao, K., & Liu, L. (2018). A decentralising attribute-based signature for healthcare blockchain In2018 27th International Conference on Computer Communication and Networks (ICCCN), IEEE (2018 Jul 30), pp. 1-9

Syed, T. A., Alzahrani, A., Jan, S., Siddiqui, M. S., Nadeem, A., & Alghamdi, T. (2019, December 4). A comparative analysis of blockchain architecture and its applications: Problems and recommendations. *IEEE Access : Practical Innovations, Open Solutions*, *7*, 176838–176869.

Taherdoost, H. (2023). Privacy and Security of Blockchain in Healthcare: Applications, Challenges, and Future Perspectives. *Sci.*, *5*(4), 41. DOI: 10.3390/sci5040041

Tandon, A., Dhir, A., Islam, N., & Mäntymäki, M. (2020, November 1). Blockchain in healthcare: A systematic literature review, synthesising framework and future research agenda. *Computers in Industry*, *122*, 103290.

Tanwar, S., Parekh, K., & Evans, R. (2020, February 1). Blockchain-based electronic healthcare record system for healthcare 4.0 applications. *Journal of Information Security and Applications*, *50*, 102407.

Vaishya, R., Haleem, A., Vaish, A., & Javaid, M. (2020, July 1). Emerging technologies to combat the COVID-19 pandemic. *Journal of Clinical and Experimental Hepatology*, *10*(4), 409–411. PMID: 32377057

Vaishya R., Javaid M., Khan I.H., Vaish A., & Iyengar K.P. (2021). Significant role of modern technologies for COVID-19 pandemic Journal of Industrial Integration and Management (2021 Mar 4), pp. 1-3

Wang, S., Wang, J., Wang, X., Qiu, T., Yuan, Y., Ouyang, L., Guo, Y., & Wang, F. Y. (2018, August 28). Blockchain-powered parallel healthcare systems based on the ACP approach. *IEEE Transactions on Computational Social Systems*, *5*(4), 942–950.

Zarour, M., Ansari, M. T., Alenezi, M., Sarkar, A. K., Faizan, M., Agrawal, A., Kumar, R., & Khan, R. A. (2020, August 27). Evaluating the impact of blockchain models for secure and trustworthy electronic healthcare records. *IEEE Access : Practical Innovations, Open Solutions*, *8*, 157959–157973.

Zhang, P., & Boulos, M. N. (2020). Blockchain solutions for healthcare Precision Medicine for Investigators, Practitioners and Providers, Academic Press (2020 Jan 1), pp. 519-524

Zhang, P., Schmidt, D. C., White, J., & Lenz, G. (2018). *Blockchain technology use cases in healthcare. Advances in Computers* (Vol. 111). Elsevier.

Zhang, P., Walker, M. A., White, J., Schmidt, D. C., & Lenz, G. (2017). Metrics for assessing blockchain-based healthcare decentralised apps In2017 IEEE 19th International Conference on E-Health Networking, Applications and Services (Healthcom), IEEE (2017 Oct 12), pp. 1-4

Zheng, K., Liu, Y., Dai, C., Duan, Y., & Huang, X. (2018). Model checking PBFT consensus mechanism in healthcare blockchain network In2018 9th International Conference on Information Technology in Medicine and Education (ITME), IEEE (2018 Oct 19), pp. 877-881

Zheng, Z., Xie, S., Dai, H. N., Chen, X., & Wang, H. (2018). Blockchain challenges and opportunities: A survey. *International Journal of Web and Grid Services*, *2018*(14), 352–3.

Chapter 4

Recent Trends in Healthcare:
Computational Intelligence, Challenges, and Opportunities

Kannadhasan Suriyan
https://orcid.org/0000-0001-6443-9993
Study World College of Engineering, India

R. Nagarajan
https://orcid.org/0000-0002-4990-5869
Gnanamani College of Technology, India

K. Deepa
Karpagam College of Engineering, India

ABSTRACT

Data are necessary for learning health systems, but feedback loops of knowledge into revised behaviour. This is dependent on knowledge application and management, both of which are reliant on efficient system development. The multidisciplinary area that covers the complete spectrum of health science, social science, information science, and technology is known as biomedical informatics. IssuesConclusions Policy makers and research funders must acknowledge the gap between the "two cultures" that currently exists and understand that in order to fully reap the social and economic benefits of data science and digital health, it is necessary to accept the interdisciplinary nature of biomedical informatics and to support a significant expansion of clinical informatics capacity and capability

DOI: 10.4018/979-8-3373-1225-5.ch004

INTRODUCTION

In the present setting, data quality in the frontline health and care system confronts two challenges. First, while effort is being done in this area, reference values and standard data sets are still not widely used. The second is poor data quality brought on by unpredictable process adherence and difficult system use. Implementing clinical terminology, such as Systematized Nomenclature of Medicine Clinical Terms (SNOMED CT) and Logical Observation Identifiers Names and Codes (LOINC), reveals to us that the complexity of these standards and our cultural context have always led to protracted debate and substantial implementation effort. Even the 'Global Digital Exemplars' have made little headway so far in fully integrating SNOMED CT. Additionally, interactions with other care settings, such as social care and mental health, add complexity, D.H Hubel (1962), et.al. The GP data is not at all reliable. Usage varies from practice to practice and from clinician to clinician. Different sectors will be used in different ways, A. Krizhevsky (2012), et.al. In the past, et.al. A system has not compelled users to standardize their practice or recordkeeping. Because of this, the data quality varies amongst GP practices, which has an impact on operational procedures as well as epidemiological research, M. D. Zeiler (2014), et.al. Numerous factors, including poor usability, unnecessarily complicated systems, a lack of data entry logic to detect mistakes, and inadequate business change leadership, contribute to the failure to enter correct data into health and care systems., R. Frank (1957), et.al.

Instead of using free text, most epidemiological studies utilizing regular clinical data employ coded data, C. Szegedy (2015) *et al.* As a result, codes used during clinical consultations are overused. Using allergy as an example, a national analysis of code usage in primary care in Scotland found that 10% of the 352 allergy codes (n = 36) accounted for 95% of usage, 21% of the codes were never used, and 50% of the codes were used in over 2 million consultations over the course of seven years J. L. Mcclelland (1987) et al. According to a comprehensive study, there are differences in the accuracy and completeness of morbidity recording among disease regions (66%–96%), D. E. Rumelhart (1988), et.al. For instance, in primary care, the recording quality for diabetes is higher than for asthma. Additionally, throughout time, changes in case definition and diagnostic standards occur across disease categories but are seldom addressed in the databases, J. Ngiam, A. (2011), et al. The choice of codes may affect outcome measures, according to a recent primary care research, Coiera E (2003). et al. For instance, the incidence rate was shown to be greater when non-diagnostic codes were used than with diagnostic codes. Since coding of data varies across general practitioner practices, there was a substantial difference in incidence rate and trends when those practices were included in the study, with a lower incidence rate and declining trends. This research emphasizes the impact of incorrect coding and categorization, Friedman (2017) et.al. Additionally, it demonstrates that missing data could not be an accident. Additionally, codes that were required during consultation and hence recorded in free text may not be available. When examining patient databases for research, all these important aspects of data coding are often overlooked, which may result in incorrect results. The underlying inconsistencies in coded data could not be sorted, no matter how much data purification was done. Confounding by indication or severity may exist, for instance, if patients with serious illnesses get more intensive care and have worse results than other patients, Heathfield HA (1995)., e.g. Clinical databases only provide information on people who used medical services. In research conducted throughout the UK, the frequency of asthma varied depending on whether it was documented via community surveys or clinical databases. Since clinical databases were not created with research as their major goal, there may also be a lack of important factors in them, such as the absence of diagnoses in outpatient hospital attendances., Rouse WB (2017), et.al. This is in addition to the quality of the data that has been coded.

We have outlined significant problems with the quality of regular data and suggested solutions that go beyond meaningless "data cleansing." We argue that in order to fully realize the social and economic benefits of digital health and data science, policymakers and research funders must accept the interdisciplinary nature of biomedical informatics and support a significant expansion of clinical informatics capacity and capability. Currently, there is a gap between the "two cultures," and this gap must be acknowledged. The use of data analytics in health informatics has increased significantly during the last ten years as a result of the enormous flood of multimodality data. Additionally, this has led to a rise in interest in the development of analytical, data-driven models based on machine learning in the field of health informatics.

In recent years, deep learning, a method built on artificial neural networks, has emerged as a potent machine learning tool that has the potential to transform the field of artificial intelligence. In addition to the technology's capacity to create automatically optimized high-level characteristics and semantic interpretation from the input data, rapid advancements in processing power, quick data storage, and parallelization have also helped to accelerate its popularity. This article provides a thorough, current assessment of studies using deep learning in health informatics and offers a critical evaluation of the relative merits, possible drawbacks, and prospects for the technology. The study primarily focuses on important deep learning applications in the areas of ubiquitous sensing, medical informatics, medical imaging, and public health. A fascinating new trend in machine learning has just emerged thanks to DEEP learning. The traditional neural network (NN) literature serves as a solid theoretical framework for deep learning. However, in contrast to more conventional applications of NNs, deep learning takes into consideration the utilization of several hidden neurons and layers—typically more than two—as an architectural benefit in conjunction with novel training paradigms. While using a large number of neurons enables thorough coverage of the available raw data, a reduced dimensional projection of the input space is produced by a layer-by-layer pipeline of nonlinear combination of their outputs. Every projection into a lower dimension correlates to a greater degree of perception. The raw data or pictures are effectively high-level abstracted as long as the network is weighted correctly.

The automated development of this feature set without human involvement has several benefits in fields like health informatics. For instance, it may provide characteristics that are more complex and challenging to detail in descriptive ways in medical imaging. Implicit characteristics may identify fibroids and polyps and describe abnormalities in tissue shape like tumors. Such traits may be used in translational bioinformatics to identify nucleotide sequences that potentially bind a DNA or RNA strand to a protein. According to the number of articles published in recent years in health informatics sub-fields such bioinformatics, medical imaging, ubiquitous sensing, medical informatics, and public health, there has been a sharp increase in interest in deep learning. Several architectures stand out in popularity among the numerous methodological deep learning versions. The number of articles using the deep learning technique since 2010. Convolutional Neural Networks (CNNs) in particular have made a significant contribution to the area of health informatics. Its design may be described as a series of feed-forward layers that implement convolutional filters interspersed with layers that perform reduction, rectification, or pooling. A high-level abstract characteristic arises at each layer of the network. The process by which the visual cortex assimilates visual information in the shape of receptive fields is similar to the architecture that was inspired by biology.

NNs with several layers, such as deep neural networks (DNNs), or recurrent neural networks (RNNs), such as those with directed cycles. Deep learning's practical adoption and acceleration have both been significantly impacted by recent advancements in graphics processing units (GPUs). In fact, while just recently beginning to gain popularity, many of the theoretical concepts behind deep learning were first put out in the pre-GPU period. By shifting the majority of common algebraic operations with dense matrices, including matrix products and convolutions, to the GPU, deep learning systems like CNNs may be massively parallelized. Numerous experimental efforts have so far used deep learning models in health informatics, often outperforming more traditional methods in terms of performance. However, there are a number of issues that need to be handled when using deep learning to health informatics. For instance, obtaining the quantity of labelled data necessary to train a deep architecture might be challenging in the healthcare industry. A significant amount of processing power is furthermore needed for deep learning, without which training could take an inordinate amount of time Rouce WB. (2024) – NHS

(2017). Finding an ideal formulation of the free parameters of the network might be a particularly difficult problem to tackle. Additional learning procedures are needed to overcome these challenges since convergence problems and overfitting may eventually impair deep learning models.

HEALTHCARE

NNs with one or more hidden layers of Perceptrons have been developed to answer increasingly challenging issues. These NNs are typically trained across a number of stages, or epochs, where each time the network receives a new input sample, the weights of each neuron are changed in accordance with a procedure known as the delta rule. The most popular type of supervised NNs employs the delta rule during training and typically does so via taking use of the back-propagation algorithm. In particular, the network weights are given random values without any previous information. The network weights are modified via an iterative training procedure to reduce the discrepancy between the network outputs and the intended outputs. The gradient descent approach, in which the network is optimized to find the minimum along the error surface, is the most used iterative training technique. The activation functions must always be differentiable in order for the approach to work. As the hidden layers capture the nonlinear interactions, adding additional hidden layers to the network enables the construction of a deep architecture that can represent more complicated assumptions. These NNs are referred to as DNNs. As soon as the mistakes are back-propagated to the first few layers, they become insignificant (the gradient vanishes), failing the learning process, making DNN training difficult. Even while more sophisticated backpropagation variation may resolve this issue, they still produce an extremely sluggish learning process.

Deep learning has made it possible to train DNN structures using new, advanced methods. DNNs may generally be taught using supervised and unsupervised learning techniques. In unsupervised learning, the training is carried out without the need for labelled data, while in supervised learning, labelled data are utilized to train the DNNs and learn the weights that minimize the error to predict a target value for classification or regression. Unsupervised learning is often used for dimensionality reduction, feature extraction, or grouping. To extract the most pertinent features for classification by using a supervised learning phase, it is usual practice for certain applications to combine an initial training approach of the DNN with an unsupervised learning step. When using deep learning frameworks, these factors need to be considered. DNNs have been unworkable for a long time because to hardware restrictions caused by high computing requirements for both training and processing, particularly for applications that call for real-time processing is shown in Figure 1.

These restrictions have since been somewhat solved by hardware improvements and the potential of parallelization due to GPU acceleration, cloud computing, and multicore processing, allowing DNNs to be acknowledged as a major advancement in artificial intelligence.

Figure 1. Challenges and opportunities of AI in healthcare

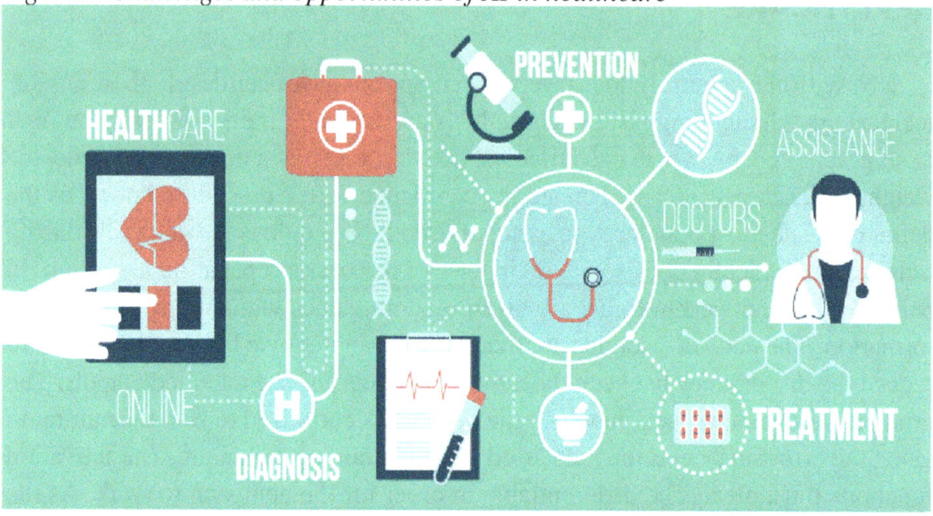

In recent years, deep learning has become more important in machine learning and pattern identification. This study describes how deep learning has made it possible to produce more data-driven solutions in health informatics by enabling the automated production of features that minimize the amount of human participation in this process. This is helpful for a variety of health informatics issues and has helped unstructured data from fields like bioinformatics, medical imaging, and medical informatics make significant strides ahead. Up until recently, the majority of deep learning applications in health informatics have required handling unstructured sources of health data. However, structured data, such as EHRs, which provide a thorough picture of the patient's history, pathology, therapy, diagnosis, outcome, and similar information, also encodes a large amount of information. When a tumor is diagnosed using medical imaging, the cytological notes may provide important details including its stage and dissemination. With the use of this knowledge, one may develop a comprehensive understanding of a patient's illness or condition and then enhance the accuracy of any conclusions drawn. In reality, artificial intelligence and robust inference via deep learning may improve the dependability of clinical decision support systems. But there are still a number of technical issues to be resolved. Obtaining patient and clinical data is expensive, and the majority of a typical health dataset consists of healthy control people. Deep learning techniques have often been used in situations where the datasets were balanced or, as a workaround, where artificial data was created to achieve fairness. The second option raises a new problem about the reliability of the manufactured biological data samples.

The methodological features of NNs must thus be reviewed in this context. Deep learning's reliance on copious quantities of training data is another issue. These criteria increase the importance of the traditional machine learning entrance hurdles, such as data accessibility and privacy. We anticipate that more ad hoc hardware platforms for neural networks and deep learning processing will be disclosed and made commercially accessible in the years to come, with reference to the problem of computing capacity. It is important to note that major IT companies (such as Google, Facebook, and Baidu), whose core businesses heavily rely on data collection, enormous storehouses, and processing power, have actively supported the development of deep learning. These companies hold a significant amount of patents in the field. Given the large number of free packages available to facilitate this study, many academics have been inspired to use deep learning to any data-mining and pattern recognition problems linked to health informatics.

On the plus side, it has encouraged a fascinating trend and raised expectations for what machine learning may do on its own. However, we shouldn't see deep learning as the panacea to every problem that health informatics presents. When compared to other fast learning algorithms that could achieve comparable performance with fewer resources, less parameterization, tuning, and higher interpretability, deep learning's need for a significant amount of training data and computational resources is still debatable in practice. As a result, we draw the conclusion that deep learning has helped NNs and connectionism come back to life thanks to the true integration of the most recent developments in parallel processing made possible by coprocessors. However, if health informatics research is consistently focused only on deep learning, this might delay the creation of new machine learning algorithms that make better use of computing resources and interpretability.

There has been an explosion of study in the disciplines of healthcare and data sciences as a result of the digital health data's rapid expansion and general availability. The traditional techniques of managing health data have had only little success because they are unable to handle the enormous amounts of complicated data that are produced at high volumes, rapid rates of change, and a wide diversity. With a methodical study of the traditional and modern approaches, this paper provides a thorough overview of the current issues, solutions, and future possibilities for computational health informatics in the big data era. Volume, Velocity, Variety, and Veracity are the four Vs that we used to categorize the issues. We also suggested a systematic data-processing pipeline for generic big data in health informatics that addresses data collection, storing, sharing, analyzing, searching, and decision support. Particularly, several machine learning algorithms and methodologies are compared and categorized. We identify and explore the key future possibilities for computational health informatics in this big data era based on the content presented here. There is growing interest in computational health informatics both within and outside of the medical sector. A variety of fields, including biomedical, medical, nursing, information technology, computer science, and statistics are all involved in this interdisciplinary subject.

Health informatics gathers and analyses data from all healthcare domains using information and communication technologies (ICTs) in order to forecast patients' health state. Enhancing Health Care Output (HCO) or patients' quality of care is the main objective of health informatics research. In recent years, the amount of medical and healthcare data has grown quickly in the sector. The development of both healthcare data and digital healthcare data. Digital health data have significantly increased in recent years as a result of the quick development of fresh technologies. Additional data sources have been made possible by new medical advancements as well as mobile applications, collecting devices, innovative sensors, and wearable technology. As a result, the healthcare sector generates a large amount of digital data by using data from all sources, including Personal Health Records (PHRs), a subset of Electronic Health Records (EHRs), and Electronic Health Records (EHRs), which include medical history, laboratory results, and medication information.

HEALTHCARE COMPUTATIONAL INTELLIGENCE

According to sources, the estimated global volume of digital healthcare data was over 500 petabytes (1015) in 2012, and according to estimates, it would rise to 25 exabytes by 2020. The structure of the digital health data is both vast in quantity and intricate for conventional software and hardware. The vast variety of structured and unstructured data, including handwritten doctor notes, medical records, medical diagnostic images (such as MRI, CT, and radiographic films) are some of the contributing factors to the failure of traditional systems to handle these datasets. Healthcare informatics has noisy, heterogeneous, complicated, longitudinal, diversified, and massive datasets.

- Difficulties in collecting, storing, processing, and visualizing such vast and complex datasets
- The need of increased processing, compute, and storage power
- The need to improve healthcare concerns that existing systems do not adequately handle, such as care quality, sharing, patient data security, and healthcare cost reduction.

Therefore, there is a need for methods to handle and analyze such large, varied, and complicated datasets in a reasonable amount of time and storage. Big data analytics, a phrase used often to refer to vast and complex datasets, are essential for handling the enormous amount of healthcare data and enhancing the standard of care provided to patients. Additionally, it offers a promising future for lowering healthcare costs, enhancing therapies, achieving more personalized medicine, and assisting medical professionals in making personalized judgements. Big data is described as "high-volume, high-velocity and high-variety information assets that demand cost-effective, innovative forms of information processing for enhanced insight and decision-making." big data in health informatics is expected to be a multidisciplinary undertaking requiring ongoing work from several topic specialists. They include, but are not limited to, engineering scientists who provide the fundamental big data infrastructure for gathering, storing, sharing, and managing big data; computer science data scientists who offer solutions for processing and analyzing high-volume, high-velocity healthcare data using a variety of data mining and machine-learning techniques; clinicians and doctors from the medical domain who provide expert healthcare data analysis, provide individualized care, and make decisions about patients' care. For this reason, it is a desired feature for an advanced big data analysis system to be able to enable input from various human specialists, exchange of viewpoints, and collaborative exploration of outcomes. Computer algorithms may find it challenging to spot patterns and analyze results at times. Additionally, there are occasions when the health sector lacks big data because there are just a few datasets or a limited number of unusual occurrences, for example, when machine-learning algorithms struggle due to a lack of training samples. In these situations, we need more than simply autonomous machine learning; we still require a person to be involved. In other words, interactive machine learning (iML) or "human in the loop" methods may be used in the field of health informatics when automated machine-learning algorithms are unable to handle uncommon occurrences on their own and need a human expert to participate in the learning process. The learning process may be enhanced by this interaction between computer algorithms and human specialists.

Big data has mostly emerged as a result of the exponential rise in computing power, the proliferation of internet-enabled data-generating gadgets, and the lowering costs of data storage itself, which make data accessible to everyone for almost no cost. One of the key industries where big data analytics has shown to be much more effective than traditional methods is the healthcare industry. Big data is primarily concerned with the storing and processing of enormous and complicated data collections, for which conventional approaches are ineffective. In order to provide readers a comprehensive understanding of the technology, methodology, and big data algorithms used for data management and healthcare decision-making, a survey on the usage of big data analytics in this field has been conducted. The findings of this survey article will be useful to academics, researchers, and businesses with an interest in big data in general and healthcare in particular.

Figure 2. Computational AI techniques in healthcare

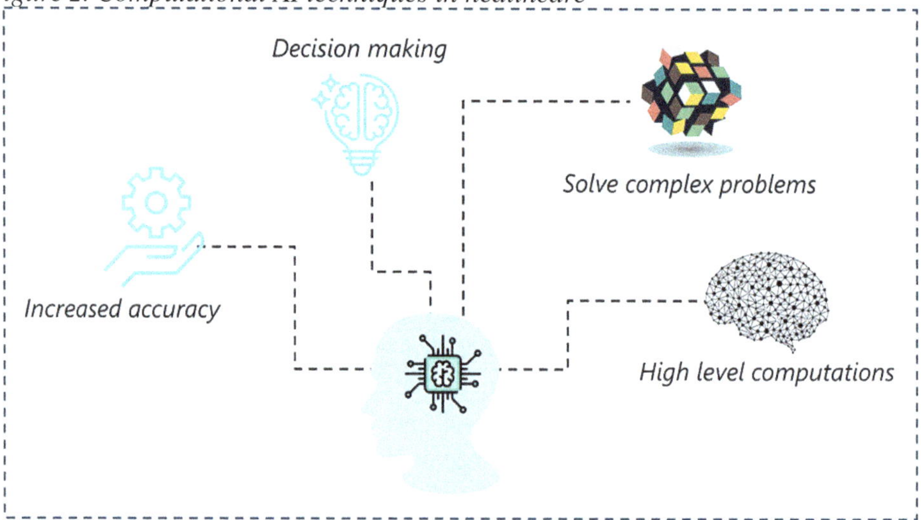

Due to record keeping, regulatory compliance, and patient care, the healthcare sector traditionally has produced enormous amounts of data. The majority of the data produced at the point of care in the past was unstructured: paper prescriptions, MRI, CT, and other images, office medical records, handwritten notes from nurses and doctors, hospital admission and discharge records. The growing digitalization of data in the healthcare sector has begun to generate data that satisfies every aspect and definition of big data. The analysis of this digital data will have a variety of positive effects on clinical procedures, illness monitoring, population health management, and other areas of the healthcare sector is shown in Figure 2. Big data in healthcare, by definition, refers to electronic health data sets that are so enormous and complicated that they are challenging (or impossible) to handle using conventional hardware and/or software, and that they are also challenging (or impossible) to manage with conventional or common data management tools and methodologies. It also includes patient information from electronic patient records (EPRs), machine-generated/sensor data, such as from monitoring vital signs, social media posts, such as Twitter feeds (so-called tweets), blogs, status updates on Facebook and other public forums, as well as clinical data from CPOE (Computerized Physician Order Entry) and clinical decision support systems (physicians' written notes and prescriptions, medical imaging, laboratory, pharmacy, insurance, and other administrative data).

CONCLUSION

The overview of big data in healthcare, its characteristics, its users, and the issues faced by healthcare informatics are all covered in this study. Despite the fact that this study presents a number of prospects and methodologies for big data analytics in healthcare, there are still many more areas that need to be investigated with regard to different elements of healthcare data, such as quality, privacy, timeliness, and so on. A new and vital research area with the potential to have a huge influence on the traditional healthcare sector is computational health informatics in the big data era. The exponential growth of digital health data will be advantageous for health informatics in the future.

REFERENCES

Coiera, E. (2003). *Guide to health informatics* (2nd ed.). CRC Press., DOI: 10.1201/b13618

Frank, R. (1957). *The perceptron: A perceiving and recognizing automaton* (Tech. Rep. No. 85-460-1). Cornell Aeronautical Laboratory. McClelland, J. L., Rumelhart, D. E., & the PDP Research Group. (1987). *Parallel distributed processing* (Vol. 2). MIT Press.

Friedman, C. P., Rubin, J. C., & Sullivan, K. J. (2017). Toward an information infrastructure for global health improvement. *Yearbook of Medical Informatics*, *26*(1), 16–23. DOI: 10.15265/IY-2017-004 PMID: 28480469

Heathfield, H. A., & Wyatt, J. (1995). The road to professionalism in medical informatics: A proposal for debate. *Methods of Information in Medicine*, *34*(5), 426–433. DOI: 10.1055/s-0038-1634627 PMID: 8713756

Hubel, D. H., & Wiesel, T. N. (1962). Receptive fields, binocular interaction and functional architecture in the cat's visual cortex. *The Journal of Physiology*, *160*(1), 106–154. PMID: 14449617

Krizhevsky, A., Sutskever, I., & Hinton, G. E. (2012). Imagenet classification with deep convolutional neural networks. In *Advances in Neural Information Processing Systems* (pp. 1097–1105).

Ngiam, J., Coates, A., Lahiri, A., Prochnow, B., Le, Q. V., & Ng, A. Y. (2011). On optimization methods for deep learning. In *Proceedings of the International Conference on Machine Learning* (pp. 265–272).

NHS England. (2017). *NHS digital academy*. https://www.england.nhs.uk/digitaltechnology/info-revolution/nhs-digital-academy/

Rouse, W. B., Johns, M. M. E., & Pepe, K. M. (2017). Learning in the health care enterprise. *Learning Health Systems*, *1*(4), e10024. DOI: 10.1002/lrh2.10024 PMID: 31245566

Rumelhart, D. E., Hinton, G. E., & Williams, R. J. (1988). Learning representations by back-propagating errors. In Anderson, J. A., & Rosenfeld, E. (Eds.), *Neurocomputing: Foundations of Research* (pp. 696–699). MIT Press., https://dl.acm.org/citation.cfm?id=65669.104451

Szegedy, C., Liu, W., Jia, Y., Sermanet, P., Reed, S., Anguelov, D., & Rabinovich, A. (2015). Going deeper with convolutions. In *Proceedings of the IEEE Conference on Computer Vision and Pattern Recognition* (pp. 1–9).

Zeiler, M. D., & Fergus, R. (2014). Visualizing and understanding convolutional networks. In *European Conference on Computer Vision* (pp. 818–833).

Chapter 5
A Blockchain-Based Framework for Secure Data Sharing in Healthcare

Usharani Bhimavarapu
https://orcid.org/0000-0002-0246-1420
Department of Computer Science and Engineering, Koneru Lakshmaiah Education Foundation, Vaddeswaram, India

ABSTRACT

All the healthcare sector problems of the past, including security, privacy, interoperability, and transparency, are addressable with blockchain technology. Because of the decentralized, tamper-resistant, and transparent nature of blockchain, it is highly appropriate to facilitate secure and effective sharing of information between healthcare professionals, patients, and stakeholders. This document details the place blockchain must occupy in enhancing the digital health system, its applications for rendering patient data secure, interoperability, ownership of health data by patients, and efficient management of healthcare supply chains. Blockchain's function in clinical trials, medical billing, eradication of fraud, and emergency response is discussed as well. While it has tremendous potential, healthcare brings to it challenges inherent in the utilization of blockchain technology, such as cost, scalability, and legality. Future development will be towards eliminating the barriers to the utilization of blockchain technology in widespread use in the health sector globally.

DOI: 10.4018/979-8-3373-1225-5.ch005

INTRODUCTION

Healthcare interoperability is the ability of different healthcare systems, technologies, and platforms to exchange and comprehend data. In today's fast digitalizing healthcare scenario, it holds a lot of value to improve patient care, workflow efficiency, and quality decision-making. The healthcare industry has not yet reached interoperability because of several reasons like siloed infrastructures, proprietary standards, and security purposes. This has resulted in fragmented delivery of healthcare and hindered proper patient information handover between institutions. Blockchain technology offers a solution to such limitations in the guise of an open, decentralized, and secure data-sharing platform. Its nature—consensus and immutability mechanisms—places it at the vanguard of tackling interoperability problems with assured data protection and confidentiality.

Decentralization in blockchain also implies that a company is not able to access the information, and it is capable of reducing the risk of unauthorized access or alteration. The old central databases where data are stored within a central area and can be broken into are no match for blockchain's system where data are stored in a number of nodes, where it is hard for hackers to taint the entire system. All the transactions performed on the blockchain are recorded in a "block" and linked to the previous block, thus creating an immutable chain. With this arrangement, it is practically impossible for anyone to alter any information without the approval of the participants within the network. In the healthcare industry, this has a unique advantage: patient data can be safely exchanged with many stakeholders without risk of data tampering, so that the information will be valid and secure.

Medical histories, laboratory test results, and individual health data are very confidential and have to be tightly secured. Blockchain provides robust protection with encryption where data can be readable or edited by only authorized individuals or systems. Stakeholders are also able to trace history and provenance of data without infringing on privacy as blockchain is transparent. To healthcare providers, it will enable them to share patient data while maintaining patient data confidentiality, just as it does in law, for instance, HIPAA (Health Insurance Portability and Accountability Act) of the United States. The use of cryptographic keys and smart contracts in blockchain technology can also be employed to seal data in a way that credentialed users will only be provided with access to segments of data.

The most useful application of blockchain for healthcare interoperability is accelerating the efficiency of exchanging data. The traditional method of exchanging patient data mostly encompasses complicated workflows, human processing, and system compatibility. Blockchain facilitates this by providing a standardized, automated process of data exchange upon which all network participants have consensus. This grants access to real-time patient information to clinicians regardless of its origin, whether from the institution or the system. Furthermore, blockchain's distributed ledger offers greater transparency with all individuals able to view and authenticate accuracy in data exchanged. It prevents more inconsistency in patient records and everyone can view the latest information.

Patient consent management is a matter of concern in healthcare data exchange. The patients must remain in charge of who will view their data and for what reason. Blockchain provides an auditable and secure approach to patient consent management. With smart contracts, the patient is able to accept, withdraw, or cancel consent at any time with all their operations recorded on the blockchain. This manner makes it transparent and auditable to everyone of the involved stakeholders in an easy way. Also, since patient consent history is unretrievable, patient consent integrity remains safe from unfair alteration or access. Patient consent integrity is safeguarded against unjust alteration or access since blockchain history can't be recovered. The system also makes patient and provider trust possible, and the patients can trust that their data are published only with their explicit consent.

Quality patient care within today's health care setting requires the coordination of several stakeholders, including research institutions, drug companies, payers, and hospitals. But since interoperable systems have never existed, coordination and how effective it is have proven to be hard to achieve. Blockchain allows information sharing between organizational boundaries, thereby making collaboration for such disparate organizations easier. Through offering a shared, common platform, blockchain renders data sharing obstacles non-existent, as various healthcare institutions and providers exchange relevant patient information in real-time. This, in turn, improves the level of care delivered since doctors are in a better position to make more discerning choices through an aggregated and real-time snapshot of a patient's medical history.

Blockchain also holds potential in clinical trials and medical research. Sharing data between institutions in a secure manner while preserving accuracy and integrity of data is one of the main issues in this area. The immutable ledger of blockchain is the best way to document clinical trials, and data entered cannot be forged or modified once entered. This lends credibility to clinical research and fraud or fiddling with data is less likely. Blockchain can potentially facilitate the real-time sharing of research findings, speeding up collaboration and decision-making towards the discovery of new treatments and therapies.

Healthcare data exchange inefficiencies are the main driver of increasing healthcare expenditure. Administrative tasks like data reconciliations, manual data entry, and patient record verification are time-consuming and costly. Blockchain automation by way of smart contracts and distributed networks has the potential to lower this cost by automating processes and eliminating intermediaries. By streamlining processes such as claims adjudication, billing, and maintaining patient records, blockchain reduces administrative burdens on health care providers and insurers. Reduced operating expenses follow, ultimately benefiting patients through the reduction of the total cost of health care services.

Although there are several advantages of blockchain technology, there are a few roadblocks to widespread adoption in healthcare. One of the first challenges is how to cross the gap between blockchain and current healthcare IT systems, perhaps not new and potentially not able to manage decentralized technology. The healthcare industry is also highly regulated, and the greatest care must be exercised to render the deployment of blockchain solutions compliant with regulations in terms of data privacy statutes and medical regulations. Scalability of blockchain networks to support the volume of data generated in an environment of healthcare is another issue. Second, there will be no universal standard of blockchain and therefore different systems would not be compatible to each other, so it will deter mass adoption.

The interoperability future of blockchain for healthcare is looking promising with the ongoing development of the technology and the regimes of regulation. With more scalable and interoperable decentralized solutions based on blockchain, the health care industry will witness widespread adoption of decentralized platforms for sharing data. Why blockchain enhances data security, automates business processes, and lowers cost is a desirable solution for health care providers, researchers, and patients. But sustained collaboration among the stakeholders such as healthcare practitioners, inventors of technology, regulators, and patients will be essential in addressing concerns on use of blockchain. In doing so, blockchain would redefine keeping and sharing of medical data to an improved, secure, and patient-focused system in the future.

Kruse et al. (2018) write about the application of Electronic Health Records (EHR) in helping population health in a systematic review. Despite that their research provides seminal data regarding EHR promises and threats, it is weakened by not delving deeply into how such systems react to innovative technologies such as blockchain. The study also focuses on traditional applications of EHRs and could be inadequate when evaluating newer health data management technology such as decentralized systems (Kruse et al., 2018).

Lehne et al. (2019) speak on digital medicine's dependency on interoperability. In pointing out interoperability as a necessity for the full potential of digital health solutions, the shortcoming of the study is not conducting sufficient inquiry of operational frameworks supporting interoperability. Nor does the article go too deeply into the likely technical and regulatory barriers to implementing such solutions across the globe, such as privacy and safeguarding of data (Lehne et al., 2019).

Agbo et al. (2019) present a brief introduction to blockchain technology in healthcare, highlighting its potential in data security management, privacy, and interoperability. The study's limitation is that it does not have any empirical testing of the application of blockchain in actual healthcare settings. It also fails to address the scalability constraints that come with blockchain when applied in large healthcare networks that may be a point of constraint to its full adoption in the industry (Agbo et al., 2019).

Sonkamble et al. (2021) propose a blockchain architecture to increase interoperability between Electronic Health Records (EHRs). While the proposed architecture is promising, the study has some limitations in that there are no pilot experiments or case studies to validate the proposed solution. Additionally, a single blockchain-based mechanism might not be sufficient to overcome the heterogeneity of technology and regulation environments of different healthcare systems (Sonkamble et al., 2021).

Menachemi and Collum (2011) detail both the benefits and the limitations of electronic health record systems. Their article gives a definition of EHR systems but not on how blockchain could be used as a solution to some of the issues that they've raised, such as data security and interoperability. The research is also more focused on the problems of the American healthcare system and may possibly not be fully representative of international variation in EHR use and functionality (Menachemi & Collum, 2011).McKibbon et al. (2012) examined in a systematic way combined health information technologies and effectiveness in stages of medication management. While their review is exhaustive in regard to the efficiency of various technologies, they fall short of the potential of the new function that blockchain technology has to bring into medication management systems' security and transparency. The study limitation is that it is confined to existing health IT systems and does not capture decentralized solutions in development (McKibbon et al., 2012).

Hasselgren et al. (2020) provide a scoping review of blockchain in health and health sciences. Even in their sweeping work on the potential of blockchain, one limitation of this research study is that it does not contain overt case studies or pilot tests demonstrating the practical effect that blockchain has on healthcare. Additionally, the overview fails to mention regulatory environments and blockchain adoption costs within healthcare systems that restrict its scope (Hasselgren et al., 2020).

McGhin et al. (2019) outline the research challenge and potential of blockchain in healthcare use. Reportings significant benefits like data privacy and openness, the study lacks a top-level theory model. It fails to carry out an in-depth analysis of technical challenges, like blockchain scalability and interoperability with the existing healthcare infrastructure, most crucial for real-world use (McGhin et al., 2019).

Gohar et al. (2022) provide a blockchain, cloud, and IoT-based patient-centric healthcare architecture for enabling semantic interoperability. While the architecture is an end-to-end one, it is marred with the limitation of few empirical studies to demonstrate its application in real-world practice. The research also lacks in describing scalability and integration challenges using the framework in diverse healthcare settings, particularly in resource-constrained settings (Gohar et al., 2022).

He et al. (2022) present a design for an integrated health information system that merges data, people, devices, and systems. Although their framework offers possibilities of greater data integration and interconnection of healthcare systems, the paper is still at the limited conceptual level at the highest level. The paper does not have detailed technical discussions and discuss issues of implementing such a system in current healthcare infrastructures such as data security and privacy issues (He et al., 2022).

A cutting-edge zero-trust blockchain-based solution for the security of electronic health records (EHRs) is put forth by Benaich et al. (2023). Even though most of the zero-trust technology adds another layer of security, the limitation of this work is that there are no specific implementation schedules or case studies to demonstrate how the system would still function in real-world health environments. It also does not take into account likely performance bottlenecks or scalability issues with zero-trust blockchain deployments in health organizations on a mass scale (Benaich et al., 2023).

Lee et al. (2020) introduce the design and deployment of a blockchain-based platform for sharing patient health records. While it is well-designed, the research is limited by the fact that it has only been tested in homogenous groups of patients and healthcare settings. In addition, although the platform supports user experience and accessibility, it fails to provide adequate technical issue-solving of implementing blockchain over current healthcare IT infrastructure in the guise of legacy systems and data migration (Lee et al., 2020).

Reegu et al. (2023) propose a blockchain-based interoperable electronic health record platform in the development of health systems. Among the shortcomings of the framework is sparse empirical evidence that justify the practicability and utility of the framework in actual healthcare environments. The study does not even explore such issues of compliance with law and regulation for applying blockchain across different countries with different laws regarding healthcare (Reegu et al., 2023).

Nan and Xu (2023) provide a literature review on FHIR-based interoperable healthcare service design. Despite the review providing high-density synthesis of existing FHIR solutions, it is inadequate in that it relies on conceptual models and does not perform rigorous analysis of real case studies. The review also fails to show how challenges of providing uniform interoperability in diverse health centers with different levels of technological capability are addressed (Nan & Xu, 2023).

Natsiavas et al. (2021) report the way that the KONFIDO project implemented secure patient summary exchange infrastructure in the EU. While the study gives explicit coverage to design and development details for infrastructure, the study is regionally specific in the EU, which can differ from conditions supplied in other locations, including developing countries with less technological infrastructure (Natsiavas et al., 2021).

Shrivastava et al. (2021) illustrate how communication standards, data privacy, and data security impact patient health data interoperability in different countries. Although the research is satisfactory for cross-border comparisons, the research is tainted in the sense that it draws from secondary sources of information and does not conduct primary research or case studies to illustrate actual challenges healthcare organizations experience in meeting such demands (Shrivastava et al., 2021).

Pathak et al. (2023) introduce SemBox, an e-health wearable device semantic interoperability solution. The study, as groundbreaking as it is, has a limited scope in that it tackles the wearables alone and not the whole domain of health technology or the problem of integration of wearable devices into existing health infrastructure. It also does not have sufficiency in the area of deployment problems and real-world issues of such technologies in real-world healthcare settings (Pathak et al., 2023).

Sreejith and Senthil (2023) propose a smart contract-based authentication mechanism for a HL7 FHIR system to enable interoperable e-healthcare systems. While the paper discusses an intriguing application of smart contracts in healthcare, its limitation is the lack of empirical testing across various healthcare environments. The research also fails to provide an in-depth analysis of security issues with the implementation of smart contracts in healthcare, notably exposure or misuses (Sreejith & Senthil, 2023).

Anitha et al. (2023) present Smart-fcd, an IoT data interoperability platform in terms of sensor-based fuzzy linked rules for cross-domain usage. While promising is the technique, research is constrained in terms of its methodology of taking into consideration sensor data within specific domains, which cannot best solve the interoperability problem of the wider healthcare environment. Moreover, application of this system to the healthcare sector, with a complex regulatory environment as well as privacy concerns, is not explored at large (Anitha et al., 2023).

Jaleel et al. (2020) propose medical data interoperability through the synchronization of healthcare devices. Despite the fact that the research presents an ideal model of device interoperability, the study is modest in that it does not provide empirical proof of practical application in multimodal healthcare environments. In addition, scalability problems and integration with existing health IT infrastructure are not properly explored, particularly regarding heterogeneity of health institutions' devices as well as technical infrastructure (Jaleel et al., 2020).

Kaur et al. (2018) provide a blockchain-based solution for cloud storage of heterogeneous Medicare data. The study is restricted to conceptual model with very little empirical evidence or real case studies to establish whether the system is operable in the real world or not. Moreover, issues pertaining to storing information in the cloud, i.e., security, healthcare regulatory compliance, and system interoperability, are not addressed (Kaur et al., 2018).

Houtan et al. (2020) provided an overview of blockchain-facilitating self-sovereign patient identity in healthcare. The paper, while giving a critical analysis, is marred with the evidence and theoretical basis of successful implementations. The realities of patient adoption, regulative requirements, and aligning such systems with the existing health infrastructure are not given appropriate consideration (Houtan et al., 2020).

Vorisek et al. (2022) take hold of the use of Fast Healthcare Interoperability Resources (FHIR) towards interoperability of health research. The review, as hopeful as it is concerning the possibilities of FHIR to solve interoperability, lacks in the sense that it cites big ideas without accompanying actionable plans. The review also does not comprehensively outline challenges towards grand-scale implementation of FHIR, particularly to smaller or less-funded healthcare institutions (Vorisek et al., 2022).

Imler et al. (2016) also provide a clear explanation of exchange and healthcare data standards. The book's weaker points, however, are its timing, to the extent of being written prior to some of the latest healthcare IT innovations like blockchain and FHIR. The study is also incapable of providing for integration complications that the health institutions are bound to encounter in an attempt to put such standards into practice (Imler et al., 2016).

Stearns et al. (2001) provide an overview of SNOMED Clinical Terms, e.g., their development history and status. While useful, the research is marred in its age, given the humongous growth that has occurred in clinical terminology since its publication. The research also fails to cover the application of SNOMED in today's standards and platforms like FHIR or blockchain platforms in modern healthcare environments (Stearns et al., 2001).

Hirsch et al. (2014) present an overview of current procedural terminology (CPT). The limitation of the study scope is that the study considers only CPT codes and not the entire environment of interoperability and integration complexity of the healthcare data with varying coding systems. The study does not emphasize the effect of new technologies, e.g., blockchain, on the future of CPT and other health standards (Hirsch et al., 2014).

Gordon and Agrawal (2018) prescribe the implementation of blockchain technology to facilitate patient-controlled interoperability. While it foresees a promising future for patient-driven data management, the study itself is limited because it is not tested empirically and lacks real-life case studies to ensure the proposed blockchain deployments. In addition, regulatory compliance, such as data protection legislation such as HIPAA, is not supported in its entirety (Gordon & Agrawal, 2018).

Daniel et al. (2016) address cross-border semantic interoperability of learning health systems in the context of the EHR4CR project. To the extent that the paper depends on crucial elements of international collaboration, the paper is limiting in taking into account the European environment which could not be easily adopted to other healthcare systems, particularly those with data privacy and security legislations. Further, project scalability in the general sense beyond the EU is not elaborated (Daniel et al., 2016).

Kasyapa and Vanmathi (2024) provide a comprehensive overview of healthcare blockchain adoption in terms of usage, performance problems, and counteractions. The drawback of this research is that it lacks a review of real issues related to the application of blockchain in healthcare settings, such as interoperability and scalability. It also lacks possible security threats of blockchain systems in the healthcare setting (Kasyapa & Vanmathi, 2024).

Duan et al. (2023) discuss the application and utilization of blockchain technology in supply chain management. While helpful, the drawbacks of this article are being concentrated on supply chain management and possibly not being suitable to the healthcare setting directly. The specific issues of healthcare organizations, such as patient privacy and regulation, are not well defined (Duan et al., 2023).

Nanda (2019) analyzes consumers' willingness to use mobile wallets. While the research provides cutting insights on the adoption of mobile wallets, it has an Achilles heel in studying consumer behavior without the technical issues of deploying mobile wallets in healthcare systems. Technical issues entailed in using mobile wallets to pay for healthcare, such as security measures and compatibility with existing healthcare IT infrastructure, are not analyzed (Nanda, 2019).

Ullah et al. (2020) give an overview of the application of blockchain technology, its challenges, and future directions in healthcare and medicine. The review is well-scoped on the majority of areas though, as it lacks sufficient scrutiny of real case studies and empirical data. The study also does not adequately account for the adoption practicalities such as cost of adoption and legacy system compatibility (Ullah et al., 2020).

Mertz (2018) depicts how blockchain technology is able to revolutionize healthcare with the optimal solution for handling data. The research is, nevertheless, limited in that it doesn't touch on the technicalities and security of employing blockchain within healthcare systems in detail (Mertz, 2018). Additionally, the legal and regulatory framework surrounding the utilization of blockchain technology within healthcare is not explored in detail (Mertz, 2018).

Khushalani et al. (2020) explain blockchain as a new way of maintaining trust in various applications. Although they pioneered blockchain as a guaranteed process, it is marred by dealing with theoretical roots without experimental evidence or actual case studies to unveil its effectiveness in everyday use. Additionally, concerns regarding blockchain scalability and adoption across sectors, particularly those that have complex regulatory conditions, are not investigated in depth (Khushalani et al., 2020).

Shicheng et al. (2023) look to the future internet revolution and wager on the revolutionary potential of next-generation technologies. The hypotheses are where the reasoning is most forceful, not in its reliance on some particular model of transition from existing technologies to new technologies accounted for in the "next internet revolution." The study does not consider the pragmatics of mass deployment, e.g., infrastructural requirements and regulation (Shicheng et al., 2023).

Omodunbi et al. (2023) propose the use of asymmetric cryptographic digital wallets in e-services for Nigeria. While research is focused on an important problem of digital wallet security, investigation is specific to the geography and does not address the problem of scalability or external validity of the solution for other regions with different technological infrastructure and regulatory requirements. Besides this, it does not present detailed empirical information on the performance of the wallet in the real world (Omodunbi et al., 2023). Suratkar et al. (2020) provide an overview of cryptocurrency wallets based on their security and features. The limitation of the paper is that it lacks references to the wide impact of cryptocurrency wallets on financial ecosystems and regulation. The critique also does not address the security concerns that are posed exactly because cryptocurrency purses are introduced in the health care or other vulnerable domains where privacy and data integrity are of critical concern (Suratkar et al., 2020).

Anonymous supply chain traceability sensitive data provision is addressed as being tackled by Glew and Tröger Schmittner (2022) through the use of blockchain. The drawback of this research is conceptual design emphasis at the expense of failing to reasonably guarantee that the solution would be functional in real-world supply chains. It also fails reasonably to compensate for the technological constraints of granting anonymity as well as traceability within a decentralized environment, especially in industries where data validation and compliance are stringent (Glew & Tröger Schmittner, 2022).

Al-Abdullah et al. (2020) suggest a GDPR compliant privacy-aware data repository system architecture for blockchain. Although the suggested architecture is a viable solution to the data privacy problem, the study is flawed by its theoretical nature and in the absence of empirical validation in actual systems. Implementation practicalities of the same in actual applications such as support of compliance across different jurisdictions and compatibility with existing infrastructures are not thoroughly discussed (Al-Abdullah et al., 2020).

Kouroubali and Katehakis (2022) discuss policies and strategies for interoperability of digital health in Europe. While enlightening as to policy setting, the research is tainted by its European-limited strategy that cannot be simply transferable elsewhere around the globe with a varying health care system and regulative framework. Whether the strategies are fitting on a global scale, particularly where there is limited resource allocation, is not tested critically (Kouroubali & Katehakis, 2022).

FAST HEALTHCARE INTEROPERABILITY RESOURCES (FHIR), A GLOBAL INDUSTRY STANDARD FOR EXCHANGING HEALTHCARE DATA ELECTRONICALLY

Fast Healthcare Interoperability Resources (FHIR) is an open standard, which was created by Health Level 7 (HL7), for the electronic exchange of healthcare data. FHIR is the solution for the interoperability issue of the healthcare industry, allowing various healthcare systems and organizations to exchange information in a standardized, efficient, and secure manner. FHIR's advent is a breakthrough in the interoperability of electronic health records (EHRs), clinical software, and other healthcare applications. FHIR facilitates real-time data interchange among vendor systems, the largest information exchange inhibitor in healthcare to date. The standard accommodates numerous types of healthcare data, including patient demographics and clinical notes and diagnostic results and medical images, for end-to-end data exchange.

FHIR is made up of a set of modular building blocks known as "resources." Any individual concrete entity in healthcare like a patient, an observation, or medication is a resource. Resources are interoperable and shareable data models. FHIR resources are extensible and light-weighted to be reused in many use cases. For instance, the Patient resource holds important details like contact, personal information, and identification numbers, whereas the Observation resource is used to transmit diagnostic findings or blood pressure. The resources are also aggregatable and can be configured to suit the particular needs of various healthcare applications. FHIR also makes standardized data exchange mechanisms like RESTful APIs possible so that interoperability and communication between healthcare systems can be made easy.

Systems interoperability has been one of the biggest challenges in healthcare. Different software solutions are used by healthcare organizations to store patient data, leading to silos and inefficiencies. FHIR accomplishes this by offering a common platform for information exchange between platforms so that different systems can communicate with each other in a standardized manner. FHIR enables systems to ask for, receive, and update data from each other unobtrusively, tearing down walls between healthcare providers, payers, and other stakeholders. Interoperability streamlines work processes, reduces errors, and enhances patient care through the presence of accurate up-to-date information whenever clinical decisions are being made by health professionals.

Through enabling efficient sharing of information, FHIR enhances patient care. It enables real-time sharing of patient records between medical centers like hospitals, clinics, laboratories, and pharmacies so that healthcare providers receive an integrated view of a patient's health record. It is specifically designed to minimize duplication of clinical errors, eliminate redundant testing, and enhance coordination among various healthcare teams. FHIR also favors patients by providing them more continuity of care since their clinical documents are accessible and modifiable by any accredited healthcare practitioner wherever they are and whatever the system. For instance, when a patient consults a specialist or is referred to another hospital, all clinical records, new diagnoses, medications, and laboratory results can be simply transferred and assist in clinical decision-making.

FHIR has strict data privacy and security controls in mind given the sensitive nature of healthcare data. FHIR leverages contemporary security mechanisms such as OpenID Connect and OAuth2 to manage user authentication and access so that only a designated user can view or modify healthcare data. FHIR also facilitates simplicity in order to be compliant with global data privacy regulations like the European Union's General Data Protection Regulation (GDPR) and the United States Health Insurance Portability and Accountability Act (HIPAA). Patient information can be protected by healthcare providers using secure encryption and security practices while sending and storing it through FHIR. The foundation architecture also supports audit trails, i.e., all interactions involving healthcare data can be monitored and logged for compliance and security reasons.

FHIR has received wide adoption since its creation in the healthcare sector. A number of healthcare associations, technology companies, and government agencies adopted FHIR as a core interoperability standard for healthcare data. U.S. Centers for Medicare and Medicaid Services (CMS) have made the use of FHIR mandatory in some of the healthcare data exchanges, such as electronic prior authorization. Also, big health IT players like Epic, Cerner, and Allscripts have implemented FHIR in their electronic health records to facilitate ease of sharing of data by medical providers. The standard has also taken big strides in the creation of mobile health applications, where patients receive their own health data through FHIR-supported applications.

Not only does FHIR support greater care interoperability, but it also supports greater data analysis and medical research. By facilitating easy retrieval and sharing of standardized data, FHIR offers researchers access to enormous amounts of data across different care environments. This type of data can be utilized for pattern-finding, tracking public health outcomes, and predictive modeling of treatment and disease prevention. FHIR also enables patient-entered data from mobile apps and wearables to be integrated into research in a form that new forms of data can be processed. As FHIR progresses, it will inevitably become a core element of data-driven health solutions such as precision medicine and AI-based diagnostic instruments.

FHIR has one of the advantages that it is patient-focused care. FHIR empowers patients to have greater autonomy over their own health data, so that they are able to provide or deny access to their data as and when they desire. With FHIR-based systems, patients are able to share their health information with other healthcare providers, specialists, or even relatives and family members and optimize coordination in monitoring their state. And through the standards ability to enable patient-facing applications, it is easy for patients to monitor their health information, make appointments, and get reminders of their treatment regimen. This makes patients more involved and participative in their care and also able to make more informed decisions regarding their health.

Although it has numerous benefits, FHIR in healthcare organizations comes with a multitude of challenges. Some of the challenges include that the healthcare institutions will have to dismantle or redesign the existing legacy systems that could be incompatible with FHIR. Although FHIR is general-purpose and scalable across a wide range of healthcare technology, it can take sweeping redesigns or even re-designings from scratch of older systems to interface with systems based on FHIR. Moreover, although FHIR provides a common framework for the exchange of data, maintaining equivalent data definitions and terminology in line with each other is not readily achievable when different terminologies or coding systems are utilized by distinct healthcare organizations. In addition, interoperability cutting across multiple systems requires cooperation between health practitioners, technology entrepreneurs, and policy-makers.

The future of FHIR in the healthcare industry is bright, with increased emphasis on increasing its application and building its capabilities. As more health care organizations adopt FHIR, the standard will drive further interoperability innovations and enable safe and smooth sharing of information across global health systems. In addition, as health care information becomes more complex, FHIR's module-based approach will enable increased scalability and flexibility. FHIR will increasingly incorporate new and emerging technologies in future development, including artificial intelligence, machine learning, and blockchain, that will increasingly enhance health care outcomes. In the long run, FHIR can build a well-networked, patient-focused healthcare setting that enhances more coordinated care, improved patient experience, and enhanced clinical decision-making.

DATA SHARING AND EXCHANGE PROCESSES

Data exchange and sharing are critical processes in healthcare that enable health professionals to share and access patient data to improve care coordination, decision-making, and results. The health setting has different stakeholders like hospitals, clinics, labs, payers, and patients who all require real-time access to right and current information. Efficient data-sharing facilities are essential in elimination of redundancy, avoidance of medical error, and ease of continuity of care across multiple providers and locations. Such systems are, however, haunted by technical, regulatory, and organizational challenges. Seamless flow and integrity of data across platforms for the purpose of efficient healthcare data exchange therefore depend on the application of standard formats, secure messaging channels, and compatible systems.

Healthcare data comes in various forms like clinical data (e.g., diagnosis, laboratory tests, medications), administrative data (e.g., insurance, billing information), and patient-generated data (e.g., patient-entered symptoms, wearables data). Various types of data come with different requirements for exchange and sharing. Clinical information would contain highest requirements for timeliness and accuracy because it is most directly associated with clinical care decision-making. Administrative information, while significant, tends to be less real-time intensive but supports billing and insurance adjudication. Patient-collected information, more easily accessed through mobile health packages of software and wearable technology, can provide situational awareness in real time about the condition of a patient but might lack the interchangeability to integrate them without special systems. Practices of sharing data have to consider the different forms, structure, and use of such heterogeneous data for such heterogeneous data to be exchanged between the involved parties.

To ensure that healthcare information is exchanged efficiently, the information must be in a standard format and protocol so that different systems are able to share information amongst themselves. Interoperability is the most practical method of accomplishing this because it is a model under which systems from different healthcare organizations will be able to exchange information regardless of whether they are created by different vendors or other technological standards. Some of the standards developed to provide a framework for the exchange of data in healthcare are Health Level 7 (HL7), Fast Healthcare Interoperability Resources (FHIR), and Digital Imaging and Communications in Medicine (DICOM). These standards support the transmission of electronic health records (EHRs), laboratory tests, and imaging studies in standard and readable form regardless of the source system. If not in a structured format, then data exchange will be cumbersome and error-prone.

Protection of healthcare data is required since it contains law-protected confidential individual health information (PHI) in nations like the U.S. under the Health Insurance Portability and Accountability Act (HIPAA). Secure data exchange mechanisms ensure that data is securely transferred correctly, being hidden from unauthorized users and intrusions. Among the common securities include encryption of data, safe communication protocols like HTTPS, and use of secure application programming interfaces (APIs). Authentication and approval controls like OAuth2, two-factor authentication (2FA), and public key infrastructure (PKI) ensure that healthcare data are accessed and modified by approved users. Such security controls find a balance between sharing and exchanging healthcare data among systems and organizations.

Among the oldest data exchange devices for health care is the electronic health record (EHR) containing a patient's complete medical history, including diagnoses, treatment plans, medications, allergies, and lab tests. EHRs are to be shared and updated among different health care providers in order to make possible continuity of care as the patient moves from one phase of care to the next and among successive health care organizations. EHRs are usually followed by health information exchanges (HIEs) that provide a safe and effective means of sharing information between clinics, hospitals, pharmacies, and laboratories. Even though the sharing of information has been significantly enhanced by the use of EHRs, the problems persist in getting different EHR systems to communicate with each other and viewing patients' information shared with proper authorization.

Health Information Exchange (HIE) networks are centralized or decentralized networks that facilitate the sharing of patient data among various healthcare organizations. HIEs allow physicians to access a patient's health data irrespective of where the patient has previously been treated so that all necessary information is available at the point of need. HIE models involve directed exchanges, query-based exchanges, and consumer-mediated exchanges. Directed exchanges are sharing some data between authorised groups, and query-based exchanges allow providers to ask and receive patient data from another organisation. Patient-controlled, consumer-mediated exchanges allow the patient to control who receives access to the patient data and shares it with healthcare providers when needed. Healthcare organisations can eliminate unnecessary services, improve care coordination, and provide more integrated care to the patient through HIEs.

Application Program Interfaces (APIs) are used for sharing data among health systems. APIs make different systems "talk" to each other and share information in real time, allowing applications to be interfaced with electronic health record systems, laboratory systems, and other health systems. FHIR, the leading standards for the exchange of health information, is constructed upon next-generation API technology that is simple to deploy within cloud environments, mobile apps, and other health IT solutions. APIs also facilitate flexibility needed in moving data between systems with different technical architecture so that they can integrate in a simpler way across the health system. As more cloud computing and mobile technology are used by healthcare systems, use of APIs will continue to increase so that faster and more effective data sharing is possible.

Telemonitoring and telemedicine are being implemented in healthcare after digital health solutions and higher demand for healthcare service outside the traditional environment. Telemedicine and remote monitoring data exchange services comprise the secure transfer of patient information from patients to healthcare professionals through electronic systems real-time or otherwise. The information can comprise clinical data, symptoms, and vital signs collected by telehealth devices or wearables. Patient information needs to be exchanged and accessed securely by the healthcare practitioner for the purposes of diagnosis and treatment to enable remote treatment. This involves the utilization of secure communication protocols, real-time data transfer technologies, and patient authorization systems to make sure data protection and privacy are maintained.

Although attempts have been made to evolve healthcare data exchange, there are certain issues which are intrinsic to the facilitation of seamless and secure data transfer. One of the greatest issues is that there are no universal data formats employed in different healthcare systems, and this can lead to loss of and incompatibility of data during transfer. Another issue is that changing regulation environments in different healthcare organizations can complicate sharing across jurisdictions. Privacy concerns are also major hindrances as patients would not give sensitive health information, and organizations would have legal problems with granting access and permission to data. The expense and complexity of offering interoperable systems and ensuring the integrity of data are additional hindrances to healthcare organizations, particularly small providers without a lot of resources.

The future for the exchange and sharing of health data is rosy with more technology and policy innovations on the horizon to address current problems. Progress on the standards like FHIR and the widespread utilization of APIs will make data transfer faster, smoother, and more secure. Aside from that, further use of artificial intelligence (AI) and machine learning (ML) technology in health information analysis will provide for faster and better decision-making on large amounts of data shared to better align patient care. With increasing and increasing integration of health care systems, the concept of "data liquidity" or the autonomy of free sharing, access, and analysis of data across the entire continuum of health care will become reality. With continued innovation and collaboration between stakeholders, health care sharing and exchange activities will become transformed to provide improved patient outcomes, more specialized treatment, and a better overall health care system.

CASE STUDIES AND PILOT IMPLEMENTATIONS IN HEALTHCARE DATA EXCHANGE

Case studies and pilot implementations are actual examples of what healthcare organizations are adopting and benefiting from new data-exchange standards and technologies. They offer actual insights into success, best practices, and challenges in implementing new healthcare solutions, particularly interoperability and data exchange. Pilot programs are applied to try theories on a small scale, demonstrate the viability of new technology, and become certified to lead giant-scale adoption. Pilot programs and case studies for medicine are great indicators of how best-in-class systems are optimized for efficiency, security, and patient care in order to enable health professionals to make data-driven decisions before applying giant-scale change.

Case Study: Implementing FHIR in a Large Health Organization

The most traditional case study for the sharing of health data is the FHIR implementation in a multi-hospital healthcare corporation. The corporation with numerous clinics and hospitals desired the sharing of data between departments and improved patient care using FHIR standards to facilitate the interoperability of data. The pilot included integrating FHIR APIs into production electronic health record (EHRs), laboratory, and pharmacy management systems. The objective was to facilitate easy and seamless sharing of patient information in real-time, between any system or vendor. Aside from the initial challenge of integrating multiple vendors' systems and resisting staff change, the project led to increased access to patients' data within the organization, reduced administrative burden, and enhanced care coordination. The pilot project was a model for other health-care organizations that would be implementing FHIR.

Pilot Deployment: Rural Health Information Exchange

Rural health care systems typically suffer from challenges that are a product of low levels of health-care resources, trained medical personnel, and secure data exchange centers. Pilot deployment to an American rural health care system to combat the challenges by establishing a regional Health Information Exchange (HIE) platform. The platform enabled hospitals, clinics, and pharmacies to securely exchange patient data even across geography. The pilot was to improve patient outcomes by making available full, up-to-date patient information to providers regardless of the location at which the patient is receiving care. The outcome was reduction in duplicative testing by considerable amounts and increased coordination among providers. But the pilot also revealed problems rural healthcare providers encounter in being connected to HIE networks due to limitations of technology and issues with data privacy and security.

Case Study: Blockchain for Interoperability and Data Security

Healthcare organizations have been increasingly looking at the value proposition of blockchain in enhancing interoperability and data security. One of the noted case studies was its application within a blockchain platform to exchange information between insurers and hospitals in a secure manner. The project was to employ an immutable ledger for patient data such that data was not tampered with or compromised during transit. The pilot was focused on safeguarding patients' access to healthcare records and maintaining confidentiality without violating data protection regulations like HIPAA. Blockchain technology, aside from guaranteeing data integrity, enabled the speed and efficiency of claim processing. While the project encountered certain scalability issues, it provided an impression of applying blockchain technology in reducing security and interoperability issues in healthcare.

Pilot Project: Telemedicine Data Exchange in Remote Areas

Where medical practitioners are in short supply, telemedicine has been the appropriate alternate means of provision of care. One of the earliest pilot telemedicine projects that exchanged information in a remote area sought to establish a platform upon which patient data, including laboratory results and history, would be safely archived to be retrieved between telemedicine experts and neighboring medical facilities. The pilot used application of encrypted communication systems and cloud storage for real-time data sharing. The pilot's result showed telemedicine to expand access to health care for rural patients in a way that maintains patient information in secure exchange. The pilot did, however, show rural internet connectivity issues, impacting on the reliance on the mechanism for data exchange. Case Study: Interoperability of EHR in the National Health Service (NHS)

In the UK, the National Health Service (NHS) has been attempting to improve interoperability of EHR so that information would be shared throughout the nation's health care system.

One of the case studies in the NHS was roll-out of an EHR system throughout the entire nation, which provided access to patient records from any one of the participating facilities to healthcare professionals. It was designed to allow clinicians to enter a patient's history, laboratory tests, and medications in real time, thereby enhancing the quality of care and reducing errors. Some of the issues faced were EHR system integration among heterogeneous providers with different technical competency statuses. But the project was able to overcome and demonstrate the advantages of central-level data access, leading to fewer duplication tests, better patient outcomes. The case study emphasizes the need for effective governance and coordination between the health professionals to achieve national interoperability. Pilot Implementation: Blockchain for Patient Consent Management

Pilot implementation of the use of blockchain technology for patient consent management in data sharing was conducted by an experiment pilot in Europe.

It aimed to put in their hands the control over who and when are able to access patients' healthcare data. The pilot pilot went ahead to create a blockchain platform where patients would grant or withdraw permission for information access by payers, researchers, or health providers safely. The platform guaranteed that the consent exchanges were documented to an irreversible ledger so the data access history was transparent and could be audited. The pilot could demonstrate that blockchain could address patient privacy and control over health data concerns. Outcomes revealed blockchain promise as a secure way to create trust among patients and healthcare professionals and compliance with data protection legislation. Case Study: Public Health and EHR Interoperability

A US case study reviewed interoperability for public health agencies and EHR systems to improve infectious disease reporting.

The pilot pilot aimed at facilitating streamlining of the reporting process via computerized presentation of patient-related data, such as codes of diagnosis and laboratory tests, from health professionals to health agencies in real-time. The system reduced administrative workload on healthcare professionals and improved response time to new public health threats. The program could improve timeliness and consistency in disease reporting, which was important in controlling outbreaks. The program did mention, however, that it must still make investments in the training of health care professionals and public health personnel so that they can use these systems to their full potential. Pilot Project: Cloud-Based Data Exchange for Rural Clinics

In the case of rural health environments, there is typically a deficit in infrastructures and resources, which impacts data exchange.

A doctor in a rural area of India developed a cloud solution for sharing patient histories to allow sharing among pharmacies, clinics, and hospitals. The cloud-enabled the care providers to be able to access the patient information anywhere and at anytime, hence enabling continuity of care even when the patient shifted from location to location. The result was positive with improved patient satisfaction and coordination of care. A areas of concern with respect to internet availability, usage of equipment, and compliance with local regulations were but indicated to be in need of improvement. The succeeding pilot tests and case studies demonstrate the promise that standards and new technologies can hold to improve data interoperability and sharing in healthcare.

The two projects provide visibility into actual-world challenges and solutions for healthcare organizations as they adopt data exchange systems. Above all, most importantly, are the most critical lessons to be learned, which include the necessity for robust stakeholder coalitions, patient and data safety, and flexible, growable technology that can scale up to accommodate the growing needs of the healthcare system. Upon their mature stage, these pilots will offer a proven model for more widespread application and guide future healthcare data exchange innovation.

CHALLENGES AND SOLUTIONS

Though the advantages of health data exchange are clear, unadulterated, safe, and effective information exchange is plagued by numerous challenges. These may include technologically rooted issues like system incompatibility and poor data quality to regulatory and patient confidentiality matters. Moreover, the pace of technological progress quickens the force of continuous adaptation on the part of healthcare organizations, and they tend to face the stumbling block of remaining in conformity with new platforms and standards. What is required to hurdle such impediments is cooperation among health providers, technology companies, regulators, and patients toward establishing a platform upon which data can exchange readily, safely, and in a format that best supports patient care and organizational efficiency.

One of the biggest of healthcare data exchange's challenges is that the systems used by health providers are non-standardized. Various Electronic Health Record (EHR) systems, laboratory information management systems (LIMS), and other health technologies have varying structures and data forms, such that the systems are unable to exchange information among them. It leads to a fragmented piece of information, such that patient information are isolated in various systems with disparate forms or protocols. The answer is the employment of universal data standards like Fast Healthcare Interoperability Resources (FHIR) and Health Level 7 (HL7), which are in predefinable formats and APIs for exchanging data. Promoting industry-wide usage of these types of standards can help minimize system incompatibility and enable the transfer of health data.

Health data itself is personal, and privacy and security of patient data are of highest priority during data sharing. The risk of data breaches or unauthorized release of patient health records is one of the major stumbling blocks for the exchange of information between health care providers, particularly between different organizations and systems. To overcome such, health care organizations have to utilize strong encryption techniques, use secure methods of communication such as HTTPS, and implement access controls allowing access to patient data only by authorized staff. Besides, blockchain technology is the only solution which can potentially protect sharing of health care information because it provides a decentralized record to record access, along with data integrity of, the information, which is tamper-evident. Data protection regulation, i.e., HIPAA in America or GDPR in Europe, also needs to be applied to provide confidentiality of the patient.

Healthcare providers are resistant to adopting new data interchange systems in their nature because of the perceived cost, complexity, and time to implement these solutions. The majority of healthcare organizations have an enormous investment in their current EHR systems, and it frightens them to switch these systems or embrace new technology. The most effective means of breaking through that resistance is to show the concrete payoff of increased data sharing, including enhanced care coordination, less duplication of testing and treatment, and better patient outcomes. Staff training and assistance are also essential to successful implementation, as is introducing new systems piecemeal in conjunction with existing processes. Having clear, stable messages regarding the value of interoperability and providing incentives for adopting such standards can facilitate such changes by health care organizations to such new technology more effectively.

Even when health care systems take standard forms such as FHIR, interoperability problems can still occur if systems are from different vendors and have to exchange information. Various packages from different vendors may implement standards slightly differently and result in data discrepancy or inaccuracy. Moreover, older systems may not be compatible with newer, more open data exchange protocols, and communication is complicated. As a work-around to the issue, middleware or interoperability platforms that can serve as an intermediary between incomplict systems is an answer. Platforms can bridge the gap by translating data in other forms so that the right data is transferred between systems. Furthermore, cloud solutions would be more likely to integrate because cloud infrastructures also have greater interoperability with other systems.

Effective data exchange further depends on the premise that data to be exchanged is current, complete, and accurate. Low data quality due to human errors, old data, or irregular data input may contribute to diagnosis and treatment errors minimizing treatment effectiveness using data sharing. To address this issue, there should be the establishment of data quality assurance procedures such as constant testing of data entered into systems, data entering process normalization, and implementation of validation checks for testing the validity of data. Machine learning (ML) and artificial intelligence (AI) technology have the potential to assist in enhancing the quality of data by scanning for and repairing errors in real time and enhancing the data's accuracy before it is shared among healthcare providers.

Data exchange in healthcare is also regulated by differences in legal and regulatory constraints, which can differ considerably geographically, nationally, and even on the basis of what types of data are being shared. For instance, HIPAA laws in the US govern use and sharing of health data, and GDPR offers strict guidelines for preserving personal information in the European Union. These types of regulations can act as a hindrance to the free movement of data across borders, wherein healthcare organizations are required to meet domestic regulations prior to accessing data across borders. Such legal issues can be addressed by healthcare organizations in collaboration with professionals in law to facilitate compliance with relevant laws and align international data exchange systems with due regard for the complexity of cross-jurisdictional data exchange. Uniform consent management procedures, through which patients can provide or withdraw consent for data sharing with ease, are also necessary in ensuring continuous compliance with privacy law.

It is expensive for low-budget health care organizations, such as small or rural health care organizations, to implement and manage interoperable data exchange systems. It is too expensive for some organizations to consolidate several systems, buy new software or hardware, and undergo employee training. One of the solutions is that the industry players or governments must offer incentives in the form of subsidy or monetary reward to convince small health providers to implement interoperable systems. Two, cloud-based systems minimize upfront maintenance and setup costs by eliminating initial capital outlays. The use of the already available infrastructure and the incremental additions on a consistent basis, rather than the rebuilding of the entire infrastructures, can also assist in keeping costs low.

Patient control over viewing their health data and when is another significant issue of healthcare data exchange. Although the healthcare providers must have access to the patient data in order to provide them with appropriate care, patients must be able to authorize or reject sharing information. This issue can be solved through the use of patient consent management systems in which patients give remote consent or refusal of access to their medical information. Another possible solution to patient consent management is blockchain technology due to the fact that it provides transparent, tamper-proof history for consent transactions. Furthermore, patient education on the importance of data sharing to be treated and having clear and understandable mechanisms of consent can enable the individual to be in charge of making decisions on their health data themselves.

The future of healthcare data exchange is via ongoing technological improvement, harmonization of the regulation, and patient-centered approaches. As emerging technologies such as artificial intelligence, blockchain, and sophisticated encryption techniques continue to improve, they will offer more secure, efficient, and productive solutions to the issue of data sharing. Moreover, as worldwide initiatives towards healthcare data format and communication protocol standardization increase speed, so will the obstacles to interoperability also disappear. Governments, health care industry leaders, and health care providers will be required to continue working together to address challenges listed above, most significantly to deliver data security, patient confidentiality, and fair access to care. With continued commitment and investment, vision for an entirely integrated, interoperable health care system will become a reality with improved care and improved patient outcomes for all persons everywhere.

INTEGRAL ROLE OF BLOCKCHAIN IN ENHANCING THE DIGITAL HEALTHCARE ECOSYSTEM

Blockchain technology has the capability to transform the healthcare industry by providing a secure, decentralized, and open environment to share and store healthcare data. As data security concerns, data breaches, and interoperability problems continue to increase, blockchain can prove to be a solution to such persistent problems. With its in-built strengths—immutability, transparency, and encryption—blockchain can enable the digital health ecosystem to become more efficient, reliable, and secure. Blockchain technology has the capability to address urgent issues like disconnected patient records, unauthorized access to private health information, and enhanced and safer sharing of information among various stakeholders in the healthcare industry.

Security and integrity of patient data are one of the key challenges of the digital health ecosystem. Centralized health databases are vulnerable to hacking, unauthorized access, and tampering, threatening patient confidentiality and trust. Blockchain, in being decentralized and having cryptographical elements, presents a solution to such problems because it offers an immutable ledger in which health data can be stored in secure and tamper-evident means. All transactions or exchanges of data on the blockchain are encrypted and linked with prior blocks in a manner that cannot be altered or erased once data has been inputted without leaving a trace. This ensures the integrity and authenticity of patient data, which ensures trust to be built between patients and healthcare providers.

Interoperability between healthcare systems is likely to be the biggest threat to the healthcare sector now. Hospitals and clinics, along with other healthcare centers, have the tendency to use diversified software systems that are incompatible and therefore lead to fragmented patient records as well as ineffective coordination of care. Blockchain can be used to enable safe and effective sharing of information among healthcare organizations so that the data of patients can be accessed in real time regardless of the platforms used. Through the provision of an interoperable and standardized architecture, blockchain allows health practitioners to access and modify patients' records securely regardless of the system being used. This improves the quality of care to patients as well as reducing errors due to flawed or incomplete patient information.

Historically, health information is maintained and owned by organizations and institutions that have collected the information, and patients have limited control over who accesses their information. Blockchain technology enables patients to have ownership over their medical records. With blockchain, patients have the control to determine who gets to view their medical history, why, and when. This is accomplished by the use of private keys and smart contracts whereby patients can withdraw or authorize as necessary. By putting patients in control of their medical information, blockchain encourages higher levels of trust, transparency, and interaction among patients and healthcare professionals.

Blockchain also revolutionizes the health supply chain, tracing in an open and unalterable form the journey of medical devices, medicines, and supplies. The supply chain for health is usually intricate, where there are multiple distributors, vendors, and administrators involved. Such intricacy may have the ability to bring about inefficiency, fake drugs, and supply chain sabotage. Blockchain facilitates every step of the supply chain to be tracked in real-time, from manufacture to delivery, to render medical products authentic, safe, and kept in appropriate conditions. Smart contracts may also be used to enact automated and regulatory compliance, further ensuring supply chain efficiency and reliability.

Clinical trials and healthcare research are the result of medicine's advancement but are typically marred with transparency, data manipulation, and unavailable data problems. Blockchain technology can enhance the integrity and transparency of clinical trials through an irreversible record of all the procedures involved in a trial, patient consent, data capture, and outcomes. Researchers can record every step of the trial process on the blockchain, and data becomes tamper-proof and verifiable. It reduces fraud, promotes responsibility, and allows research findings to be based on trustworthy and accurate facts. Blockchain allows researchers and institutions to collaborate to be enhanced by providing a safe platform for data sharing and knowledge.

The process of billing and payment in healthcare is susceptible to be complex with multiple stakeholders such as patients, payers, and health care providers. Complications could lead to misstatements, delayed remittance, and disagreements over billing correctness. Blockchain can simplify billing and payment by deploying smart contracts that can execute transactions in an optimal way. Smart contracts can authenticate directly, make prompt payments, and reduce fraud cases. By providing an open, immutable record of every transaction, blockchain establishes trust between patients, providers, and insurers with fewer administrative loads and the entire billing process streamlined overall.

Abuse and fraud are huge issues in healthcare, where the sector loses billions of dollars annually due to fraudulent claims, misrepresentation of treatment, and overbilling. Blockchain will help reduce fraud by providing an open book, auditable record of every health care transaction. Each step along the process, from the patient check-in and treatment to billing and payment, is recorded into the blockchain, and it would be practically impossible to tamper with or forge information without detection. Additionally, the ability of blockchain to execute processes automatically using smart contracts ensures that only approved actions are carried out in the first place, limiting the scope for abuse and deceit. This not only protects healthcare organizations from loss of funds but also ensures that patients are given the treatment they deserve without overpayment. In emergency medicine, rapid access to a patient's medical record is crucial in a bid to do the best one can in terms of treatment. In traditional health care, the patient records are stored in various locations, and chances are it may be difficult for the emergency staff to retrieve the crucial information at a given time. Blockchain can rectify the situation by building up a decentralised, centrally located database of patient records that authenticated healthcare providers can view from anywhere online. This can be very helpful during crisis situations where time is a factor because it provides health care professionals with instant access to patients' entire medical history, allergies, medications, and past treatments, leading to better and timely decision-making.

As technology in blockchain improves, its use in health care will further increase with even more possibilities to make the digitized health care platform even more enhanced. Together with other new technologies, such as artificial intelligence (AI), machine learning, and the Internet of Things (IoT), blockchain generates more intelligent and more effective healthcare systems. AI, for instance, can be used to verify health data driven by blockchain and produce actionable intelligence that enhances patient outcomes. In addition, as more and more is being adopted of blockchain technology, policy for using it in the healthcare industry will be even more standardized, and how it is integrated into the healthcare system will be more and more streamlined. Lastly, blockchain's transparent, decentralized, and safe nature makes it a treasure for creating a better, efficient, patient-centered, and reliable healthcare system.

FUTURE WORK IN BLOCKCHAIN-ENABLED HEALTHCAR

Future developments in blockchain-based healthcare include ongoing innovation in the interoperability of several healthcare systems globally. Blockchain has already achieved some improvements to increase interoperability for local or national health systems, yet complete interoperability remains a problem at the universal level. The future research will aim to develop cross-universal protocols and standards which can overcome the gap between incompatible healthcare systems among nations and regions. This includes integrating blockchain-enabled healthcare platforms into common global standards like Fast Healthcare Interoperability Resources (FHIR) and making sure that information exchange is standardized as well as safe worldwide. Blockchain adoption

Blockchain integration with emerging technologies like AI, ML, and IoT is also one of the areas of future growth with significant potential. Blockchain has the ability to authenticate health data for AI and ML to improve decision-making because it becomes accurate, transparent, and verifiable. AI and ML, for example, can utilize blockchain-verified patient data and use it to learn patterns and forecast future health status. IoT devices such as wearable health trackers, similarly, may feed real-time health data into the blockchain where it may be saved safely and accessed by medical professionals. The intersection of blockchain with these technologies has immense promise for creating smarter, more efficient, and automated medical systems.

Whereas blockchain has been promising in pilot projects and case studies of small scale, one of the greatest challenges facing future research is scaling up blockchain solutions so that they can handle the big data that global health systems currently generate. With more use of electronical health records (EHRs) as well as other electronic healthcare platforms, the volume of data to be processed, stored, and transferred will increase exponentially. Blockchain networks need to scale optimally without compromising their fundamental properties of decentralization, security, and transparency. Blockchain architecture and consensus protocols for large-scale health data capabilities will be research areas in the future without compromising performance or security. This may include using newer blockchain architectures such as sharding or layer-2 solutions for scaling.

Another vital field of activity in the future is developing regulatory guidelines for blockchain use in healthcare. Use of blockchain in healthcare currently is still under regulatory uncertainty in most countries, most significantly in respect of data privacy, security, and patient consent. Future work will involve collaboration with regulatory bodies to establish strong and uniform rules that address these. The promise of blockchain to make it possible to share data securely and transparently is enormous but has to be harmonized with current legislation and regulation, e.g., HIPAA in the US or GDPR in the EU. An international regulatory framework for blockchain in healthcare will be pivotal in bringing about acceptance and adoption worldwide.

Patient ownership and consent of data are also major issues in the sharing of healthcare data, and future studies will be compelled to push ahead with how patient ownership of their health data can be maximized using blockchain. Blockchain's ability to form an incorruptible and visible record of patient consent is enormous in expanding on the management of health data. The future can learn more advanced versions of patient consent, such as dynamic consent, where patients are able to switch their consent options quickly and in real-time. Nothing would be under the control of health professionals; patients would be in charge of who has access to their data, when they require it, and why, which will enhance trust and keep the patients in charge. In addition, work has to be made towards maintaining patients' rights to data privacy and not sharing their information without express consent.

One of the greatest challenges that blockchain for healthcare is currently encountering is the fact that it appears to be expensive, particularly infrastructure to be deployed when rolling it out as well as transaction fees. Subsequent research will seek to lower the price tag of blockchain applications and make them accessible to small health cohorts, clinics, and developing countries. This can involve developing lightweight blockchain solutions with little or no computing or hardware needs, as well as researching cost-cutting innovations such as off-chain storage or layer-2 solutions. By lowering the expense of blockchain solutions, blockchain can be deployed to healthcare organizations in volumes and interoperable and secure systems can reach all.

Enabling provenance for health data and audit trails for healthcare transactions is a critical function of healthcare data management. The inherent transparency and immutability of Blockchain offer an extremely powerful method of following the complete life cycle of healthcare data from its initial creation and modification to sharing and storage. The future will involve creating systems that can trace every interaction with a patient's health information in the blockchain so that all data exchanges are fully traceable and auditable. This will not only increase transparency and accountability but will also avoid fraudulent cases, such as health data tampering. By providing auditable audit trails, blockchain can assist in ensuring the integrity of health data throughout its lifecycle.

With increasing healthcare organizations adopting health blockchain technology across the health sector, public and patient awareness will become increasingly important. To convince the patients and use blockchain-based healthcare systems, they should be aware of how the technology works, the people who get access to their information, and the benefits it poses. Educational resources and courses in the future will be created to inform patients and physicians how blockchain will improve the provision of healthcare. These programs should address privacy, consent, and security concerns around data with a focus on the benefits of blockchain, such as increased control over one's own health data and enhanced care coordination.

One possible research direction in the future is exploring the long-term impact of blockchain technology within healthcare settings. While blockchain provides a tangible solution to most of the issues in healthcare today, it is highly necessary to investigate how its mass use would impact the healthcare system in general. This involves studying its potential impact on healthcare costs, outcomes of patient health, provider operations, and healthcare policies. More research would be welcome on the potential future role of intermediaries such as pharma and insurance and how blockchain will affect or alter prevailing models of healthcare business. Identification of these broader impacts will guide future policy and business planning in healthcare.

Finally, blockchain technology has potential to aid global health initiatives, particularly within the settings of resource constraint in which the infrastructure of health is fragile. Future studies will investigate how blockchain can improve access to healthcare, make it easier to manage health records for under-resourced communities, and optimize the impact of global health initiatives. With the promise of providing a secure, affordable, and scalable way to store health information, blockchain is poised to revolutionize healthcare systems across developing countries. In addition, the ability of blockchain to provide transparency and accountability will also revolutionize global health activities to be more efficient with the guarantee that the funds and resources get to the intended recipients. The future of blockchain and its applications in healthcare isn't only promising but also intimidating. With the advancement of technology, the potential for transforming the healthcare system is being unveiled day by day. With scalability, interoperability, regulatory adherence, and empowerment of patients on its horizon, blockchain can potentially have a massive effect on managing, sharing, and protecting health data. Through continued research and collaboration, blockchain can potentially enhance not just the digital health system but also the quality and outcomes of care worldwide.

CONCLUSION

Blockchain technology brings a paradigm solution to the ages-old problems of the healthcare industry. The fact that it can have secure, transparent, and immutable records brings an opportunity for better patient care, improved stakeholder confidence, and seamless data exchange between different health systems. While the technology has already indicated potential in various pilot studies and case studies, it also must address problems with scalability, regulatory, and cost hurdles. With further development of blockchain, its use combined with new technologies like AI, ML, and IoT will make healthcare systems even smarter with increased efficiency. With a possibility of providing more autonomy to patients in controlling their own health data, making the clinical trials transparent, and supply chain efficient, blockchain technology can revolutionize the healthcare system. Increased collaboration between healthcare practitioners, technology firms, and regulators will be required in terms of unlocking the full potential of blockchain technology for healthcare.

REFERENCES

Agbo, C. C., Mahmoud, Q. H., & Eklund, J. M. (2019). Blockchain Technology in Healthcare: A Systematic Review. *Health Care*, *7*, 56. PMID: 30987333

Al-Abdullah, M., Alsmadi, I., AlAbdullah, R., & Farkas, B. (2020). Designing privacy-friendly data repositories: A framework for a blockchain that follows the GDPR. *Digit. Policy Regul. Gov.*, *22*, 389–411.

Anitha, K.; Balasubramani, M.; S, V.P.K. (2023). Smart-fcd: Iot data interoperability using sensor based fuzzy linked rules for cross domain applications. Malays. J. Comput. Sci., sp2023, 54–64.

Benaich, R., El Mendili, S., & Gahi, Y. (2023). Advancing Healthcare Security: A Cutting-Edge Zero-Trust Blockchain Solution for Protecting Electronic Health Records. HighTech. *The Innovation Journal*, *4*, 630–652.

Daniel, C., Ouagne, D., Sadou, E., Paris, N., Hussain, S., Jaulent, M.-C., & Kalra, D. (2016). Cross border semantic interoperability for learning health systems: The EHR4CR semantic resources and services. *Learning Health Systems*, *1*, e10014. PMID: 31245551

Duan, K., Pang, G., & Lin, Y. (2023). Exploring the current status and future opportunities of blockchain technology adoption and application in supply chain management. *J. Digit. Econ.*, *2*, 244–288.

Glew, R., Tröger, R., & Schmittner, S. E. (2022). A solution approach for the anonymous sharing of sensitive supply chain traceability data. arXiv preprint arXiv:2204.00317.

Gohar, A. N., Abdelmawgoud, S. A., & Farhan, M. S. (2022). A patient centric healthcare framework reference architecture for better semantic interoperability based on blockchain, cloud, and IoT. *IEEE Access : Practical Innovations, Open Solutions*, *10*, 92137–92157.

Gordon, W. J., & Agrawal, A. (2018). Blockchain Technology for Healthcare: Facilitating the Transition to Patient-Driven Interoperability. *Computational and Structural Biotechnology Journal*, *16*, 224–230. PMID: 30069284

Hasselgren, A., Kralevska, K., Gligoroski, D., Pedersen, S. A., & Faxvaag, A. (2020). Blockchain in healthcare and health sciences—A scoping review. *International Journal of Medical Informatics*, *134*, 104040. PMID: 31865055

He, W., Zhang, J. Z., Wu, H., Li, W., & Shetty, S. (2022). A Unified Health Information System Framework for Connecting Data, People, Devices, and Systems. *Journal of Global Information Management, 30*, 2022.

Hirsch, J. A., Leslie-Mazwi, T. M., Nicola, G. N., Barr, R. M., Bello, J. A., Donovan, W. D., & Manchikanti, L. (2015). Current procedural terminology; a primer. *Journal of Neurointerventional Surgery*, *7*(4), 309–312.

Houtan, B.; Hafid, A.S.; Makrakis, D. (2020). A Survey on Blockchain-Based Self-Sovereign Patient Identity in Healthcare. IEEE Access 2020, 8, 90478–90494.

Imler, T. D., Vreeman, D. J., & Kannry, J. (2016). Healthcare Data Standards and Exchange. In Finnell, J. T., & Dixon, B. E. (Eds.), *Clinical Informatics Study Guide: Text and Review* (pp. 233–253). Springer International Publishing.

Jaleel, A.; Mahmood, T.; Hassan, M.A.; Bano, G.; Khurshid, S.K. (2020). Towards Medical Data Interoperability Through Collaboration of Healthcare Devices. IEEE Access 2020, 8, 132302–132319.

Kasyapa, M. S. B., & Vanmathi, C. (2024). Blockchain integration in healthcare: A comprehensive investigation of use cases, performance issues, and mitigation strategies. *Frontiers in Digital Health, 6*, 1359858. PMID: 38736708

Kaur, H., Alam, M. A., Jameel, R., Mourya, A. K., & Chang, V. (2018). A Proposed Solution and Future Direction for Blockchain-Based Heterogeneous Medicare Data in Cloud Environment. *Journal of Medical Systems*, *42*, 156. PMID: 29987560

Khushalani, J., Chandwani, S., Shaikh, A. S., Talreja, B., & Hande, R. Blockchain: The Novel Way to Secure Confidence! In *Proceedings of the International Conference on Electronics and Sustainable Communication Systems (ICESC)*, Coimbatore, India, 2–4 July 2020; IEEE: New York City, NY, USA, 2020; pp. 754–759.

Kouroubali, A., & Katehakis, D. G. (2022). Policy and Strategy for Interoperability of Digital Health in Europe. In *MEDINFO 2021: One World, One Health–Global Partnership for Digital Innovation* (pp. 897–901). IOS Press.

Kruse, C. S., Stein, A., Thomas, H., & Kaur, H. (2018). The use of Electronic Health Records to Support Population Health: A Systematic Review of the Literature. *Journal of Medical Systems*, *42*, 214. PMID: 30269237

Lee, H.-A., Kung, H.-H., Udayasankaran, J. G., Kijsanayotin, B., Marcelo, A. B., Chao, L. R., & Hsu, C.-Y. (2020). An architecture and management platform for blockchain-based personal health record exchange: Development and usability study. *Journal of Medical Internet Research*, *22*, e16748. PMID: 32515743

Lehne, M., Sass, J., Essenwanger, A., Schepers, J., & Thun, S. (2019). Why digital medicine depends on interoperability. npj. *Digital Medicine*, *2*, 79. PMID: 31453374

McGhin, T., Choo, K.-K. R., Liu, C. Z., & He, D. (2019). Blockchain in healthcare applications: Research challenges and opportunities. *Journal of Network and Computer Applications*, *135*, 62–75.

McKibbon, K. A., Lokker, C., Handler, S. M., Dolovich, L. R., Holbrook, A. M., O'Reilly, D., Tamblyn, R., Hemens, B. J., Basu, R., & Troyan, S.. (2012). The effectiveness of integrated health information technologies across the phases of medication management: A systematic review of randomized controlled trials. *Journal of the American Medical Informatics Association : JAMIA*, *19*, 22–30. PMID: 21852412

Menachemi, N., & Collum, T. H. (2011). Benefits and drawbacks of electronic health record systems. *Risk Management and Healthcare Policy*, *4*, 47–55. PMID: 22312227

Mertz, L. (2018). (Block) Chain Reaction: A Blockchain Revolution Sweeps into Health Care, Offering the Possibility for a Much-Needed Data Solution. *IEEE Pulse*, *9*, 4–7. PMID: 29757744

Nan, J., & Xu, L.-Q. (2023). Designing Interoperable Health Care Services Based on Fast Healthcare Interoperability Resources: Literature Review. *JMIR Medical Informatics*, *11*, e44842. PMID: 37603388

Nanda, A. (2019). Consumers' Intention to use Mobile Wallets. *AIMS Int. J. Manag.*, *13*, 143.

Natsiavas, P., Mazzeo, G., Faiella, G., Campegiani, P., Dumortier, J., Stan, O., Nalin, M., Martinez, D. M., Theodouli, A., & Moschou, K.. (2021). Developing an infrastructure for secure patient summary exchange in the EU context: Lessons learned from the KONFIDO project. *Health Informatics Journal*, *27*, 14604582211021459. PMID: 34142613

Omodunbi, T., Akindutire, A. S., Awoyelu, T. M., Ikono, R., & Gambo, I. (2023). Integrating Asymmetric Cryptographic Digital Wallet for Online Services in Nigeria. *Int. J. Inf. Eng. Electron. Bus.*, *3*, 29–40.

Pathak, N., Mukherjee, A., & Misra, S. (2023). SemBox: Semantic Interoperability in a Box for Wearable e-Health Devices. *IEEE Journal of Biomedical and Health Informatics*, *27*, 2306–2313. PMID: 35439151

Reegu, F. A., Abas, H., Gulzar, Y., Xin, Q., Alwan, A. A., Jabbari, A., Sonkamble, R. G., & Dziyauddin, R. A. (2023). Blockchain-Based Framework for Interoperable Electronic Health Records for an Improved Healthcare System. *Sustainability*, *15*, 6337.

Shicheng, W., Lin, H., Gan, W., Chen, J., & Yu, P. (2023). The Next Internet Revolution. arXi, arXiv:2304.06111.

Shrivastava, U., Song, J., Han, B. T., & Dietzman, D. (2021). Do data security measures, privacy regulations, and communication standards impact the interoperability of patient health information? A cross-country investigation. *International Journal of Medical Informatics*, *148*, 104401. PMID: 33571743

Sonkamble, R.G.; Phansalkar, S.P.; Potdar, V.M.; Bongale, A.M. (2021). Survey of Interoperability in Electronic Health Records Management and Proposed Blockchain Based Framework: MyBlockEHR. IEEE Access 2021, 9, 158367–158401.

Sreejith, R., & Senthil, S. (2023). Smart Contract Authentication assisted GraphMap-Based HL7 FHIR architecture for interoperable e-healthcare system. *Heliyon*, *9*, e15180. PMID: 37089400

Stearns, M. Q., Price, C., Spackman, K. A., & Wang, A. Y. (2001). SNOMED clinical terms: Overview of the development process and project status. *Proc. AMIA Symp.*, •••, 662–666. PMID: 11825268

Suratkar, S., Shirole, M., & Bhirud, S. Cryptocurrency Wallet: A Review. In Proceedings of the 2020 4th International Conference on Computer, Communication and Signal Processing (ICCCSP), Chennai, India, 28–29 September 2020; pp. 1–7.

Ullah, H. S., Aslam, S., & Arjomand, N. Blockchain in Healthcare and Medicine: A Contemporary Research of Applications, Challenges, and Future Perspectives. arXiv 2020, arXiv:2004.06795.

Vorisek, C. N., Lehne, M., Klopfenstein, S. A. I., Mayer, P. J., Bartschke, A., Haese, T., & Thun, S. (2022). Fast Healthcare Interoperability Resources (FHIR) for Interoperability in Health Research: Systematic Review. *JMIR Public Health and Surveillance*, *10*, e35724. PMID: 35852842

Chapter 6

Application of AI and IoT in Blockchain-Based Healthcare

Manas Kanti Saha
https://orcid.org/0009-0009-4273-0435
Brainware University, India

Subhojit Ghosh
https://orcid.org/0009-0003-2040-6251
Brainware University, India

Senjuti Mondal
https://orcid.org/0009-0002-7039-6525
Brainware University, India

ABSTRACT

This chapter describes the integration of AI, IoT, and blockchain with healthcare, with a focus on transformative impact. AI supports predictive analytics, data security, and workflow automation, whereas IoT enables real-time monitoring of patients and data transmission without interruption. Blockchain focuses on data integrity, transparency, and security and thereby addresses issues such as interoperability and scalability. Remote monitoring, decentralized clinical trials, and drug supply chain management will improve safety and efficiency. It will discuss the challenge of data privacy, ethical concerns, and regulatory complexities while calling for responsible implementation. The envisioned next-generation healthcare system would leverage such technologies to make care efficient, secure, and centered on the patient, supporting global collaboration and innovation to build a more equitable healthcare ecosystem.

DOI: 10.4018/979-8-3373-1225-5.ch006

INTRODUCTION

Overview of AI and IoT in Healthcare

Contemporary health issues approached synergistically have led to noticeable breakthroughs in patient diagnosis, care, and management that result from the disruptive technologies that AI and the Internet of Things have introduced into the health sector. Systems become more effective and patient-centered when approaching modern health issues synergistically. AI has transformed the healthcare sector significantly with the capability to process vast volumes of data and generate perceptive insights. Machine learning algorithms help doctors diagnose diseases at an early stage by using test results, histories of patients, and medical images. For instance, an AI system can detect abnormalities in radiological scans or very early warning signs of long-term conditions such as cancer or diabetes. The concept of individualized medicine is also helped by AI. For instance, to enhance the outcome and also minimize side effects, it allows for a treatment plan which is tailored based on an individual's genetic profile. Beyond mere diagnosis, AI eliminates tedium such as scheduling and billing that contributes to operational inefficiencies in health institutions.

It connects several devices which collect and share patient data in real-time; therefore, IoT helps bring the gulf between patient monitoring and delivery closer together (Samad, 2022).

Vital indications including heart rate, oxygen saturation, and glucose levels are recorded by wearables like fitness trackers and biosensors, enabling ongoing patient monitoring even in far-off places. This is particularly effective in the management of chronic illnesses, because early intervention might prevent consequences. By employing smart devices to monitor inventory, control medical equipment, and make the most use of available resources, IoT also assists hospitals in managing their operations. Together, the advantages of AI and IoT grow, and a solid basis for predictive, preventive, and individualized healthcare is established. AI analyzes the vast volumes of data generated by IoT devices to identify patterns, predict how diseases will develop, and provide real-time treatment (Samad, 2022). For example, AI-based data analytics of IoT can inform doctors about early signs of heart failure so that they can take timely interventions before that. In a nutshell, AI with IoT rejuvenates healthcare by elevating precision, accessibility, and efficiency levels (Samad, 2022). This potential is so vast that it cannot yet be exhausted by any imagination to shift the paradigms governing global health systems.

Blockchain Technology in Healthcare

Blockchain technology is revolutionizing the healthcare sector with safe, open, and effective ways of handling private patient information (Haddad, Habaebi, Islam, Hasbullah, & Zabidi, 2022). Because its decentralized structure ensures data exchange and storage with unmatched security, blockchain technology represents an invaluable tool in dealing with issues in health systems, such as data breaches, inefficiencies, and interoperability (Haddad, Habaebi, Islam, Hasbullah, & Zabidi, 2022).

In other words, blockchain is basically an unalterable and permanently locked ledger. This ensures a secure sharing of patient data across a patient, hospitals, lab centres, insurance companies, among many medical providers (Alabdulatif, Khalil, & Rahman, 2022). Blockchain cuts through intermediaries: the processes are streamlined with lowered costs for administration. Patients' access to health data ownership gives permission or denial to certain stakeholders for accessing the information needed.

Figure 1. Blockchain in Healthcare technology

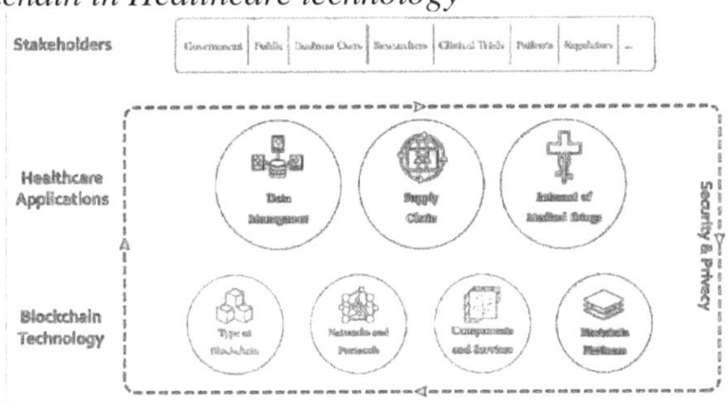

Blockchain will have the most essential usage in healthcare in providing data integrity. Incomplete or false records of patients are frequently a reason for medical errors. Inequities are decreased, and diagnosis and treatment precision are increased by maintaining one record, current and on-demand across all platforms with the use of blockchain (Alabdulatif, Khalil, & Rahman, 2022). A whole history of a patient's medication would make sure doctors take timely, informative decisions about it, instead of being delayed and ignorant due to incomplete information on traditional systems (Haddad, Habaebi, Islam, Hasbullah, & Zabidi, 2022).

There has also been a transformation regarding blockchain and its use especially with managing supply chains in the healthcare domain in the pharmaceutical sector. Since it guarantees authenticity, these technology-related schemes keep counterfeit drugs off store shelves. The blockchain chronicles each transaction from inception to delivery, allowing instantaneous tracking and validation.

Another blockchain component is smart contracts, which automate procedures like clinical trials and insurance claims. For example, once certain requirements are fulfilled, like finishing treatment, smart contracts can verify and carry out insurance reimbursements. Blockchain also promotes ethical research procedures in clinical trials by guaranteeing transparency and traceability in data collection and analysis (Haddad, Habaebi, Islam, Hasbullah, & Zabidi, 2022).

Blockchain use in healthcare is nevertheless hampered by issues like scalability, energy consumption, and regulatory concerns, despite its potential. Unlocking its full potential will require addressing these problems with regulatory frameworks and technical breakthroughs.

In conclusion, blockchain technology can lead to an improvement in safety, efficiency, and confidence among healthcare systems (Haddad, Habaebi, Islam, Hasbullah, & Zabidi, 2022). With rising adoption, it will radically transform the way health-care data is managed, shared, and used to have better patient outcomes and optimal operational excellence.

ROLE OF AI IN BLOCKCHAIN-BASED HEALTHCARE

Figure 2. Blockchain impact on healthcare

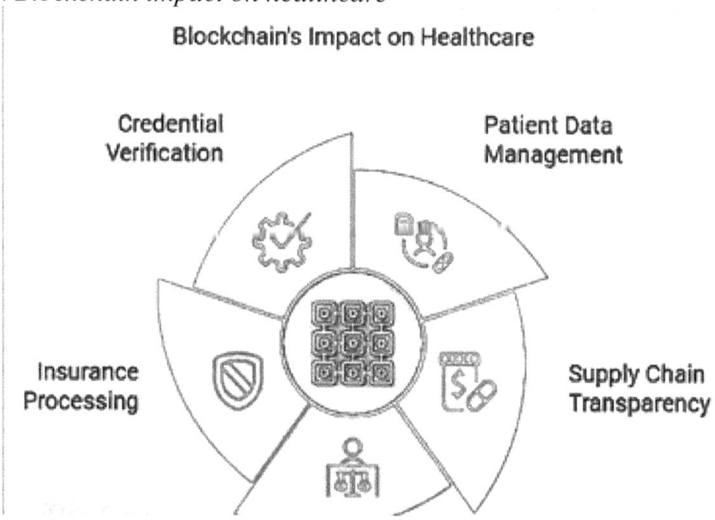

AI for Predictive Analytics

AI has the most revolutionary role in predictive analytics when combined with blockchain technology in the health sector (Gul, Paul, Rho, & Kim, 2020). This way, extensive datasets stored safely in a blockchain network could be analyzed to make precise predictions for the outcome of health, thereby ensuring proactive intervention and efficient utilization of resources in providing improved care to patients with greater efficiency.

Blockchain Security Enables Prediction of Early Diseases

AI systems are able to recognize early indicators of diseases including diabetes, cancer, and heart problems by using genetic information, patient histories, and medical imaging. Blockchain technology increases the security and transparency of the projections provided. It is possible for AI models to work with precise and unaltered data due to blockchain's assurance of the integrity and immutability of patient data (Haddad, Habaebi, Islam, Hasbullah, & Zabidi, 2022). Blockchain-based decentralized records provide highly accurate AI-based predictions that help doctors diagnose and treat diseases at the earliest stages (Samad, 2022).

Personalized Risk Assessment and Data Integrity

AI-based predictive models assess the health risks of an individual based on lifestyle, genetic, and medical data securely stored on blockchain networks (Gul, Paul, Rho, & Kim, 2020). Blockchains enable patients to own their health data but to make it accessible for AI-based analysis. For example, in the management of chronic diseases, AI can analyze data stored in blockchains to predict complications and personalize interventions. Such a combination will not only facilitate risk stratification but also ensure privacy while complying with the regulatory frameworks such as HIPAA and GDPR.

Smart Resource Optimization with Clear Analytics

AI integrated with blockchain will predict any kind of demand, whether it is the admission to hospitals or demand for medications. Since blockchain is a decentralized system, all the stakeholders such as hospitals and insurers will get access to AI-validated predictions in real time (Gul, Paul, Rho, & Kim, 2020). Thus, this transparency will help better plan the resource allocation from staffing to chains of medical supplies during the time of public health crisis.

In summary, AI for predictive analytics when integrated with blockchain in the health sector provides unmatched benefits related to accuracy, security, and efficiency. Combining blockchain's ability to ensure data integrity with AI's analytical capabilities, health systems can provide proactive patient-centric care while protecting sensitive information. This synergy promises great potential for advancing global healthcare (Gul, Paul, Rho, & Kim, 2020).

Enhancing Data Security with AI

Enhancing data security requires artificial intelligence, particularly in the healthcare industry where sensitive data must be safeguarded. Advanced AI algorithms guarantee data integrity, threat detection, and breach prevention.

Identifying and Preventing Threats in Real Time

AI is perfect to be kept running constantly to scan and correct security threats in advance. The machine learning model can trace the anomalies of a network, for instance, which may result in unauthorized accesses or anomalous data transfer patterns (Gul, Paul, Rho, & Kim, 2020). For instance, AI-enabled systems can promptly respond to the ransomware attack by 'isolation of compromised areas minimizing damage'. This proactive posture is of utmost importance in healthcare because EHRs and data of the patient need protection.

Data Protection with Encryption and Behavior Analysis

AI improves encryption protocols by dynamically managing encryption keys to ensure that only authorized people have access to sensitive information. It also monitors user behavior within systems to detect possible insider threats. Unusual activities, such as repeated failed login attempts or accessing large amounts of data outside typical hours, are flagged by AI and prevented from being misused. This combination of encryption and behavioral analytics significantly boosts the security of healthcare data.

Blockchain Integration for Data Integrity

The role of AI in blockchain-based healthcare systems strengthens security further. Since blockchain is immutable, there cannot be any data manipulation while AI analyzes the transactions for detecting fraudulent activities (Haddad, Habaebi,

Islam, Hasbullah, & Zabidi, 2022). Such a synergy protects the patient information with transparency and accountability among the stakeholders.

Figure 3. Ensuring of data integrity of blockchain

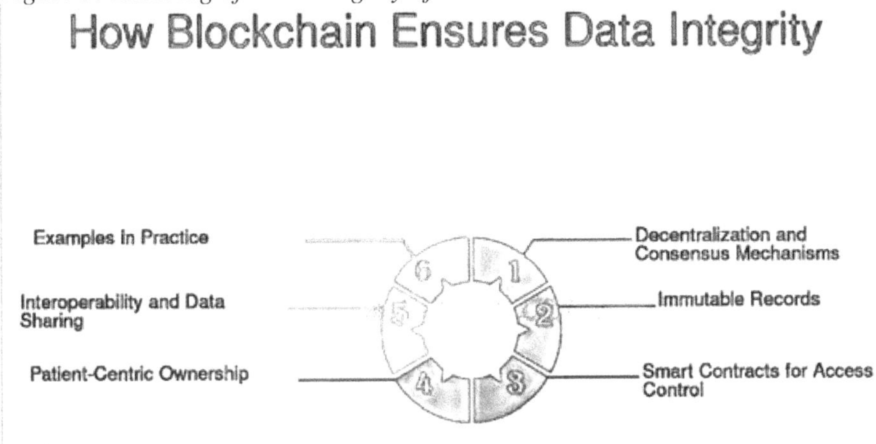

In conclusion, AI will enhance data security through real-time threat detection, strong encryption, and easy integration with technologies such as blockchain. Its proactive capabilities in the prevention of breaches and safeguarding sensitive information are what transform data security in the healthcare sector, allowing for trustworthy and compliant care in this digital age.

AI in Smart Contracts for Healthcare

AI and smart contracts are revolutionizing the healthcare industry by automating procedures, increasing their efficacy, and guaranteeing safe, transparent transactions (Gul, Paul, Rho, & Kim, 2020). Blockchain-powered smart contracts execute predetermined activities when specific circumstances are satisfied; artificial intelligence gives these processes intelligence, allowing for more dynamic, adaptable, and effective results.

Automating Claims Processing and Payments

AI-integrated smart contracts streamline the claims and payments process in the healthcare system. This process is cumbersome as it takes too much time and always causes disputes because of mistakes. AI technology will help to develop smart contracts that automatically validate claims by cross-verifying patient data, treatment records, and policy information on a blockchain. For instance, once the patient's treatment is over, an AI algorithm will validate a claim by checking diagnosis, care rendered, and terms of insurance coverage. Once validated, this causes the smart contract to autonomously trigger a payout so delays, administrative overhead and also fraud risks are all minimised. This system protects and benefits both patients and service providers through prompt and secure transactions.

Consent and Secure Sharing of Data

This aspect of AI improves managing patients' consent and making secured data sharing. Patients would be able to point to the conditions under which such healthcare data is accessed and distributed, and smart contracts do enforce such rules (Gul, Paul, Rho, & Kim, 2020). The algorithms can read the requests to access the data and comply with patient-defined terms and also HIPAA or GDPR regulations. An example could be researchers accessing anonymized patient data to use for studies. This is allowed by smart contracts where they will check the preset conditions of a request and open up to authorized parties while ensuring privacy of the patient.

Facilitating Personalized Health Services

Smart contracts with AI pave the way to a more personalized healthcare experience. AI analyzes patient data, suggesting treatments or changes in medication, which can then be securely communicated through smart contracts to pharmacies, labs, or clinicians. For example, a smart insulin pump for a diabetic patient could use AI monitoring of glucose levels to initiate a contract to order automatic refills. This integration reduces human intervention and ensures timely and personalized care delivery.

AI is enhancing smart contracts to automate, secure, and intelligent healthcare processes. From claims processing and data sharing to individualized care, this synergy makes healthcare a more efficient, transparent, and patient-centric system.

IOT INTEGRATION IN BLOCKCHAIN-BASED SYSTEMS

In recent decades, wireless communication plays a vital role in the medical industry's growth, smart cities, vehicular and transportation systems using IoT networks (Haddad, Habaebi, Islam, Hasbullah, & Zabidi, 2022). The wireless nodes are dispersed in the observing field for collecting the related data and further transmitting it towards the cloud paradigm. The application users use the internet and access the needed information directly on their smartphones and computing machines. Almost all critical applications need an on-time response from the sensing objects and facilitate their users. The architecture of wireless networks consists of small, less expensive, and low-powered intelligent sensors distributed either uniformly or randomly in various fields, i.e., military, agriculture, healthcare, smart cities, and grids for information observing. The sensory data is collected based on particular events or periodic intervals and transmitted to centralized servers. In medical applications, the medical experts access the patients' information from centralized or distributed servers using the internet through some developing next-generation wireless techniques. However, the traditional data analysis techniques are incompatible to extract useful health information; therefore, most academics are focusing on intelligent methods with the internet of medical things for a precise and thorough exploration of patients' sensitive data. Health services widely adopt the internet of medical items due to its significant impact on diagnosing disease and facilitating treatments with the least communication cost (Haddad, Habaebi, Islam, Hasbullah, & Zabidi, 2022). The medical applications consist of three main phases. In the first phase, wearable sensors collected the patients' data and forwarded them to a local administrator or coordinator. The second phase communicates the patients' data to the server or sinks node with the intermediate devices over the wireless transmission system. Finally, the medical data is stored on some cloud service providers; thus, medical professionals judge the patients' condition and provide suitable actions. In the flat-based structure with the same processing, receiving, forwarding, and storage capabilities (Haddad, Habaebi, Islam, Hasbullah, & Zabidi, 2022).

Figure 4. IoT for integration in blockchain based system

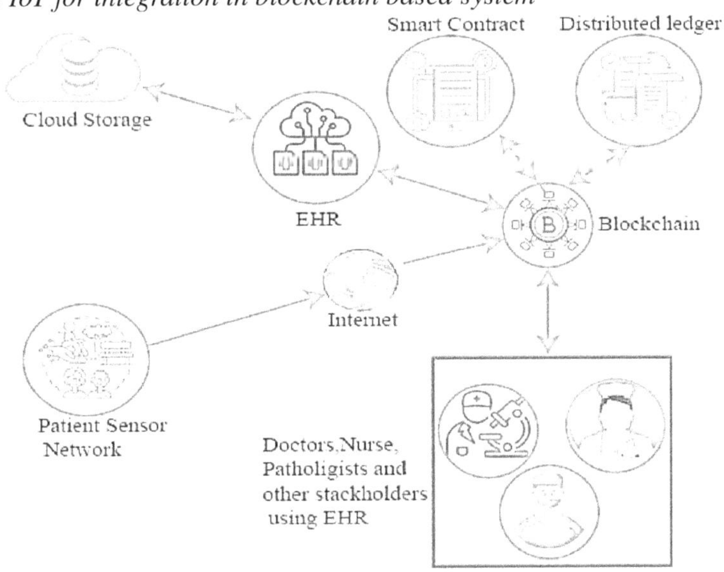

The Internet of Things has transformed health care, where patients can be monitored in real-time and improved quality and effectiveness in care. With the IoT, information regarding a patient's health can be captured from devices and transmitted to give health care providers constant monitoring with proactive responses.

Continuous Monitoring with Early Intervention

Patients will continue to be monitored by IoT using wearable devices. Embedded biosensor and wearable sensors Vital signs that are part of daily monitoring include blood pressure, heart rate. oxygen saturation and blood sugar levels This allows for a regular assessment of the patient's health. Especially chronic diseases such as diabetes or heart disease. For instance, this will inform the medical staff of an abnormal heart rhythm, where they can respond quickly in an attempt to prevent disaster. In addition to that, it minimizes hospital readmissions and expenses of hospital readmissions.

Remote Monitoring and Telemedicine Integration

IoT makes it possible for remote monitoring which bridges patients with the health caregivers particularly in rural or poorly served areas (Mistry et al., 2021). Devices send data into the cloud, which these healthcare service providers access without having to visit patients every now and then.

For example, after surgery, patients can upload recovery to physicians' devices through Internet of Things-enabled tools and thus adjust the recovery treatments on time. This may further integrate well into telemedicine, assisting doctors to study real-time data and raise the diagnosis accuracy and care quality through virtual consultations.

Secure IoT Data Sharing through Blockchain

The IoT and blockchain combination is changing the face of healthcare as it enables safe, transparent, and efficient data sharing. This is because IoT devices are constantly generating a huge amount of patient data, which creates a massive challenge in ensuring security and integrity while sharing this information (Haddad, Habaebi, Islam, Hasbullah, & Zabidi, 2022). Blockchain addresses the challenge in the form of decentralized and tamper-proof frameworks that can manage sensitive health information.

Figure 5. Secure internet of medical things

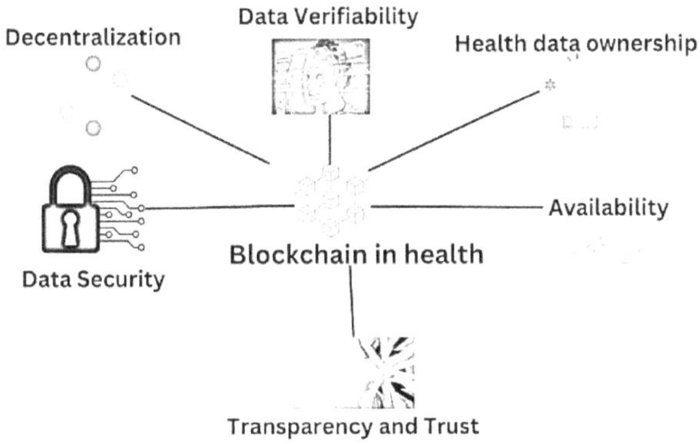

Reliable Data Integrity and Security

Blockchain makes the data of IoT "write once" and unreadable, unerasable, and uninterruptible. Each of the pieces of information in the form of vital signs, diagnostic, and treatment reports is ciphered and formed as blocks that are maintained in chains. Every block is timestamped, and through the linking procedure to the preceding block makes alteration impossible or virtually detected. For example, blockchain can securely transmit data from IoT devices in remote patient monitoring systems to healthcare providers so that it will be accurate and untampered. This is crucial for trust in critical applications, such as chronic disease monitoring or medication adherence tracking (Haddad, Habaebi, Islam, Hasbullah, & Zabidi, 2022).

Controlled and Transparent Data Access

Blockchain improves the data-sharing process by giving patients control over their information. Using smart contracts, patients can define specific conditions under which their data can be accessed. For example, a patient undergoing a clinical trial can permit researchers to access only anonymized data while keeping personal identifiers private. IoT devices, integrated with blockchain, ensure that all data access is recorded transparently, enabling auditability and compliance with regulations like HIPAA or GDPR (Samad, 2022).

Supporting Interoperability Across Stakeholders

Blockchain enables interoperability among the IoT systems and stakeholders of healthcare. With this technology, hospitals, labs, insurance companies, and patients can share data safely without depending on any central intermediary. This would bring greater efficiency, more cooperation, and faster decision-making for in-patient care (Haddad, Habaebi, Islam, Hasbullah, & Zabidi, 2022).

In fact, with the recent COVID-19 pandemic, IoT played an important role in combating diseases. However, IoT devices are tiny, with limited capabilities (Mistry et al., 2021). Therefore, IoT systems lack encryption, insufficient privacy protection, and are subject to many attacks. Accordingly, IoT healthcare systems are extremely vulnerable to several security flaws that might result in more accurate, quick, and precise diagnoses.

IoT Devices and Interoperability Challenges

Among the many devices that have exploded in the healthcare industry as a result of the Internet of Things or IoT, wearables such as sensors and smart medical devices (Samad, 2022). These can gather huge amounts of data for caring for patients but have an interoperability problem associated with them within the healthcare system. For optimization in patient outcomes as well as operational efficiency, seamless communication and data transfer must take place between many different kinds of IoT and healthcare systems (Haddad, Habaebi, Islam, Hasbullah, & Zabidi, 2022).

Figure 6. Challenges in IOT devices and interoperability

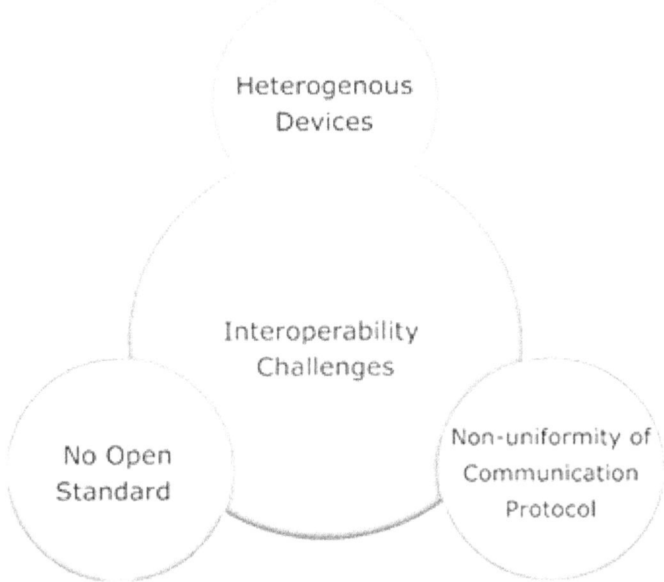

Non-Standardized Protocols in IoT Devices

The other major challenge to achieve interoperability in relation to IoT is the presence of non-standardized protocols in various devices (Samad, 2022). Standardized communication standards, format of data, and network architecture, vary in the usage pattern of different manufacturers in their devices. A firm may come up with a heart rate monitor, but that heart rate monitor does not necessarily communicate well with a glucose monitoring system developed by some other firm. This may break the data (Haddad, Habaebi, Islam, Hasbullah, & Zabidi, 2022). The non-standardized nature of doing things makes health data sharing and aggregation across different platforms problematic hence does not support IoT implementation in the health sector.

Data Compatibility and Integration

IoT devices in healthcare generate varied types of data, including biometric readings, environmental information, and treatment data. At times, these data formats do not match the ones prevailing in existing healthcare systems, like EHRs or HIS (Samad, 2022). It gets complex because it has to enter centralized systems without being compromised in its integrity or accuracy. If seamless integration is not possible, even for health care providers, there would be a tough job to access all information associated with the patient, hence causing late diagnosis or treatment.

Security and Privacy Concern

The two main concerns about the interoperability of IoT devices are security and privacy. Since several health-related systems and different equipment exchange patient-related sensitive information, the information needs the highest security. Most of the IoT devices are highly vulnerable to cyber-attacks; thus, access to the health information can be accessed, hence violating the privacy of the patient. In addition, interoperability among the IoT devices has to follow very stringent requirements like HIPAA and GDPR (Samad, 2022). It is therefore a very challenging integration process.

Scalability Issues

Scalability is a huge issue as more IoT devices are integrated into healthcare organizations. It becomes very difficult to support an increasing number of devices without compromising performance, security, or data accuracy (Samad, 2022). Specifically in a large-scale deployment, it requires an infrastructure that can be used for managing the enormous amounts of data produced by these devices. It requires an immense investment in platform, protocol, and system updates, which is necessary for staying with the growing IoT ecosystem (Samad, 2022).

Conclusion Despite how much promise that IoT devices bring for the future in revolutionizing health care delivery, it can only reap fully from their presence only when issues related to interoperability have been answered. Issues about standardization, integration of data, security, and scalability issues will answer the problem, making IoT much more efficient and effective in healthcare.

SYNERGY OF AI AND IOT IN BLOCKCHAIN

AI-Driven Insights from IoT Data

Artificial Intelligence is releasing the power of IoT healthcare data. It's turning the way patient information is gathered and used on its head. IoT devices include all sorts of wearables, medical sensors, and monitoring systems that collect health information continuously (Haddad, Habaebi, Islam, Hasbullah, & Zabidi, 2022). AI algorithms may process such a massive amount of data to deliver value that enhances decision-making while improving the outcomes for patients.

Real-Time Health Monitoring and Early Detection

AI-powered analytics can instantly extract information about health trends and disorders from Internet of Things data. For example, wearable technology monitors blood pressure. heart rate and oxygen saturation as a result, a database is continually being built, which AI models analyze in real time to identify early indicators of health problems, such as respiratory problems. arrhythmia or a sudden spike in blood sugar (Mistry et al., 2021).

Predictive Analytics for Personalized Care

AI models will be able to predict health outcomes in the future with the help of historical data from IoT related to medical histories of patients. These predictive insights are necessary for personalizing healthcare, specifically for patients with chronic diseases. For instance, AI is able to identify patterns of data to predict a risk of hypoglycemia in a diabetic patient or forecast the likelihood of rehospitalization in a patient with heart failure.(Haddad, Habaebi, Islam, Hasbullah, & Zabidi, 2022). Foreseeing these events will assist healthcare providers in devising individualized treatment plans that will allow them to intervene immediately, thus optimizing patient care while reducing hospital visits. In summary, AI-driven insights from IoT data greatly improve healthcare systems in real-time monitoring, early detection, and predictive analytics (Haddad, Habaebi, Islam, Hasbullah, & Zabidi, 2022). These technologies allow health providers to be more personal, efficient, and proactive in providing better care for their patients.

Automated Workflows in Healthcare Systems

One of the major components of workflow automation is important for improving operational efficiency while cutting back on human errors and to eventually make possible quality patient care (Samad, 2022). The administration in healthcare systems, combined with AI, machine learning, and robotics, can now streamline administrative tasks so the professionals have more time spent on direct patient care.

Reduction of Administrative Tasks

Perhaps the most significant advantage of automation in healthcare is that it saves time in administrative work. All such activities can be performed through software systems, such as scheduling a patient, billing, and verification of insurance. These processes save time but also reduce the chances of human error. For example, scheduling with AI will automatically assign the patient to the healthcare provider available. This means a lower degree of intervention required. Automated billing ensures that the claims get processed correctly and quickly, ensuring that the reimbursement happens as early as possible and there is a lower administrative cost overhead.

Clinical Decision Making

Automation facilitates clinical decision-making in a timely manner with accurate, data-driven insights being offered to healthcare professionals. The AI algorithms analyze data from patients from various sources such as EHRs and IoT devices to identify patterns, make outcome predictions, and make treatment recommendations. These automated insights can help clinicians make rapid decisions, which results in improved patient outcomes. Automated alerts can automatically notify a doctor of changes in a patient's condition, calling the doctor to intervene soon enough (Mistry et al., 2021). These streamlined decisions have resulted in efficient time management and quality care.

Optimization of Resource Utilization

Automated workflows are best suited for managing healthcare resources, like the fact that AI systems can predict inflow. In this sense, hospitals can use up staff and equipment appropriately with supplies kept automatically inventoried, thus making sure updated stocks are always available, minimizing waste and shortages (Samad, 2022). With emergencies, automation also maximizes critical cases, directing resources to the areas where more need is shown.

The introduction of automated workflows to healthcare systems brings tremendous improvements in operational efficiency and clinical decision-making as well as resource management. Automation eliminates administrative burdens and enhances processes in the care of the patient while ushering into a new era of health care innovations.

Personalized Healthcare Delivery

Personalized health care delivery is transforming the character of health care through individualized treatment plans, taking into consideration the patient's specific needs. Using technologies like Artificial Intelligence (AI), genomics, and data analytics, personalized health care has come out of the ordinary one-size-fits-all health care approach and has taken on the responsibility of tailoring care according to a person's health conditions, genetic makeup, and lifestyle. This change has been effective in bettering the outcome of patients, boosting their satisfaction levels, and strengthening health care systems.

Data-Driven Treatment Plans

Personalized medicine heavily relies on the combination of big chunks of patient data. Be it EHRs, wearable health devices, or any other means, the data is continuously being captured and gives a real-time view of the health condition of a patient (Samad, 2022). AI and ML algorithms interpret this data and formulate personalized treatment plans for every patient. For example, in oncology, AI may scan the genetic information of a patient and his or her medical history to provide the best available cancer treatment. In such a way, AI-based recommendations will reduce the traditional trial-and-error approach in treatments and make them more personalized based on the genetic, environmental, and lifestyle factors of the patient, leading to higher efficacy and fewer adverse effects. Additionally, with wearable devices, it will be possible to continuously monitor the health condition, which then would be responded to and treatment plans adapted in a real-time setting. Chronic diseases such as diabetes could, for instance, involve real-time processing of the level of glucose and adjustment recommendations regarding medication or diet due to individual needs, therefore avoiding complications and improving general management.

Figure 7. Data driven treatment revolution

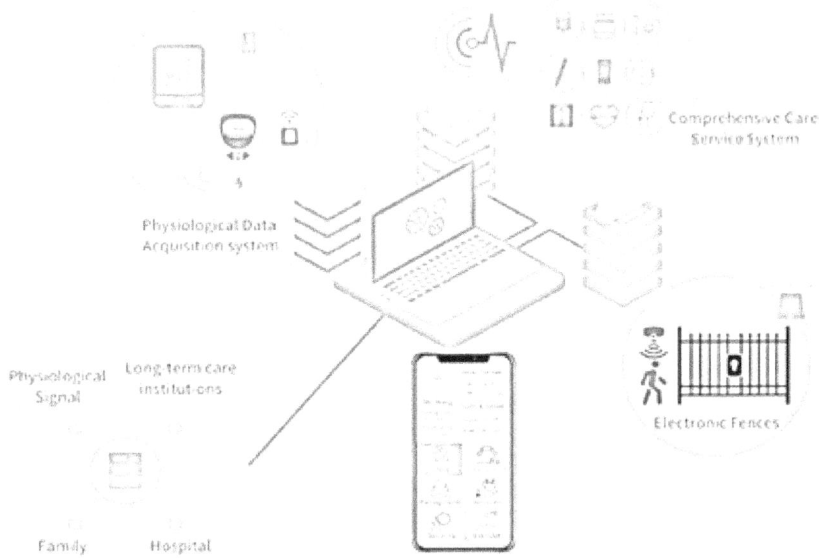

Precision Medicine and Genomic Insights

Another important component of personalized care is precision medicine. This will adjust the treatment plan according to the patient's genetic characteristics. With the success of genomics This allows doctors to now have access to the most comprehensive genetic information available. This can be used to predict a patient's susceptibility to specific diseases. Optimal response to treatment and side effects of drugs.

By integrating this genomic information into the care process Healthcare providers can design highly targeted treatments. For example, pharmacogenomics ensures that drugs to be used in a particular patient would probably work given the said genetic makeup of the individual. It therefore eliminates unhelpful treatment and less adverse reactions. Conclusion: The personalized delivery of healthcare alters the traditional health delivery process using data, AI, and genomics while devising a treatment program specific to a patient's case. Precision medicine and data-driven care make a difference in the outcomes for patients and help reduce the cost while making the experience more comprehensive for healthcare.

APPLICATIONS AND USE CASES

Remote Patient Monitoring

One of the recent innovative models of modern health care is RPM, where a clinician monitors the health conditions of a patient from remote locations with the support of sophisticated technologies such as IoT devices and telemedicine platforms. This model enhances care delivery to the patient and decreases hospital visits and fosters efficient health care for patients, mainly chronic and post-acute care services.

Continuous Monitoring of Health

RPM tracks patient vital signs through wearable devices, biosensors, heart rate, blood pressure, glucose levels, oxygen saturation, etc. All these devices should be able to communicate their status to the healthcare provider. To be able to monitor remotely in various locations. For instance, a hypertensive patient might have a connected blood pressure monitor that periodically forwards a report to his or her doctor. Real-time data allows timely intervention, among which are adjustment of medications dosages, preventing complications, and reducing the rate of emergency hospitalizations.

Expanded Access to Care

The telemedicine technology of RPM links the patients and service providers, especially in distant rural or underserved populations. Patients can get high quality care without having the geographic barriers by removing frequent visits in-person. The RPM-based telemedicine platforms enable the physicians to access this information remotely and conduct virtual consults. For example, the patients can transfer recovery metrics to their doctors after surgery through the devices of RPM (Samad, 2022). Thus, the doctors can track and give feedback while maintaining their distance. This is quite convenient for the patients, and it reduces the workload on healthcare facilities.

Better Management of Chronic Diseases

For patients suffering from chronic conditions like diabetes, heart failure, or COPD, RPM offers individualized care through constant data collection and AI-driven analytics. Health metrics are tracked, allowing for preventive adjustments in treatment plans.

An example would be an AI system analyzing the data from RPM that detected early signs of heart failure, thus calling for instant action before the condition worsened. This proactive approach to patient care improves patient results while concurrently reducing the cost burdens of care associated with hospital readmissions. In a nutshell, Remote Patient Monitoring transformed healthcare delivery systems by establishing continuous oversight for patients' conditions, enabling access, and improving management of chronic diseases. Leveraging on technology, the RPM platform empowers not only patients but also health providers for better health results and living quality (Samad, 2022).

Decentralized Clinical Trials

DCTs is a paradigm shift in conducting clinical research by using digital technologies and remote methods (Alshehri & Muhammad, 2020). It is unlike the old trials, where patients must visit centralized sites, allowing for data collection, monitoring, and interaction with the patient to be conducted from remote locations, thus making the process more efficient, accessible, and engaging for the patients.

Improved Accessibility and Patient Involvement

DCTs eliminate geographical and logistical barriers as more diversified participation in clinical research becomes possible (Alshehri & Muhammad, 2020). The classic trials enroll only people living next to the location of a site of trials and many a times underrepresented the diverging populations. DCT allows participants to access the trials from their nearest available places by virtue of its electronic modalities, including cell applications (Alshehri & Muhammad, 2020), wearable devices, or remote medicine platforms. Therefore, for example, such monitors can send their monitored signs straight to the scientists with no need to access physical sites.

This increased access is particularly important for patients who are immobile, in rural areas, or at work and cannot take a day off to visit sites regularly. As a result, DCTs offer more convenience to patients and increase the diversity and generalizability of clinical trials, thus making them more representative and generalizable.

Better Collection and Efficiency of Data

DCTs make use of advanced technologies to enhance data collection, monitoring, and analysis. Real-time capture of data can be done through IoT devices, mobile sensors, and electronic diaries, allowing for continuous and accurate monitoring of the participants' health. Often, blockchain technology is implemented to secure and streamline the sharing of data, hence ensuring data integrity and patients' privacy (Alshehri & Muhammad, 2020).

Furthermore, AI-driven analytics becomes significant for analyzing huge data generated in DCTs. For instance, AI algorithms may be able to find early warnings of adverse events or pattern analysis on the patient responses that can be used later on for timely interventions and adaptive trial designs. This model also is a logistical cost saver in physical trial sites and makes research cheaper without any compromise on quality.

Additionally, An Artificial Intelligence (AI)-enabled and blockchain-driven Electronic Health Record (EHR) maintenance system has a tremendous potential to facilitate reliable, secure, and robust storage systems for EHRs. Such an EHR system would also facilitate researchers, doctors, and government authorities to access data for research, perform analytics, and help in making well-informed decisions. The Artificial Neural Network (ANN) is employed to classify the patients as potentially COVID-19 positive and potentially COVID-19 negative based on the clinical reports and reports of CT-scan. The data of potentially COVID-19 positive patients is stored on blockchain employing InterPlanetary File System (IPFS) protocol. The accessibility of EHR can be done by authorized entities post verification and validation of entities (Mistry et al., 2021).

Blockchain for Drug Supply Chain Management

This will enable better transparency, traceability, and security in pharmaceuticals by the blockchain technology in a drug supply chain. Most processes of drug supply chains involve stakeholders that can range from the manufacturer to the pharmacy through various distributors. Blockchain ensures all transactions are recorded securely by creating an immutable and decentralized ledger; this boosts efficiency while reducing the risk factors of counterfeit drugs and inefficient supply chains (Haddad, Habaebi, Islam, Hasbullah, & Zabidi, 2022).

Enhanced Traceability and Transparency

Blockchain allows the traceability of drugs end to end from the supply chain. Every step, such as manufacturing, packaging, transportation, or delivery, is recorded as a block in the blockchain. Thus, an auditable record is created, which cannot be tampered with by the journey of the drug, so that stakeholders may authenticate its authenticity. In some of them, a QR code might be attached to every batch so as to give every one complete detail of where the origin is, date of production, storage, and when shipped. This ability has found tremendous usage in dealing with the major portions of pharmaceutical markets- counterfeited drugs. Blockchain provides a transparent view of the supply chain. This increases trust between stakeholders. and ensures that only genuine products reach consumers (Samad, 2022).

Increased Productivity and Lower Expenses

The blockchain automatically makes the drug supply chain simpler by removing some middlemen and automating some procedures. Smart contracts, a blockchain feature, automate transactions as well as enforce specific predefined conditions. Thus, payments to suppliers will automatically begin once the drugs have been authenticated at their destination.

More important, blockchain reduces the fuss of paper-based documentation that pertains to invoices, customs forms, and compliance reports. It has minimal chances of error, has reduced processing time, and saves the cost that entails manual record-keeping. Better operational efficiency gives ample time for pharmaceutical companies for innovation and quality assurance activities.

Higher Security and Compliance with the Norm

The pharmaceutical supply chain is really vulnerable to data tampering and theft. Such situations make it susceptible to any security breach. Technology underpinned by the Blockchain is very secure, firstly because it is a system that is decentralized; the data stored on the ledger gets encrypted and gets to be distributed across the nodes. The network instantly would recognize and reject a piece of record modification.

Blockchain helps support the needs of pharmaceutical corporations to uphold regulatory standards such as laid down by organisations like FDA or EMA (Samad, 2022). Information regarding drug batch numbers could be given which would eventually help in making checks and allowing approval much easily without long delays. It simplifies transparency and helps ensure better safety together with having stronger collaboration that creates more cohesion and helps make this system much stronger.

CHALLENGES AND LIMITATIONS

This section explores the unsolved issues and research challenges in smart healthcare systems that harm patients' health during remote monitoring.

Smart healthcare lacks security standardization because current health safety rules are too old-fashioned and outdated. They also can't stand up to modern security threats. The medical field needs standards to cut down on mistakes, boost patient safety, and make a big difference in how patients experience care (Jabarulla & Lee, 2021). Also, security problems from remote patient monitoring can hurt patients' health and make them not want to take medicine from that healthcare provider. This can damage the hospital management's reputation, which might lower their overall earnings.

Scalability Issues

Scalability is established as the one important aspect to be controlled whenever wireless communication takes place between the patient and the doctor in remote treatment setups. Based on the symptoms presented by the patient, health providers may have to incorporate various implantable sensors and medical devices to gather health data of a patient to make decisions regarding the appropriateness of further therapy (Jabarulla & Lee, 2021). In the smart health systems, network bandwidth needs to be effectively optimized for medical diagnosis, so that low-scalability communication between patients and medical experts does not delay treatment, causing patients to deteriorate, or even pass away.

Data Privacy Concerns

While the healthcare industry is proactive and concerned with safeguarding such sensitive patient data from breaches, illegal access, and improper use, such data privacy concerns assume greater importance when health institutions adopt cutting-edge technologies such as blockchain, the internet of things, and artificial intelligence. The main concerns are:

Breaches of Private Data

Healthcare is a prime target for a cyberattack since health-related information has substantial personal and medical ramifications (Elhoseny et al., 2021). Data breaches can lead to identity theft, financial fraud, and even a credibility blow to the patients. For example, a compromised EHR system may leak thousands of patient records, with severe consequences for both patients and physicians.

Inadequate Control of Information

Too often, patients have little or no say as to who collects, stores, and shares their data. Ethical and legal concerns arise when third-party agencies use data obtained from patients for marketing and research purposes without their consent (Elhoseny et al., 2021). The capability of a patient to dictate where their data goes is thus critical for the perpetuation of patient confidence in the otherwise venerable healthcare systems.

Poor Methods of Encryption

Some healthcare companies still protect sensitive data with outdated or ineffective encryption methods. A consequence of that is making their systems open to illegal access and hacking. Adaptive network protocols combined with recent encryption methods are vital to safeguarding data during transport and storage.

Compliance with Privacy Laws

Healthcare systems must operate within rigid privacy regulations such as CCPA, GDPR, and HIPAA. Noncompliance leads to massive fines and loss of reputation. Managing vast data sets across multiple platforms while adhering to these regulations is taxing and takes a considerable amount of effort.

Interoperability and Risk of Data Sharing

At the time the healthcare system merged, privacy concerns were raised in regards to sharing patient data across the various platforms (Elhoseny et al., 2021). Complications are introduced by the careless execution of data-sharing agreements or improperly configured technologies that allow for unintentionally exposing patients' information.

In short, the concerns surrounding data privacy in the healthcare sector highlight an individual need for robust security protocols, an empowering patient experience, and strict adherence to privacy regulations. Addressing these challenges arms healthcare systems with the ability to protect sensitive patient data and build trust (Rajawat et al., 2022).

Regulatory and Ethical Challenges

Along with the numerous other advantages, the incorporation of modern technologies like blockchain, IoT, and AI into healthcare presents various sets of ethical and legal dilemmas (Kumar et al., 2022). For safe, fair, and efficient applications of these technologies, such problems need to be addressed. Important challenges include:

Data Security and Privacy

As healthcare tech handles sensitive patient information, compliance with CCPA, GDPR, and HIPAA cannot be overstressed. Processing, sharing, and storing patient data in a secure manner while keeping the data transparent remains one of the greatest challenges (Rajawat et al., 2022).

Informed Consent

Patients must fully understand how their information would be used, particularly in connection with artificial intelligence or blockchain applications. Obtaining informed consent becomes more complicated because these advanced technologies can sometimes be more complex than the average patient might easily comprehend.

Algorithmic Bias and AI Fairness

Often introduced from the training datasets, AI algorithms bequeath biases toward unfair and discriminatory outcomes (Kumar et al., 2022). In the context of this topic, an example might be diagnostic tools trained on a non-diverse dataset, performing poorly for certain demographic groups thus calling into play the ethical issue of equitable care.

Responsibility and Liability

It remains a gray area as to who takes responsibility in case of errors or failures of AI or automated systems. For instance, if an AI diagnoses a condition incorrectly, it is ambiguous whether liability rests on the developer, the healthcare provider, or their system.

Interoperability Standards

The lack of standardized algorithms defining how various healthcare technologies can integrate creates regulatory and operational hurdles. Creating a seamless intercommunication process between IoT devices, EHRs, and blockchain and other technologies is integral to efficiency and compliance.

Ethical Data Use

Obtaining the informed consent of individuals after they have united, or later attempted to unite, with their data has, at various times, led to issues also being raised in the face of concerns about the implementation of detailed, practical data-sharing and data-mining initiatives (Kumar et al., 2022). The balance between advancing patient care based on data and allowing for independent patient autonomy and rights with regard to their data is one never-ending battle (Rajawat et al., 2022).

Cost and Accessibility

The high costs of implementing and keeping advanced technologies may deter one from adopting them in the setting to do so, thus raising cases of ethical concerns whereby issues revolving access to medicine get into place.

Global Regulatory Disparities

Different regulations of healthcare technologies from one country to another": that is why it is not easy for international partnerships and deployments as a matter of fact. Such criteria should be aligned for cross-border healthcare solutions.

To summarize, privacy, justice, accountability, and access must all be carefully scrutinized in view of the ethical and regulatory issues around healthcare technology

(Tagde et al., 2021). Through addressing these issues, technology might improve patient care while retaining confidence.

FUTURE PROSPECTS

Next-Generation AI and IoT in Blockchain

With blockchain, next-generation technologies such as AI and IoT are transforming a good number of industries, among them health care. Such a powerful combination opens up the possibility of more dependable systems that can solve all the pressing issues of security, efficiency, and scalability (Haddad, Habaebi, Islam, Hasbullah, & Zabidi, 2022). These technologies together bring creative answers in the four primary domains as listed below:

Enhanced Data Security and Privacy

This ensures that patient records, IoT sensor outputs, and AI-generated insights about the environment, which contain sensitive data, are completely safe (Kumar et al., 2022). The next-generation IoT devices have more advanced algorithms of AI that generate tremendous amounts of real-time data. Blockchain helps to store the data across the network of distributed nodes and thereby encrypts the data; hence, any kind of unauthorized tampering is very much impossible. In health care, for instance, data breaches could have dangerous consequences. In addition, AI-based anomaly detection in blockchain systems is able to identify potential threats or unauthorized access attempts thereby reinforcing the security framework.

Improved Interoperability and Integration

The smooth integration of IoT devices with AI and blockchain overcomes interoperability challenges in complex systems. Blockchain provides a universal framework for securely storing and sharing data from diverse IoT devices (Kumar et al., 2022). AI enhances this by interpreting the data, identifying patterns, and generating actionable insights. For instance, in healthcare, IoT devices in wearable formats collect vital signs while blockchain technology guarantees secure data transmission. AI will then study these trends to predict probable risks and adverse health effects. Thus, the collaborative approach creates consistent data and interoperability across devices and platforms.

Real-Time Decision Making

Real-time processing of IoT data is the hallmark of next-generation AI systems, which provide swift decision-making in critical scenarios. When combined with blockchain, these decisions can be recorded transparently and audited later for accountability. For instance, when there is an emergency in healthcare, IoT devices may transmit patient vitals to an AI system that would recommend immediate interventions. The blockchain ensures that these recommendations and actions are securely logged, fostering trust among the stakeholders while improving response times (AlGhamdi et al., 2022).

Scalability for Complex Systems

Blockchain, AI, and IoT together solve the scalability challenge. It optimizes the use of resources. The number of repeated operations in the blockchain network decreases through AI algorithms; on the other hand, wide applicability can be observed with IoT devices as the latter continuously feed into the system the suitable information (Kumar et al., 2022). For example, the automatic transactions on the blockchain platform among the IoT devices, which might be ordering medical supplies according to the actual levels of inventory, means less human involvement is needed to obtain scale without degrading the system performance (AlGhamdi et al., 2022).

In a nutshell, with the integration of next-generation AI and IoT with blockchain, the data security, interoperability, decision-making, and scalability of the systems will be revolutionized. In this context, these technologies together bring smarter, safer, and more efficient systems, especially in critical sectors like healthcare, thereby ensuring innovation drives better outcomes for all stakeholders in the future (Rajawat et al., 2022).

Potential Impact on Global Healthcare Systems

Figure 8. Impact in adoption in healthcare

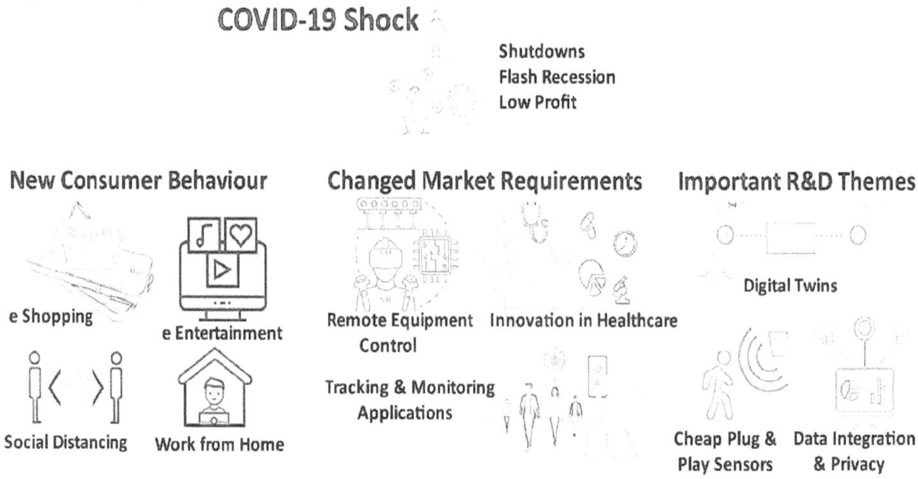

With emerging technologies such as AI, IoT, and blockchain, the global health system has a chance to change utterly (Jabarulla & Lee, 2021). These innovations will offer a response to the problems of access, efficiency, and equity and thus create an ideal foundation for a data-driven and patient-centered healthcare system. Some three areas where the application of these technologies is important are as follows:

Access to Quality Care

Technological advancements enable healthcare services to be delivered across a distance by removing the barriers of geography and making access to care equitable. IoT-enabled monitoring devices, telemedicine services, and AI-driven diagnosis allow healthcare providers to serve the underserved in the rural or remote setting. Blockchain ensures that the patient data is shared across borders safely and seamlessly, therefore continuing the care (AlGhamdi et al., 2022).

For example, a patient in a rural village can monitor their vital signs with the aid of IoT devices while AI analysis will help them make early diagnoses (Singh & Singh, 2020). Blockchain ensures the safe storage of the records and allows the specialists from urban centers or even abroad to access the records of the patient. Such an approach not only helps enhance the outcomes for the patient but also decongest overburdened health facilities in urban centers.

Lower Costs and More Efficiency in Operations

By removing waste and inefficiencies present in the conventional system, AI, IoT, and blockchain increase the effectiveness of the health system (Bibhu, Das, Rana, Sharma, & Salagrama, 2023). For instance, AI analytics makes a hospital's operations efficient because it predicts how many patients will arrive during a certain period or the number of staff members required. IoT can make inventory monitoring and equipment monitoring automatic processes. Blockchain secures financial transactions and eliminates fraud (Kumar et al., 2022).

For instance, blockchain-based smart contracts can automate insurance claim processing, thus avoiding lengthy delays and disputes in administration. AI systems analyze real-time IoT data to predict medical equipment maintenance needs, therefore minimizing downtime and ensuring a continuous care delivery system (Bibhu, Das, Rana, Sharma, & Salagrama, 2023). This efficiency brings with it considerable cost savings for health care providers and patients alike.

Fastest Research and Innovation

The rising number of chronic patients and the aging of the population render the avoidance of diseases an important requirement of healthcare. Prevention is not only defined by regular exercise, nutrition, and periodic preventive controls as a way to sustain a healthier environment but also as a method of keeping serious conditions from becoming worse. The future health sector must tackle an increasing number of chronic problems and the scarcity of treatments to satisfy patient demands. COVID-19 has recently highlighted the importance of quick, comprehensive, and accurate eHealthcare and intelligent healthcare involving different types of medical and physiological data to diagnose the virus (Mistry et al., 2021).

The use of emerging technology in protective policies and behavioral systems can help identify potential health conditions early and enable the scheduling of appropriate steps, such as concurrently monitoring treatments and preparing new assessments. The world's smart health market is forecast to reach USD 143.6 billion in 2019, which will expand by an average growth rate of 16.2% between 2020 and 2027 (AlGhamdi et al., 2022).

Smart healthcare refers to platforms for health systems that leverage devices such as wearable appliances, the Internet of Things (IoT) (Alabdulatif, Khalil, & Rahman, 2022), and the mobile Internet to easily enter health documents and link people, resources, and organizations. Intelligent medical treatment includes diverse actors, including physicians, staff, hospitals, and research bodies. It comprises a dynamic framework with many facets, including disease prevention and identification, assessment and evaluation, management of healthcare, patient decision-making, and medical research. Elements of intelligent healthcare involve automated networks like the IoT, mobile Internet, cloud networking, Big Data, 5G, and artificial intelligence (AI), along with evolving biotechnology.

The combination of AI, IoT, and blockchain promotes speedy and accurate clinical research with innovation in treatment and development of drugs (Bibhu, Das, Rana, Sharma, & Salagrama, 2023). Speeding up the analysis of large datasets, AI is able to recognize the most probable patterns or even the therapy targets. In the real-time, IoT devices collect real-world information from diverse populations for even more representative clinical studies. Blockchain guarantees the integrity of all the research data while making such collaboration among global stakeholders easier and secure.

For example, Internet of Things and Blockchain clinical trials distributed allow for the real-time gathering of information from contributors anywhere in the world; AI analyzes that for trends or outcomes and accelerates the time it takes to discover medicine. Through collaboration towards innovation and bringing the latest treatments to patients faster (Tagde et al., 2021).

In a nutshell, with AI, IoT, and blockchain, there is huge potential to revolutionize the world's healthcare systems in regard to opening up more access, boosting efficiency, and accelerating innovation. As they address all critical challenges to deliver more equitable, efficient, and patient-centered care toward the future of health globally, they do that.

CONCLUSION

These three technologies are expected to change the face of patient care and make healthcare operations more efficient, along with being secure in terms of data. AI is highly crucial in predictive analytics, such as early detection of health issues by analyzing patient data and forecasting potential health risks (Singh & Singh, 2020). It also enhances data security through identifying anomalies and preventing cyber threats within blockchain-based systems. Moreover, AI-based smart contracts will also implement the health processes without human malpractices and hence improve efficiency in workflow generally (Wazid et al., 2020).

Data from devices such as wearable and remote monitoring tools from IoT are real-time and can keep track of patients' health over time (Shinde et al., 2024). This, if combined with blockchain, is sure to adopt the properties of blockchain technology, that is, immutability, security, and decentralization, towards ensuring the integrity and transparency of health data. However, the major challenge is interoperability between the IoT devices and systems (AlGhamdi et al., 2022). Therefore, overcoming these issues would ensure that communication and data exchange are seamless among various platforms and healthcare institutions.

AI and IoT may, together, form a synergy to provide complete coverage while at the same time making monitoring, personal care, and treatment of patients improved. Large volumes of data from IoT would be processed by AI and provide actionable insights on improving the decision-making power of healthcare professionals (Jabarulla & Lee, 2021). The automation of workflows will bring about a reduction in administrative burden on healthcare providers and improved efficiency within the system. Patients are being assisted through accurate diagnoses, personalized treatment plans, and improved health outcomes.

Many of these applications are currently being implemented within healthcare systems. Remote monitoring of the patient is aiding patients diagnosed with chronic illness to continually receive care through fewer clinic visits. Clinical trials data sharing between different researchers enables blockchain to promote security and transparency (Rajawat et al., 2022). In terms of supply chain management within drugs, blockchain ensures medicines are not counterfeit and tracked throughout supply chains so they can offer safe and efficient treatments.

While such huge potential exists, the issues that surround it include scalability, data privacy, and regulatory issues. The scaling efficiency of Blockchain is still posing challenges to its adoption widely. Concerns over data privacy and ethical use about the patient also need to be addressed with care. With respect to the technological revolution happening in the world of patient safety and data protection, the regulatory framework should progress at the same rate as well.

This presents a transformational opportunity when AI, IoT, and blockchain come together in the healthcare system. Overcoming the challenge of scalability, privacy, and regulation are important aspects that will lead to their full utilization in the sector. These technologies, implemented responsibly, are capable of reshaping health systems in the world so that they are more efficient, secure, and available to all (Tagde et al., 2021).

Vision for Blockchain-based Healthcare

Blockchain-based healthcare systems hold great promise for the transformation of healthcare globally (AlGhamdi et al., 2022). The concept will improve security, access, efficiency, and patient-centered care in these systems. Some of the key aspects are shown below:

Improved Data Security and Privacy

Blockchain technology provides a decentralized and immutable framework safeguarding healthcare data against altering, fraud, and improper access (Rajawat et al., 2022). The blockchain facilitates the transparency of patient medical records, histories, or treatment details in a non-accessible manner only through authorized personnel (Alabdulatif, Khalil, & Rahman, 2022). It means that data integrity is maintained, and patient confidentiality ensured while adhering to a strict regulatory compliance of standards such as GDPR and HIPAA.

Inherent Data Interoperability

A blockchain-based healthcare system would allow the seamless interoperability of all the different platforms, systems, and devices in use in healthcare (Alabdulatif, Khalil, & Rahman, 2022). With distributed ledger in blockchain, real-time sharing of patient information is possible without any barriers across different health care providers and systems, thereby breaking silos (Rajawat et al., 2022). More coordination would be there among different health care providers, as well as a better quality of care will be established, especially during emergencies or when patients move between geographically divided regions.

Efficiency in Health Operations

Blockchain will remove the administrative burdens and long delays that occur in a healthcare process. The intelligent contracts and automated workflows execute on blockchain, making the management of patient records, handling of insurance claims, as well as billing operations smoother. Automated systems eliminate processes that are done manually leading to errors and delay so that operational efficiency and cut down healthcare costs for the advantage of both providers and the patients (Mistry et al., 2021).

Power to Patients on Deciding Their Health Data Control

One of the basic visions for blockchain in the health sector is giving absolute control to patients on controlling their health data. A block network can allow medical records of a patient to be accessed and managed and to share with him according to his preference (Alabdulatif, Khalil, & Rahman, 2022). This can lead towards higher patient engagement and further customized care, as such patients can opt to provide access to their data to varying healthcare providers or researchers who could better diagnose and subsequently treat them.

Increased Transparency in Drug Supply Chains

Through a blockchain mechanism, the drugs will achieve better transparency and traceability along the supply chain for authenticity, storage, and transportation (Alabdulatif, Khalil, & Rahman, 2022). It helps avert counterfeit drugs, fraud, and errors by putting a record of every transaction along the supply chain into operation, creating better medicine for patients and a much more responsible pharmaceutical industry.

Decentralised and Inclusive Clinical Trials

The future vision of blockchain will be decentralized clinical trials, whereby participants' data will be shared and monitored in real-time with total security (Bibhu, Das, Rana, Sharma, & Salagrama, 2023). Blockchain makes data integrity possible because its very nature is transparent. Since it's decentralized, anyone around the world can participate, so more people are included to get a diverse set. That accelerates medical research and brings new treatments faster into the market.

Thus, blockchain for healthcare would envision an atmosphere of security, efficiency, and patient empowerment. So long as the present inefficiencies and problems are present in the health industry, this face of healthcare will be changed worldwide with respect to security, transparency, and a more patient-oriented service.

REFERENCES

Alabdulatif, A., Khalil, I., & Saidur Rahman, M. (2022). Security of blockchain and AI-empowered smart healthcare: Application-based analysis. *Applied Sciences (Basel, Switzerland)*, *12*(21), 11039.

AlGhamdi, R., Alassafi, M. O., Alshdadi, A. A., Dessouky, M. M., Ramdan, R. A., & Aboshosha, B. W. (2022). Developing trusted IoT healthcare information-based AI and blockchain. *Processes (Basel, Switzerland)*, *11*(1), 34.

Alshehri, F., & Muhammad, G. (2020). A comprehensive survey of the Internet of Things (IoT) and AI-based smart healthcare. *IEEE Access : Practical Innovations, Open Solutions*, *9*, 3660–3678.

Bibhu, V., Das, L., Rana, A., Sharma, S., & Salagrama, S. (2023). AI Model for Blockchain Based Industrial Application in Healthcare IoT. In *AI Models for Blockchain-Based Intelligent Networks in IoT Systems: Concepts, Methodologies, Tools, and Applications* (pp. 163–184). Springer International Publishing.

Elhoseny, M., Haseeb, K., Shah, A. A., Ahmad, I., Jan, Z., & Alghamdi, M. I. (2021). IoT solution for AI-enabled PRIVACY-PRESErving with big data transferring: An application for healthcare using blockchain. *Energies*, *14*(17), 5364.

Gul, M. J. J., Paul, A., Rho, S., & Kim, M. (2020, December). Blockchain based healthcare system with Artificial Intelligence. In *2020 International Conference on Computational Science and Computational Intelligence (CSCI)* (pp. 740-741). IEEE.

Haddad, A., Habaebi, M. H., Islam, M. R., Hasbullah, N. F., & Zabidi, S. A. (2022). Systematic review on ai-blockchain based e-healthcare records management systems. *IEEE Access : Practical Innovations, Open Solutions*, *10*, 94583–94615.

Jabarulla, M. Y., & Lee, H. N. (2021, August). A blockchain and artificial intelligence-based, patient-centric healthcare system for combating the COVID-19 pandemic: Opportunities and applications. [). Mdpi.]. *Health Care*, *9*(8), 1019. PMID: 34442156

Kumar, P., Kumar, R., Garg, S., Kaur, K., Zhang, Y., & Guizani, M. (2022, December). A secure data dissemination scheme for IoT-based e-health systems using AI and blockchain. In *GLOBECOM 2022-2022 IEEE Global Communications Conference* (pp. 1397-1403). IEEE.

Mistry, C., Thakker, U., Gupta, R., Obaidat, M. S., Tanwar, S., Kumar, N., & Rodrigues, J. J. (2021, June). MedBlock: An AI-enabled and blockchain-driven medical healthcare system for COVID-19. In *ICC 2021-IEEE International Conference on Communications* (pp. 1-6). IEEE.

. Rajawat, A. S., Bedi, P., Goyal, S. B., Shaw, R. N., Ghosh, A., & Aggarwal, S. (2022). Ai and blockchain for healthcare data security in smart cities. *AI and IoT for Smart City Applications*, 185-198.

. Samad, A. (2022). Internet of things integrated with blockchain and artificial intelligence in healthcare system. *Research Journal of Computer Systems and Engineering, 3*(1), 01-06.

Shinde, R., Patil, S., Kotecha, K., Potdar, V., Selvachandran, G., & Abraham, A. (2024). Securing AI-based healthcare systems using blockchain technology: A state-of-the-art systematic literature review and future research directions. *Transactions on Emerging Telecommunications Technologies*, *35*(1), e4884.

Singh, P., & Singh, N. (2020). Blockchain with IoT and AI: A review of agriculture and healthcare. [IJAEC]. *International Journal of Applied Evolutionary Computation, 11*(4), 13–27.

Tagde, P., Tagde, S., Bhattacharya, T., Tagde, P., Chopra, H., Akter, R., & Rahman, M. H. (2021). Blockchain and artificial intelligence technology in e-Health. *Environmental Science and Pollution Research International*, *28*, 52810–52831. PMID: 34476701

Wazid, M., Bera, B., Mitra, A., Das, A. K., & Ali, R. (2020, September). Private blockchain-envisioned security framework for AI-enabled IoT-based drone-aided healthcare services. In *Proceedings of the 2nd ACM MobiCom workshop on drone assisted wireless communications for 5G and beyond* (pp. 37-42).

Chapter 7
Virtual Healthcare in the Metaverse Leveraging XAI and Blockchain for Secure and Personalized Care

Usharani Bhimavarapu
https://orcid.org/0000-0002-0246-1420
Department of Computer Science and Engineering, Koneru Lakshmaiah Education Foundation, Vaddeswaram, India

ABSTRACT

Healthcare is in a paradigm shift with technology adoption like Artificial Intelligence (AI), Explainable AI (XAI), and Blockchain (BC) in the metaverse. The article presented the use, limitation, and effect of adoption of these technologies to bring about a transformation in healthcare delivery. Blockchain and XAI-based health metaverse is an emerging paradigm to improve patient treatment, secure data, and optimize. XAI improves the interpretability and explainability of AI-based health decisions, while blockchain allows for distributed control of patient data securely. Healthcare in the Metaverse can be provided within virtual space, thus allowing remote visits, treatment plans customized to individual patients, and secure sharing of medical data. All these technologies together create new possibilities of health delivery innovation regarding accessibility, efficiency, and trust. There are numerous issues still to be addressed, though, such as ethics, regulation, and how doctors will take advantage of new technology. This report ends with some analysis of how the technologies as a whole will shape the future of healthcare.

DOI: 10.4018/979-8-3373-1225-5.ch007

INTRODUCTION

The convergence of the metaverse and blockchain technology is making it possible for one to build the infrastructure of the virtual paradigm shift in healthcare. The security, decentralization, and transparency of the blockchain are providing a paradigm choice of storing and exchanging the healthcare process and data in the virtual world. The shared virtual world, the metaverse, is giving the healthcare yet another level of interactivity and immersion. With AI and ML implemented on this platform, we can utilize blockchain and metaverse to maximum extent to provide effective, secure, and customized health care services. AI networks can handle huge amounts of data being produced in virtual health care environments, and blockchain provides secure and immutable management of patient data. Such converging technologies will simplify the system, make it more accessible and efficient, a care receipt and delivery revolution.

Blockchain technology's secure, open, and tamper-evident data exchange capability is most appropriate for virtual use in healthcare. Decentralized storage of the Metaverse health information is feasible so that there is never any point of full control over the patient's confidentiality information. Not only is it safe, but patients' trust also increases since patients are given transparency and control over their own health information. Other than that, self-executing smart contracts with rules encoded within themselves or smart contracts are applied to enable automatic administrative tasks like billing, consent, and claim management. Blockchain facilitates the creation of interoperability between health care systems to enable roaming without compromising data integrity and data confidentiality. Blockchain decentralizes control and leads to patient-centered, secure, and cost-efficient virtual health care.

Artificial intelligence and machine learning underlie pervasively present health care from predictive modeling to personalized medicine. Health AI can operate on vast sets of data, recognize patterns, and direct predictions entered into advanced decision-making. Theoretical machine learning technology can be trained to operate with large health data like medical images, patient data, and genomic data in order to facilitate diagnosis, drug discovery, and tailored treatment plans. Virtual health and AI will make the doctors more efficient and precise in their treatment, and the patients will be treated on their individual records. Besides this, AI will also enhance the metaverse health system because it will prevent redundant work, errors, and enhance the treatment of patients.

And while blockchain and AI together are being applied in virtual worlds of health, interoperability is so huge that apart from delivering quality of security, it delivers quality of intelligence. Blockchain authenticates data in transit in the metaverse and renders it tamper-proof, and AI processing can query the data and garner useful information out of it. For instance, healthcare patterns can be scanned by artificial intelligence and patient outcomes forecasted based on blockchain data. Anomaly scans or tampering scans can also be performed through machine learning, and security can be enhanced. With blockchain and AI, the healthcare information is not only made secure but also utilized to the fullest so that health care professionals can provide wiser, smarter, and patient-centered care to the users of metaverse.

Metaverse medicine can be procedure-independent and patient-specific and provide patient-specific experience and treatment to the patient. Virtual reality would enable patients to interact with health care providers through fully immersive modes, e.g., as 3D avatars or virtual consultation. AI can be used to enable such interaction as personalized health advice in the context of real-time analysis of data. For instance, there have been chatbots based on AI that have conducted initial consultations, diagnosis of symptoms, and follow-up advice. Every patient message is encrypted in blockchain, and patient data are recorded and stored confidentially, and health record owners are patients themselves. Not only is it cheap, but also it provides ownership and privacy to the owners of health information, and that's a very important element of the metaverse.

The most fascinating virtual metaverse medical application of AI is AI diagnosis. Machine learning is capable of learning medical data in real time and providing virtual medical professionals accurate diagnostic tools that currently do not exist in the world. The AI will also be capable of interpreting medical images like X-rays or MRIs and scanning tumors, breaks, or other abnormalities with precision. The devices in the metaverse are used for online consulting in that doctors can visit patients virtually and diagnose them within minutes. The ability of AI to gather and analyze information from unseen sources, e.g., wearables or health apps, ensures the quality and extent of diagnosis is improved. It is not just improved on the front of delivery of care but also is the best in terms of patient outcomes because AI will be in a position to identify health hazards prior to their becoming a threat to life. Security and confidentiality of patient information come top in virtual medicine, and that is why blockchain is introduced. Blockchain stores all the patient records in the metaverse encrypted and dispersed so that no single employee member of the small team can lay their hands on or change them. Blockchain smart contracts can also determine who can access a patient's file and when, and patients own their healthcare information. Virtual communication in the metaverse with medical data can remain confidential, blockchain integrity and transparency maintain confidentiality of the patient. Blockchain can be used to enhance AI through discrepancy checking and patterns of forgery or authentication of medical history. They present a secure and solid foundation for one another regarding the management of medical records, and virtual treatment can be more normalized and secured.

The biggest advantage of the use of blockchain and AI in virtual health care is that it opens up greater access to health care. The metaverse enables health care workers to offer health care services to individuals who live in remote or medically underprivileged regions and extend them equal quality care as their city-dwelling peers. Telemedicine solutions provided through artificial intelligence, including virtual consultations and diagnostic devices, enable the patient to receive healthcare from his or her remote site without going to a clinic. Blockchain provides the ability to issue guarantees that information shared through the like sessions will be secure and confidential. The metaverse also offers the ability to design virtual health environments where patients are navigated by learning material, are provided with health information, and are given peer support in a virtual environment. Such technologies enhance care access to a world population, diminish barriers to care, and enhance world health equity.

AI predictive capabilities can be an asset in preventing disease and early diagnosis in virtual health environments. AI would be able to traverse extremely large volumes of data and detect patterns with a high likelihood of certain diseases or illnesses. With AI being used in the metaverse, it would be able to track patients' health records in real time and also flag any abnormalities requiring treatment or intervention. For instance, artificial intelligence can utilize heart rate variability or blood glucose levels to forecast the development of heart disease or diabetes even before such has exhibited even a glimmer of disease. Blockchain keeps such information safely and offers it to the stakeholders and AI develops actionable insights. This marriage of AI vision and the safety of blockchain can make it possible for health care professionals to work towards disease avoidance and improved patient health outcomes in the virtual delivery model of health care.

Future use of AI and blockchain is very promising but plagued with many issues that must be addressed. Maybe one of the biggest challenges will be how they are implemented into current health care systems. To witness mass adoption, health care providers will require blockchain and AI technical infrastructure, standards, and education investment. Regulatory compliance and ethics will also be required in this context, i.e., patient consent and data protection. As the metaverse expands, these technologies will have to become optimized and secured as they expand. But their potential advantages—improved patient care, improved efficiency, and improved treatments—spark interest to augment AI and blockchain in virtual medicine. Each of them potentially can complement the other to reshape the provision of health care in the metaverse one day into one which becomes an experience for everyone as a safer, improved, and more convenient one.

Although Joshua's refusal of computationally-instilled stress in Neal Stephenson's Snow Crash provides some insight into psychological effects of virtual reality, it does not necessarily constitute an argument regarding real-world applications and concerns with bringing such ideas to reality for health care or the metaverse (Joshua, 2017). The work is theoretical and speculative and therefore not easily linked back to contemporary health care innovation within the metaverse. It is neither case-based nor empirical in its evidence to advocate for either of the health technologies.

Thomason's article addresses the overlap of metaverse technologies and non-communicable disease but more traditionally theory-led to how rather than when it happens (Thomason, 2022). The article does not have an empirical illustration and does not include statistics and would hence not be of particular utility to stakeholders that are interested in scaling out interventions grounded in metaverse for healthcare. The article does not ever truly bring to the forefront the technical and infrastructural issues that would bedevil the interaction between token economies and virtual space and health as the target of the health intervention.

Yang and authors offer insightful expert opinion on metaverse for health care but the paper does not afford full serious consideration to actual technical, ethical, and regulatory concerns of bringing the metaverse to health care (Yang et al., 2022). In creating expert opinion, it does not fully consider scalability or practicability of such platforms for actual health care settings.

The research issues of the metaverse in education go as far as artificial intelligence but to school environments instead of healthcare environments (Hwang & Chien, 2022). There is less direct transfer to healthcare environments, and the implication may not be in the area of providing health care or taking care of patients in the metaverse.

Gursoy and colleagues discuss the metaverse in the field of hospitality and tourism in providing a general overview of trends not medical (Gursoy et al., 2022). Restricting the paper to the non-medical areas restricts the usefulness of the paper to the health care industry, and it says nothing about how precisely the metaverse technologies will benefit the patients, hospitals, or healthcare practitioners.

Virtual training of agriculture flexible new technology through learning metaverse does not sufficiently explain how the same technologies could be redirected or translated to the healthcare sector (Khunsulivong et al., 2022). While as much fun as it does provide some keen observation on usage of learning, it does not take into consideration some healthcare demands like patient confidentiality, data security, or procedural controls in exercising in virtual health worlds.

Shin's metaverse game affordance actualization theory is game contextually rooted and less pragmatically applicable for use in healthcare settings (Shin, 2022). Constraints on gaming affordance research make it less pragmatically applicable to apply in metaverse healthcare environments where clinical fidelity, security concerns, and empowering needs for patients are vital.

Jungherr and Schlarb's examination of game engine firms and applying the metaverse in extended reality is not considering the health implications of the emergence of the metaverse (Jungherr & Schlarb, 2022). While the research is not on the tech, ethics, and policy dimensions of healthcare, even though it is on the broad field of the metaverse.

Kraus et al. simply call Facebook the first to construct the metaverse without addressing the question of whether health care organizations would be offered new challenges when implementing such technology (Kraus et al., 2022). Their business model innovation orientation does not make the result general to the health care industry, whose challenges are patient care, data privacy, and regulation.

Fortnite being a videogame developed by Epic Games is itself an entrepreneurial gaming world and never passes the correct information to the metaverse of medicine which must be exclusively medically accurate and patient-centered (Games, 2017). It has no health background and therefore it is not possible to develop strong lessons for health organizations ready to utilize the metaverse in teleconsulting, surgery, or medical training.

Wiederhold explains that medical care may be enhanced using metaverse games but has no empirical evidence or organized case histories to show that virtual worlds are going to transform the provision of medical care (Wiederhold, 2022). The presentation is highly speculative and disregards the sheer magnitude of technical, ethical, and practical challenges to applying the metaverse for medical care.

Tan et al. and others talk about the future and future limitations on the use of metaverse in ophthalmology but talk about only one line of medicine in one article (Tan et al., 2022). Conclusions made in articles cannot be translated directly to practice in medicine on a daily basis and limitations imposed within their construction cannot be transferred to other uses of the metaverse to medicine. Apart from that, research is not strictly demonstrating the adoption of blockchain or XAI technology in virtual healthcare systems. Abbott and Shaw's input as virtual nursing avatars is more directed towards how the ideas and nurse roles need to be adopted in virtual settings (Abbott & Shaw, 2016).

There are few enough empirical research and actual case studies where results would prove difficult to apply in practice in the healthcare sector. The research does not give us technological or infrastructural implications of virtual nursing avatar scale-up such as protection of data, privacy, or interaction with already existing health infrastructure. Your and Gui's article on AI symptom checkers developed with chatbots has some qualitative findings on the user experience but does not talk about other boundaries of medicine in AI, i.e., ethics, vulnerability to bias, or dependability of AI platforms in diagnosis (You & Gui, 2020). Secondly, integration was not examined in the research in less technologically integrated care environments or rural settings. Garavand and Aslani's systematic review of healthcare literature on synthesizing the metaverse is all-encompassing but not an exhaustively inquiring discussion of how health issues of the metaverse technology should be addressed (Garavand & Aslani, 2022).

No reference to challenges like access to vulnerable populations, application cost, or technology for secure and safe virtual spaces for healthcare can be found in the review. No straightforward and apparent direction of the health care professionals toward adoption of such technologies is present in the review. Wu and Ho's critique of metaverse use in emergency care only talks about potential uses but hardly speaks of implementation facts with metaverse technology in emergency health care environments (Wu & Ho, 2023).

The article does not speak to subtleties of emergency or intricacies of regulation on how to integrate metaverse technology into emergency medicine situations where rapid decision and rapid follow-through action are most relevant. Jeong and co-authors describe an area of commerce in the metaverse but use it as a discourse on commerce instead of health care (Jeong et al., 2022). It is not possible to directly extrapolate the findings to health care and, for health-related matters such as confidentiality of patients, sound medical information requirements, or ethical issues of AI-based health decision-making in the metaverse, no such domains have been investigated in the study. Cai, Jiao, and Song take us to the metaverse of education and how to implement it, issue and possibility, but how the concept could be implemented in healthcare (Cai et al., 2022). None of the things mentioned in the article regarding special needs consideration in healthcare, for instance, integration of medical information systems, patient safety, and regulatory matters. The article does not inform us about how to train the physicians and how improved care can be provided to the patient in virtual healthcare environments. Allam et al.'s article (2022) addresses the potential of the metaverse being a virtual city of a smart city but not medicine. Though the work will be helpful to city planners, they are not designed for the very specific, more stringent needs of health centers, i.e., patient care, protecting data, and incorporating virtual space into traditional medical planning. Um et al. have in mind planning a metaverse tourist destination with no healthcare applications (Um et al., 2022). It does not say anything about clean issues of using metaverse technology to the medical field, i.e., medical ethics, patient empowerment, or changing delivery of healthcare to virtual space. It does not say anything about whether health professionals are to be trained specially to practice in virtual space or not.

Skalidis et al. 2023 give the explanation of metaverse use in cardiology, which is a hard topic. The publication fails to note the process of use of metaverse-guided therapy in cardiology as technology (Skalidis et al., 2023). The publication fails to make a proper analysis of regulative, data protection, or ethical questions which must be solved at realization of new technology in medical activity.

AI blockchains in cardiovascular medicine article presents novel hypotheses but not an entire review of the real activity of the implementation of AI and blockchain technology to existing cardiovascular care networks (Krittanawong et al., 2022). It fails to emphasize the risk taken, i.e., the cybersecurity risk, privacy intrusion risk, or algorithmic bias risk in clinical decision-making.

Koo's article on virtual training for lung cancer surgery in the metaverse contains some recent facts about virtual training systems but cannot tell us anything about matters behind the application of such systems in actual healthcare practice (Koo, 2021). Matters such as how much money one spends on technology, requirements of specialty equipment, and some probable problems with healthcare professionals using virtual reality systems are not spoken of sensibly.

Zeng et al. provide mention of the application of the metaverse in cancer treatment but is not able to provide a summary of elaborating on logistics, technical, and budgetary matters to the application of the metaverse in traditional cancer treatment (Zeng et al., 2022).

It does not responsibly inform of the development of virtual worlds to assist geographically distant patients and clinicians from the multiregional areas and does not report the resultant concomitant health disparities occasioned by unequal access to such technology.

Porras et al.'s (2018) virtual reality review in rehabilitation is insightful to know of possibilities of applying virtual reality to walking and balance rehabilitation but not of scaling virtual reality technology for application among populations. The review is mum on issues surrounding the inclusion of virtual reality systems in existing healthcare systems or regulation challenges concerning the deployment of such technology into patient care.

METAVERSE ARCHITECTURE AND CONSTRUCTION BLOCK TECHNOLOGIES

Metaverse is a coherent virtual world where physical and virtual coexist. It is not a platform but an architecture that is a mix of technologies providing shared experience in a virtual universe. The metaverse architecture can be described as comprising numerous layers in such a manner that each layer does exist for a particular reason to construct and maintain the virtual world. The elements of the metaverse are constructed based on technologies such as virtual reality (VR), augmented reality (AR), blockchain, artificial intelligence (AI), and the Internet of Things (IoT). Their intersection is the basis of immersive experience, socially interactive interaction, and secure transactions in the metaverse. Metaverse architecture provides a new economic model for economics, society, and learning to interaction with unlimited possibility for interaction, innovation, and creativity.

The most fundamental of the two components of the metaverse are augmented reality and virtual reality, both a new virtual sense of space. VR surrounds human beings with fully virtual worlds, usually through a headset with a 360-degree vision field, and AR places digital information on top of the real world and provides the user with a sense of reality. AR and VR provide an incredible range of alternate experiences in the metaverse, such as entertainment and games, education, and well-being. AR and VR are employed in metaverse development for immersive avatars, interactive worlds, and world interaction. VR and AR provide depth to the user experience with sensory inputs simulating or enhancing real experience and empower users with the capability to interact, collaborate, or learn through an immersive virtual world.

Blockchain builds the virtual building blocks of the metaverse infrastructure enabling decentralization, security, and transparency. Blockchain offers the metaverse a decentralized ledger system for the storage of assets, transactions, and identities. Blockchain gives data the capability of making, e.g., virtual ownership, immutable and stationary, and user-held virtual assets. Blockchain may be applied in virtual property, digital art, and cryptocurrency with the capability to track and authenticate ownership and origin. Smart contracts, or smart self-executing blockchain contracts, can be used to enable programmed transactions like digital commerce, content creation, and trade throughout the metaverse. Blockchain's decentralized character is well-suited to the open, interoperable model of the metaverse in an attempt to make trust and secure digital economies easier.

Machine learning (ML) and deep learning (DL) are applied in an attempt to build responsive and dynamic experiences throughout the metaverse. AI is employed to build intelligent user experience, personalized content, and intelligent avatars or personal assistants in a bid to give immediate responses to questions. For example, artificially intelligent avatars within virtual reality can interact with the users of the game as a regular human person and improve over time. Machine learning algorithms can be trained to learn to recognize stupendous amounts of user experience data sets so that they can fine-tune the systems and develop more engaging and interactive virtual worlds. Further, AI facilitates simple moderation automation, security, and content in the metaverse while making it possible for more advanced and scalable virtual worlds. Both AI and ML are making the metaverse intelligent and more intelligent, and the metaverse is a more intuitive, a smarter, a more personalized, and a more responsive experience for the user.

Internet of Things (IoT) is one of the technologies which allows things physical to enter the internet in an attempt to make it easier to interface between the virtual and the physical. IoT in the metaverse facilitates the duplication of physical systems, sensors, and intelligent devices into virtual space. For instance, IoT devices like wearables or home automation devices can be duplicated in the metaverse, and the user can control them or see them real-time in virtual space. IoT smart cities and smart infrastructure can similarly be duplicated in the metaverse with a virtual replica of real space. With the inclusion of IoT in the metaverse, physical and virtual items are accessed directly by the user in physical space in real-time, thus making it more immersive and interactive in virtual space. Real-time feedback loops between virtual space and physical space made available by IoT is the most significant functionality that makes metaverse experience more integrated and real.

High-definition 3D rendering and visualization are critical to building visually rich and immersive metaverse worlds. They facilitate photorealistic virtual worlds, high-fidelity avatars, and interactive objects. Ray tracing and real-time rendering features enable greater rendering horsepower for realistic light, shadow, and texture to create the immersed-in-virtual-worlds experience. 3D visualization software also allows users to explore and engage with virtual objects and virtual worlds in an intuitive, natural manner. Graphics rendering of the metaverse brings the virtual cities, landscapes, and buildings to life so that humans can experience and inhabit fully immersive virtual space. Ongoing technological development in high-end graphics engines like Unreal Engine and Unity continues to enhance reality and quality of metaverse experiences.

Cloud and edge computing are the foundational technologies to make scalability and performance possible in the metaverse. Cloud computing offers storage, calculation, and sharing of immense data at different parts of the global's fragmented points of computation to facilitate computation for developing enormous virtual worlds. Cloud computing in the metaverse facilitates real-time synchronization of data and interaction between various users in order to facilitate adaptive and dynamic virtual worlds. Edge computing does bring the user closer to computer infrastructure in terms of processing information and reducing latency and improving real-time interaction. This is essentially needed by the metaverse as the user experience must ideally be seamless and low-latency performance. Cloud and edge computing both allow for a seamless and interactive experience of the metaverse to the world user.

Digital identification evidence and identity management are the most significant elements of the metaverse to support interaction as well as transactions. Provable identities are required by the inhabitants of the virtual world so that they can engage with the other inhabitants, use services, and secure their information. Blockchain is applied here that belongs to the citizens and from which the citizens can secure their information. Decentralized identifiers (DIDs) and self-sovereign identities (SSIs) enable users to have control over their identity without any central authority's need. Further, biometric authentication along with artificial intelligence (AI) like facial recognition or voice recognition could make the metaverse more convenient and secure. All these technologies will securely authenticate the virtual identity of users and they can communicate confidentially and anonymously in the metaverse safely.

To denote metaverse users as a collective, special hardware like VR headsets, AR glasses, motion controllers, and haptic feedback devices are fast becoming the necessity of the times at a very fast rate. Virtual reality headsets like Oculus Rift and HTC Vive provide total immersion by turning off the real world and immersing participants in a virtual 3D environment. AR glasses like Microsoft HoloLens provide an immersive mixed reality experience by bringing virtual objects into the real world. Motion controllers enable the user to touch and interact with virtual objects and rooms through hand tracking. Haptic feedback devices provide resistance or vibration feedforward in pressure or touch to simulate real touch in the virtual world. These hardware infrastructures for computers are combined with software technologies such as VR and AR to provide us with an interruption-free and immersive experience of the metaverse.

The metaverse is still in its infancy, and the future of the metaverse will be defined by next-generation technological advancements in major technologies. VR, AR, AI, blockchain, and IoT will continue to evolve and embed the metaverse in an even more interconnected, interactive, and intelligent world. Technologies like 5G, quantum, and space computing will continue to empower the metaverse to become even faster, faster, and more engrossing virtual worlds. Open protocols and standards will develop to enable interconnectivity of numerous independent virtual worlds and enable seamless switching among them. New industries and new applications will develop from metaverse creation that will transform education, medicine, entertainment, and business processes. The metaverse will become the virtual place of living, social place, and innovation center and achieve unlimited potential for customers and businesses.

STRUCTURE OF HEALTHCARE METAVERSE ENRICHED BY EXPLAINABLE ARTIFICIAL INTELLIGENCE (XAI) AND BLOCKCHAIN (BC)

Metaverse is a virtual universe, generated by computer where patient information, medical treatment, and caregivers are remodeled into interactive virtual universes. Metaverse is designed on such new emerging technologies as explainable artificial intelligence (XAI) and blockchain to construct an open, secure, and participative world. XAI is artificial intelligence that provides machine learning models in healthcare as accurate, human understandable, and explainable and therefore provides trust and accountability. Blockchain decentralizes ownership of the data to the point of patients' data and transactions being encrypted by applying an immutable ledger. Blockchain and associated technologies are the foundation to a health metaverse with safe, transparent, and personalized patient outcomes and treatment and delivery of health care.

A conceptual model of a health metaverse based on XAI and blockchain is composed of some fundamental layers: virtual worlds, UI, data management layer, AI and XAI systems, and blockchain infrastructure. The UI is composed of real-time interactive virtual interfaces like VR headsets and AR devices where doctors and patients interact in real-time. The virtual environment layer provides medical simulation, telemedicine consultation, and health education courses. Blockchain data management layer provides secure storage of patient history, medical records, and other healthcare data. XAI and AI-based systems are combined and utilized to process and analyze the information and give suggestions, insights, and predictions. Eventually, digital health assets such as medical history and freely stored secure and transparent patient data are owned by the blockchain platform. Blockchain is a metaverse healthcare platform with freely stored secure and transparent patient data. Blockchain uses distributed ledgers in order to facilitate secure storage of such medical history in a way that neither the information nor even its modification can be accessed. Blockchain places all of the histories of the patients on a blockchain network where it gets encrypted using cryptography keys and smart contracts. Blockchain also facilitates sharing of information by the various caregivers and organiaisn providers but with control and confidentiality of consent. Blockchain offers more stringent management of patient access to information by the patient, revoking and granting as patient whim made simple. Transparency is most important to create trust in the healthcare metaverse if security and integrity of health data are needed.

Explainable Artificial Intelligence (XAI) is the unsung backroom hero in this respect since it makes sure that artificial intelligence models applied in healthcare metaverse are not just accurate, but also transparent and explainable. In clinical practice, AI comes in treatment recommendations, diagnosis, and predictive algorithms. XAI enables doctors and patients to know why a certain decision is being made by an AI system so that they are able to trust the technology. In other words, an AI system can forecast the probability of a patient to develop a certain disease, and XAI methods will dissemble the explanation of the forecast into, say, part of the patient's medical record or lifestyle. By generating clear explainable answers, XAI bridges the knowledge gap between clinical decision-making and black box AI systems such that medical clinicians are able to validate AI suggestions and reason about them.

Artificial intelligence-driven decision-support systems are metaverse of health care backbone and assist health care personnel with real-time processing of patient information. Artificial intelligence-driven decision-support systems are patient data analysis support and metaverse of health care backbone. They are able to read lab reports, imaging reports, and medical history and provide evidence-based recommendations. XAI: XAI provides explanations in simple language such that the clinicians know why the AI suggested that. For instance, a machine may suggest a certain treatment for a patient, and XAI details why it's the optimal treatment for a patient based on his/her condition, his/her history, etc. It not only improves clinical decision-making in terms of accuracy but also prepares the clinicians for such information in a way that they are prepared to make decisions without diminishing patient confidence.

Metaverse medical facilitates remote treatment of patients such as telemedicine consultation, remote monitoring, and focused health interventions. Physicians and patients can also interact with each other in avatar and virtual space and can perform diagnostic testing or consultation using virtual equipment. XAI can be utilized to monitor patient data in real-time as a patient is treated, offering physicians real-time feedback regarding the health information of a patient. Blockchain safeguards patients' data during telemedicine therapy by maintaining it on distributed encrypted ledgers. Blockchain smart contracts also facilitate simple processing of administrative tasks such as billing and scheduling to make telemedicine more convenient. XAI deployment and blockchain-virtual metaverse patient care is an improved, scalable, and secure way of carrying out geographically-based care.

Its most exciting application in medicine is that it can provide tailored treatment. AI is able to sift through mountains of patient information in attempting to create tailored treatment advice based on your disease history, genetic makeup, and life style. XAI blocks explanation of why the personal treatment suggestion has been generated by making what the why is understandable and interpretable. Medical professionals can thus verify and customize the recommendations. Personalization is also enabled by blockchain technology since patients will be the owners and they will be keeping their medical records safely and they will be getting more personalized and apt treatment according to their present medical history. The effectiveness in implementing proper treatments in blockchain and AI driven metaverse medicine can change health care delivery in a significant way, enhancing outcome and satisfaction.

Traditional healthcare organizations are beset by one of their biggest weaknesses when information that does not fit within other facilities becomes a follow-up issue. Blockchain offers the answer because it allows safe and efficient transfer of data among various agencies and care providers. Patient information can be passed from one virtual healthcare site within the metaverse to another without divulging confidentiality and security using blockchain's decentralized platform. The patient can authorize access to his or her record using cryptographic keys, and whatever is entered gets onto the blockchain, and everyone can see that. This is the kind of interop that will be required to provide high-quality, coordinated care, especially in a metaverse where there can be a myriad of different kinds of providers who are coming from everywhere with multiple levels of skill and must be able to communicate back and forth amongst each other to coordinate care for an individual patient.

Simplistically implementable contracts, or smart contracts, whereby terms of the contract are programmatically expressed in a literal sense form the basis for automating medical transactions in the metaverse of health care. These can also be used to automate transactions such as patient authorization, payment, and claims. For example, payment can be verified by smart contract upon completion of a medical procedure or upon filling of a prescription. Not only is electronic transfer faster, but it also eliminates human intervention or tampering. In that regard, smart contracts can enable all stakeholders of a healthcare transaction - providers, payers, or patients - to agree to open and transparent terms. Through automating in the health metaverse, it ensures services are being delivered in a secure and timely fashion, with higher patient satisfaction.

As pleasant as the union of blockchain and XAI to the metaverse for health care is, there are a few negatives to it. One of the biggest negatives is getting these technologies on board and incorporating them in existing health care environments, which is a Goliath technology and employee-training cost. A second disadvantage is the expense of expensive technology, which has the propensity to increase costs. Also expressed is concern about data security, confidentiality, and uses of AI in health, because policy on how to regulate them has not been developed and healthcare professionals have to interpret them. As technology gets more matured and standards are being established, the metaverse of healthcare will keep on evolving to make healthcare more individualized, secure, and comfortable to deliver. Quantum computing, 5G and next generation AI algorithms can also provide the metaverse with another spur to push healthcare even further. Then all the technologies mentioned above can intersect and make healthcare an even more patient-centric, open, and efficient system.

CASE STUDIES OF HEALTHCARE METAVERSE WITH EXPLAINABLE AI (XAI) AND BLOCKCHAIN (BC)

1. Blockchain Virtual Reality Surgery Simulation for Safe Data Handling

US top-ranked healthcare service group had developed a healthcare metaverse platform based on virtual reality (VR) for simulating surgery. It had utilized XAI to generate explainable records of each step of the surgery end-to-end so that the students are aware of why certain procedures are performed. Blockchain also came in handy to safely store the records of the simulation, i.e., the trainee performance record and correct technique utilized for each simulation. Using blockchain, the health organization was guaranteed data were not going to be tampered with and trainers could see and certify the trainee's progress during the course. It facilitated better determination of trainee skills and allowed safe storage for hosting and processing exclusive training information.

2. AI-Assisted Diagnostic Assistance in a Virtual Clinic

A Japanese healthcare system integrated AI-assisted diagnostic assistance with an online clinic on VR technology in the metaverse. Physicians could consult patients via avatars in virtual consultation rooms. Trained software systems with vast medical information were employed to assist doctors in making diagnoses from patient history, symptoms, and laboratory tests. Explainable AI (XAI) was employed to permit doctors to see the reasoning behind the AI diagnosis, be more confident, and make authoritative clinical decisions. Blockchain was employed to render the patient's medical history safe, decentralized, and accessible to qualified health professionals in cyberspace. Accurate diagnosis was achieved by the system, fewer mistakes were committed, and required sharing of information by patients and healthcare physicians was simplified.

3. Blockchain for Safe Exchange of Health Information in a Global Metaverse Network

There existed a global health metaverse network developed by a team of European physicians as an insured exchange platform of health information between clinics, research institutions, and hospitals across the world. Blockchain technology provided safe, inter-facilitated exchange of information, encrypting the patients' information to be accessed by only access authorities. Blockchain was used here as the platform for patient data management where no invasive data and free exchange of health data were being done. Explainable AI was used in helping doctors to explain data to be used in clinical research as well as medical studies. Real-time prediction of potential trends and epidemics of poor health was being enabled on the basis of AI models, and XAI framework provided the methodology on which the medical professionals were able to justify and explain the predictions. The platform enabled global collaboration and protected patient data and saved it securely.

4. Virtual Health and Wellness Support in Chronic Disease Care

One of the health insurers in the UK introduced a virtual health and wellbeing support web portal in the metaverse to take care of patients suffering from chronic conditions like diabetes and hypertension. Artificial intelligence-powered, the web portal gave patients lifestyle change suggestions based on their medication adherence, lifestyle, and clinical history. Explainable AI (XAI) educated patients why they were implementing particular lifestyle modifications, patient activation and medication compliance in the process. Explanation. Blockchain secured the patients' healthcare data like the daily blood glucose and the blood pressure levels from interception and made it viewable only to trained caregivers. The platform further facilitated real-time telemedicine consults within an online environment, enhancing accessibility and enabling timely personalized interventions. This use of the healthcare metaverse resulted in enhanced disease control, enhanced patient satisfaction, and reduced utilization of hospital resources.

5. Blockchain and AI-Based Decision Making Critical Care Remote Monitoring

Canada's largest hospital had built a metaverse platform as well as remote monitoring devices and AI for accelerating patient care. The critically ill patients with heart failure were tracked with IoT sensors too, and their information was fed into the blockchain-driven system in the hospital at all times for safe storage and real-time analysis. Machine learning algorithms processed the data to make predictions regarding patient deterioration and assist doctors with treatment. Explainable AI enabled the reason behind why the AI had predicted it to be explained such that physicians could cross-check the recommended process. Blockchain made the patients' data immutable and accessible to only genuine healthcare professionals. The system facilitated earlier and more accurate intervention in critical care patients and improved patient care in general.

6. Metaverse Virtual Mental Health Therapy

An Australian mental health clinic developed a therapy platform on the foundation of virtual reality in the metaverse for the provision of experiential mental health care to patients. The website offered one-on-one as well as group therapy, where the patients interacted with the therapists and similarly tilted patients through a virtual platform. AI technology tracked speech, emotion, and physical activity to build up emotion knowledge and give real-time feedback. XAI gave therapists feedback in the format of what the AI was doing with the data so that treatment could be adjusted accordingly. Blockchain concealed patient conversation and documents from sight but made them available for those who needed to access them. The platform increased access to mental health, decreased help-seeking stigma, and gave end-to-end visibility for therapists on patient performance.

7. AI-Powered Personalized Health Coaching and Blockchain-Based Data Monitoring

A UAE wellness business introduced a health metaverse platform with personalized health coaching to customers founded on their medical data. AI tracked fitness states, nutritional states, and well-being emotional states and sent feedback in the form of customized advice and fitness regimens. Explainable AI gave explanations on how the suggestions were calculated so that the users would be able to see the parameters that were inputting into their personal plans. Blockchain kept all the user information, such as health histories and coach histories, safe from storage and access by the user and chosen health coaches alone. Secure transmission of information between the health professionals and the users to enable collaborative work and other counseling services was also enabled through the use of blockchain technology. The website encouraged proactive care by compelling the users to decide on information and develop healthier habits.

8. Blockchain for Secure Vaccine Supply Chain and AI for Demand Forecasting

During the COVID-19 pandemic, a global health firm debuted a metaverse platform on blockchain to manage the secure supply chain of vaccines. Blockchain tracked stocks, distribution, and delivery of vaccines in an open-source setting to prevent counterfeiting. AI also predicted demand for vaccines in real-time and forecasted where outbreaks were going to happen, adjusting distribution plans accordingly in the process. XAI approaches maintained the company's employees in sync in the manner of determinants of demand forecasting, thus making decisions achieved with the help of AI more organic. Metaverse capability allowed medical professionals to work with one another across various virtual settings, and coordination and decision-making were simplified. The platform not only facilitated easy distribution of the vaccine but also logistics, saving time wastage and vaccines reaching destinations on time.

9. XAI and Blockchain-based Remote Surgery Support

The remote surgery platform has been developed by a Singaporean hospital in the metaverse with a vision to enable master surgeons to conduct complex surgeries remotely in real-time between locations.

The physicians utilized VR helmets to see real-time 3D images of the patients, while AI devices offered instant feedback and comments on scanning the operating field. Explainable AI allowed surgeons to see and understand AI recommendations, which improved surgical decision-making. Blockchain facilitated enabling protection of patient data like pre-surgery scans and procedures in such a manner that access to confidential data was granted only to authorized personnel. This remote surgery platform not only increased confidentiality of access to expert surgical experience but also reduced the risk elements of remote medical procedures.

10. AI-Based Predictive Analytics for Population Health Management

AI-based predictive analytics on a metaverse platform by a large South Korean health care system improved population health management. The platform forecasted future health patterns in specific groups based on vast amounts of data from wearables health monitoring devices, electronic health records (EHRs), and environmental data. XAI methods enabled clinicians to observe why the prediction was being generated, i.e., risk disease groups for chronic diseases.Blockchain made the health data secure and decentralized across institutions without going into patient privacy. Evidence-based practice enabled the healthcare provider to implement preventive intervention before the development of any health problem and thus ensured health outcomes in the population while reducing future health care expenditures. The case studies would be transformed if blockchain and XAI are used in the healthcare metaverse for the application of maximum maximized patient care, transparency, security, and operational efficiency. With these developments within our reach, we should also expect more developments and opportunities in health care on the horizon.

IMPLICATIONS OF HEALTHCARE METAVERSE BY EXPLAINABLE AI (XAI) AND BLOCKCHAIN (BC)

1. Improved Patient Care and Outcome

Applications of blockchain and XAI in healthcare metaverse can improve patient care and outcome. Clinicians can gain with improved fact-based decision-making with decision support by applying AI-based reasoning. AI explainability guarantee that the doctor will be able to comprehend why the recommendation is provided is more reassuring and instills confidence and trust for clinical decision. Customized care plans on AI-assessment-based and blockchain-based secure and open data management individualized the care. By tracking information in real-time and placing it under constant inspection, precise interventions are guaranteed to be offered at the appropriate time to the patients, and overall healthcare outcomes can be optimized.

2. Enhanced Trust and Transparency in the Healthcare Sector

Blockchain's greatest impact on healthcare metaverse systems is enhanced transparency and trust with information. Blockchain's decentralized and tamper-proof ledger keeps patient data safely, accurately, and tamper-proof from anyone who shouldn't have it. It is that openness that builds even more trust between physicians and patients because individuals are aware when and with whom they are seeing their medical records. XAI also builds this trust with even more interpretable and explainable medical recommendations offered from AI. As patients and physicians get to know the reasons for AI models, there is greater room for adoption and following AI recommendations.

3. Data Privacy and Confidentiality Threats

Using blockchain to protect healthcare information but also to raise confidentiality and information privacy risks. Decentralized nature of blockchain gives data protection from attack at a single point but makes it harder to maintain individual data in confidence. For example, sacrificing privacy in order to facilitate data exchange across healthcare metaverses is not an easy choice. Second, while XAI facilitates transparency in decisions, there must be protections to prevent AI models from inadvertently revealing sensitive personal information when explaining. Proper balancing of security, privacy, and accessibility will be among the central forces underlying how these technologies ultimately come to be deployed in a way that they are available to the health care community.

4. Expanded Access to HealthCare Services

The XAI and blockchain-based health metaverse can dramatically expand access to health care services, particularly for rural or disadvantaged communities. Teleconsultation with a doctor, telemonitoring, and use of immersive technologies like VR and AR can limit physical consultations in an effort to close the gap between doctor and patient. Blockchain makes patients' health data accessible anywhere across the world, thus having full control over their health data. Greater access has the potential to usher in smoother access for patients, especially those who reside in distant or economically weaker parts of society, to best care, leading towards health equity.

5. Ethical Implications of AI in Medicine

AI application in medicine, more so decision-making, carries serious ethical implications. Vulnerability of AI systems, especially towards discrimination against weaker sections of society or minorities, can actually lead to variance of health outcomes. This is avoided through the incorporation of XAI, hence making the decision-making by AI explainable and transparent. There also needs to be continuous monitoring on and updating of the AI models in order to train them using diversified and representative data. Besides that, use of AI to core regions like diagnosis and treatment needs to be regulated so that it does not encourage more dependence on machine recommendation and human intelligence must remain at the center of clinical decision-making.

6. Regulatory and Legal Challenges

Application of blockchain and AI technologies to healthcare metaverse poses a set of regulatory and legal challenges. For example, medical records are protected under rigorous privacy laws like HIPAA (Health Insurance Portability and Accountability Act) in the US or the GDPR (General Data Protection Regulation) in the EU. Decentralized blockchain is hard to comply with such a law if patient information is copied across different nodes spread over multiple jurisdictions. Secondly, the health care AI technology will have to follow ethical norms and regulations so that it is safe and effective. The governments and the health care centers will have to communicate with one another for developing appropriate regulation policies on how to use such technologies in the metaverse.

7. Health Care Provider Training and New Technology Adoption

Blockchain and AI deployment in healthcare involves vast training of doctors to enable them to work with the systems. Explainable AI judgments may bridge the gap between sophisticated AI software packages and doctors. Doctors need to continue learning how to utilize the technologies, however. Doctors will need to be trained not only in the technology of blockchain and AI but also how to balance ethics, privacy, and legality in its application. Training modules for facilitation will thus be necessary in order to put an AI and blockchain-capable healthcare system in place.

8. Healthcare Cost Savings and Increased Operating Efficiency

Use of blockchain and AI technology in the health metaverse can minimize healthcare spending by as much a percentage as possible by making the process optimizable to its maximum potential. Use of blockchain smart contracts in automating the process and optimizing the data can save unnecessary administrative cost, avoid fraud, and maximize proper billing. Artificial intelligence decision-support systems also justify clinical practice in real time and disease diagnosis or medication prescription prevention as time-wasting activities. Hospitals and healthcare centers reduce costs by avoiding inefficiencies, which are transferred to the patient and make the health sector economically viable.

9. Innovations in Healthcare Delivery Model

The combination of blockchain, AI, and the metaverse opens new avenues for healthcare delivery models in the future. Virtual clinics based on AI, for example, can conduct consultations, track patient status, and even offer mental health care without having to set up a physical clinic. Blockchain enables secure and cheap exchange of health information between providers and systems, which equates to more integrated and coordinated care. These technologies hold out the promise of revolutionizing decentralized health systems in which the patient is facilitated to take charge of his/her own health and the health professionals are poised to provide more patient-led, responsive care. Healthcare workers also train through cross-professional collaboration with other healthcare workers worldwide, leading to more sharing of information as well as collaboration, through the metaverse.

10. Future of AI and Blockchain in Healthcare

Its future with blockchain and AI in medicine is promising but will take ongoing research, innovation, and cooperation to reach its potential. The more advanced the AI algorithms become, the more advanced the medical applications will become, with improved diagnostics and more tailored treatment protocols. Blockchain will increasingly be utilized in safe and clear health data management without compromising patients' privacy and autonomy. Moreover, as the metaverse is created, the health care system will be decentralized and virtual forms of care which can be delivered to even more patients. The intersection of these technologies will revolutionize the provision of health care, which will create new fronts in patient outcome optimization, cost savings, and access to health care worldwide. Globally, blockchain-based healthcare metaverse and XAI impact is vast with various benefits like improved patient care, safe data, and easy accessibility. The sectors in which the effort must be made before applying the technologies in the healthcare industry are ethics, regulatory delays, and training staff. Being a new technology, healthcare metaverse can revolutionize the healthcare sector, considering patients as individuals, making healthcare effective and just.

Blockchain and XAI-based healthcare metaverse will be a highly promising area of expansion for healthcare services. With ongoing research, development, and implementation, the technologies have unlimited scope to redefine the delivery of health care towards making it personalized, efficient, and equitable. The future can be nothing but bright if the systems are properly integrated and implemented in the right direction, towards a healthy, safe, and patient-focused system of healthcare.

CONCLUSION

Blockchain (BC) and Explainable AI (XAI) convergence of the health care metaverse has the possibility to reshape health care delivery and regulation as a whole. Open, evidence-based, and secure decision-making using the convergence of such technologies addresses most of the pitfalls of the conventional health care systems such as data security, patient confidentiality, and requirements of personalized medicine. XAI offers explainability to clinical AI-driven decisions, and potentially it can enable clinicians and patients to be able to understand more clearly why treatment and diagnostic decisions were made, thus easier to instill trust and collaboration. Blockchain is the foundation for security behind patient information, utilized data being decentralized, imputable, and readable only by access-limited individuals authorized to read it. Other than that, the metaverse also offers the home-based care platform, virtual consultation, and even interprofessional interprofessional team collaboration among the healthcare providers, hence taking the healthcare to the people wherever they are. But to harness these technologies on a mass level in the healthcare industry will rectify a whole range of issues. These will include repairing the ethical issues, tackling the health levels, and providing training and assistance to the medical staff such that the AI and blockchain networks become a success. Despite all these challenges, the possibility of more health benefit, lower cost, and greater accessibility makes convergence of XAI, blockchain, and metaverse very intriguing future healthcare landscape.

REFERENCES

Abbott, M., & Shaw, P. (2016). *Virtual nursing avatars: Nurse roles and evolving concepts of care*. OJIN Online J. Issues Nurs.

Allam, Z., Sharifi, A., Bibri, S. E., Jones, D. S., & Krogstie, J. (2022). The Metaverse as a Virtual Form of Smart Cities: Opportunities and Challenges for Environmental, Economic, and Social Sustainability in Urban Futures. *Smart Cities*, *5*, 771–801.

Cai, S., Jiao, X., & Song, B. (2022). Open another door to education—Applications, challenges and perspectives of the education metaverse. *Metaverse*, *3*, 11.

Games, E. (2017). *Fortnite*. Epic Games.

Garavand, A., & Aslani, N. (2022). Metaverse phenomenon and its impact on health: A scoping review. *Informatics in Medicine Unlocked*, *32*, 101029.

Gursoy, D., Malodia, S., & Dhir, A. (2022). The metaverse in the hospitality and tourism industry: An overview of current trends and future research directions. *Journal of Hospitality Marketing & Management*, *31*, 527–534.

Hwang, G.-J., & Chien, S.-Y. (2022). Definition, roles, and potential research issues of the metaverse in education: An artificial intelligence perspective. *Comput. Educ. Artif. Intell.*, *3*, 100082.

Jeong, H., Yi, Y., & Kim, D. (2022). An innovative e-commerce platform incorporating metaverse to live commerce. *International Journal of Innovative Computing, Information, & Control*, *18*, 221–229.

Joshua, J. (2017). Information Bodies: Computational Anxiety in Neal Stephenson's Snow Crash. *Interdisciplinary Literary Studies*, *19*, 17–47.

Jungherr, A., & Schlarb, D. B. (2022). The Extended Reach of Game Engine Companies: How Companies Like Epic Games and Unity Technologies Provide Platforms for Extended Reality Applications and the Metaverse. *Social Media + Society*, *8*, 20563051221107641.

Khansulivong, C., Wicha, S., & Temdee, P. Adaptive of New Technology for Agriculture Online Learning by Metaverse: A Case Study in Faculty of Agriculture, National University of Laos. In Proceedings of the 2022 Joint International Conference on Digital Arts, Media and Technology with ECTI Northern Section Conference on Electrical, Electronics, Computer and Telecommunications Engineering (ECTI DAMT & NCON), Online, 26–28 January 2022; IEEE: Piscataway, NJ, USA, 2022.

Koo, H. (2021). Training in lung cancer surgery through the metaverse, including extended reality, in the smart operating room of Seoul National University Bundang Hospital, Korea. *Journal of Educational Evaluation for Health Professions*, *18*, 33. PMID: 34965648

Kraus, S., Kanbach, D. K., Krysta, P. M., Steinhoff, M. M., & Tomini, N. (2022). Facebook and the creation of the metaverse: Radical business model innovation or incremental transformation? *International Journal of Entrepreneurial Behaviour & Research*, *28*, 52–77.

Krittanawong, C., Aydar, M., Virk, H. U. H., Kumar, A., Kaplin, S., Guimaraes, L., & Halperin, J. L. (2022). Artificial intelligence-powered blockchains for cardiovascular medicine. *The Canadian Journal of Cardiology*, *38*(2), 185–195. PMID: 34856332

Porras, D. C., Siemonsma, P., Inzelberg, R., Zeilig, G., & Plotnik, M. (2018). Advantages of virtual reality in the rehabilitation of balance and gait: Systematic review. *Neurology*, *90*, 1017–1025. PMID: 29720544

Shin, D. (2022). The actualization of meta affordances: Conceptualizing affordance actualization in the metaverse games. *Computers in Human Behavior*, *133*, 107292.

Skalidis, I., Muller, O., & Fournier, S. (2023). CardioVerse: The cardiovascular medicine in the era of Metaverse. *Trends in Cardiovascular Medicine*, *33*(8), 471–476. PMID: 35568263

Tan, T. F., Li, Y., Lim, J. S., Gunasekeran, D. V., Teo, Z. L., Ng, W. Y., & Ting, D. S. (2022). Metaverse and Virtual Health Care in Ophthalmology: Opportunities and Challenges. *Asia-Pacific Journal of Ophthalmology*, *11*, 237–246. PMID: 35772084

Thomason, J. (2022). Metaverse, token economies, and non-communicable diseases. *Global Health Journal (Amsterdam, Netherlands)*, *6*, 164–167.

Um, T., Kim, H., Kim, H., Lee, J., Koo, C., & Chung, N. Travel Incheon as a Metaverse: Smart Tourism Cities Development Case in Korea. In Proceedings of the ENTER22 e-Tourism Conference, Tianjin, China, 11–14 January 2022; Springer: Berlin/Heidelberg, Germany, 2022.

Wiederhold, B. K. (2022). *Metaverse Games: Game Changer for Healthcare?* Mary Ann Liebert, Inc.

Wu, T. C., & Ho, C. T. B. (2023). A scoping review of metaverse in emergency medicine. *Australasian Emergency Care (Online)*, *26*(1), 75–83. PMID: 35953392

Yang, D.; Zhou, J.; Chen, R.; Song, Y.; Song, Z.; Zhang, X.; Wang, Q.; Wang, K.; Zhou, C.; Sun, J.; et al. Expert consensus on the metaverse in medicine. Clin. eHealth 2022, 5, 1–9.

You, Y., & Gui, X. (2020). Self-Diagnosis through AI-Enabled Chatbot-Based Symptom Checkers: User Experiences and Design Considerations. *AMIA ... Annual Symposium Proceedings - AMIA Symposium. AMIA Symposium*, *2020*, 1354–1363. PMID: 33936512

Zeng, Y., Zeng, L., Zhang, C., & Cheng, A. S. (2022). The metaverse in cancer care: Applications and challenges. *Asia-Pacific Journal of Oncology Nursing*, *9*, 100111. PMID: 36276879

Chapter 8
Blockchain and Metaverse Revolutionizing Healthcare Systems:
Transforming Healthcare for a Secure and Patient-Centric Future

Jyoti Rani
https://orcid.org/0000-0002-5577-7808
Parul University, India

ABSTRACT

The convergence of blockchain technology and the metaverse presents transformative potential for healthcare, addressing challenges like data security, patient privacy, and decentralized medical services. Blockchain ensures secure, transparent, and efficient management of sensitive health data, enhancing patient-centric care, streamlining processes via smart contracts, and enabling decentralized identity management. Emerging technologies like Artificial Intelligence (AI), the Internet of Medical Things (IoMT), and Non-Fungible Tokens (NFTs) expand possibilities in virtual healthcare delivery. However, challenges such as scalability, cost-effectiveness, regulatory hurdles, and ethical concerns require sustainable solutions. A comprehensive research roadmap emphasizing interdisciplinary collaboration is critical to fostering a secure, efficient, and patient-empowered healthcare system in the digital era.

DOI: 10.4018/979-8-3373-1225-5.ch008

INTRODUCTION

It is a transformative frontier in digital health, merging blockchain, metaverse and healthcare to create innovative solutions for patient care, data management, and healing. These technologies are being integrated with the aim of improving the efficiency, security, and accessibility of healthcare services. The metaverse, a virtual space where physical and digital realities converge, has the potential to transform healthcare by enabling immersive experiences and transforming patient engagement and care delivery. In this digital ecosystem, blockchain technology is the key to guarantee trusts and secure data. Key aspects of this intersection are examined in detail below.

Metaverse in Healthcare

- The metaverse features a graphical environment in which healthcare practices can be virtually undertaken, improving surgical precision and therapeutic strategies facilitated by technologies such as AI, VR, and AR (C. Wang et al., 2024).
- Renowned involvement in for medicine systems virtual hospitals and clinics can be used to change clinical workflows and expedite diagnosis and treatment of diseases (mental health, cardiology, etc.) (Curtis & Brolan, 2023).
- Validators of social prescribing, the metaverse enables healthcare providers to reach patients through novel modalities, while focus on human-o-human connections and ethical implications (Nadarasa, 2024).

Role of Blockchain

- In the metaverse, blockchain technology secures the health data providing its privacy and integrity. It allows for a distributed system for data controlling, leading to increased faith & trust in patient-provider relationship (Ali et al., 2023).
- First and foremost, Blockchain-enabled Internet of Everything (BIoE) will help manage this connectivity and also secure the metaverse applications, which require interactions between physical (physical + digital) entities (Rafique & Qadir, 2024).
- In addition, Blockchain and AI integration within the metaverse supports disease forecasting and diagnosis through explainable AI models that foster greater trust and transparency in healthcare decisions (Ali et al., 2023).

Privacy and Security Concerns

- The volume of health-related data generated in the metaverse requires robust privacy and security measures to protect sensitive information from data collection and processing.
- Plus, ethical factors are paramount, as the metaverse may also reinforce problems such as data misuse and discrimination if they are a not strictly monitored, regulated, and implemented (McCourt, 2024) (Curtis & Brolan, 2023).
- Informed consent and protecting patient data during metaverse interactions and safeguarding confidentiality represent significant challenges that must be addressed to build trust in the acceptance of metaverse-enabled healthcare services.

CONSTRAINTS AND FUTURE DIRECTIONS

- To support different healthcare applications, network demands, such as network quality in terms of fast speed, that's why there should be focused metaverse-based healthcare services, despite network requirements including higher bandwidth and lower latency (Q. Wang et al., 2023).
- Governance frameworks that address ethical and social dimensions of metaverses must be comprehensive in scope to ensure equitable access and prevent discrimination (Curtis & Brolan, 2023).
- Further studies can be conducted to integrate AI, blockchain, and similar technologies into metaverse so that healthcare can be delivered most optimally to the patients.

As exciting as the merging of blockchain, metaverse, and healthcare may be, this premise will also bring a plethora of challenges to be faced head-on. Nonetheless, there are important ethical concerns, data privacy issues, and inequitable access that need to be considered to ensure that these technologies benefit all stakeholders in the healthcare ecosystem. It is important that as digital innovations evolve further, we must continue to focus on human experience during these processes to avoid dehumanization of care and to elevate the capabilities of these emerging technologies to serve the best need of all.

Current advancements and limitations in integrating blockchain in metaverse healthcare applications.

Metaverse applications of healthcare have the potential to become more secure overall through blockchain technology integration and more patient centric delivery of service with data that is immutable on the blockchain. The decentralised structure of blockchain ensures secure data management - especially for sensitive health information as it is exchanged in immersive metaverse environments. But nevertheless, various challenges and obstacles still remain, preventing the smooth incorporation of blockchain into metaverse health care applications.

Progress In Blockchain Integration

- Data Security and Privacy: The Metaverse can be constructed over blockchain which allows the user to have better security in managing EHRs and other sensitive data. It provides for data integrity and restricts unauthorized access; thus, it is essential for maintaining the confidentiality of patients (Liu et al., 2024) (Ali et al., 2023).
- Interoperability and Trust, the metaverse hosts multiple online worlds and virtual environments, making interoperability key for the integration of blockchain technology. It enables the transfer of data and provides credibility among stakeholders by ensuring the accuracy and accountability of transactions (Rafique & Qadir, 2024) (Ali et al., 2023).
- Patient-Centric Care: Blockchain puts FHE on data to patients, they no longer just have control over their health data. In a tech-enabled metaverse, tailoring care delivery and leveraging personalized services is essential for placing patients first (Liu et al., 2024).
- Demand forecasting: By using data analytics, healthcare providers can dissect the demand for services with more accuracy. Modeling supply chains is, as we will see, one of the killer apps of the metaverse; where virtual and physical supply chains intersect (Bak et al., 2023).

Limitations and Challenges

- Scalability Problems: There are scalability issues when using blockchain on metaverse healthcare applications, due to the amount of computational overhead and constrained resources available from blockchain (Ali et al., 2023) (Bak et al., 2023).
- Interoperability and Standardization: Even when the system function, it often hinders the integration of blockchain due to the interoperability challenge and lack of standard information elements in a variety of healthcare systems and metaverse platforms (Bak et al., 2023).
- Buffered Challenges: New challenges in implementing blockchain technology based on having to conduct this under conditions of resource constraints come along within developing countries. An other challenge which stems

under this umbrella is the absence of technologic infrastructure and the requirement of customized solutions to adjust to local circumstances (Liu et al., 2024) (Bak et al., 2023).

- Concerns regarding Ethics and Privacy – Ethical issues around data privacy and the risk of dehumanization of care in the metaverses Aidaptation: However, the normative deployment and anthropocentric dimension should remain always relevant (Nadarasa, 2024) (Ali et al., 2023).

However, these benefits are countered with some of the disadvantages of the metaverse and its connection to blockchain. Scalability, interoperability, and ethics should be the main topics in future research to derive scalable solutions, improve interoperability among applications/services, and address potential jurisdictional and ethical issues related to the use of blockchain in the metaverse. One other area to consider is the combination of blockchain with other emerging technologies such as AI and IoT, which could expand the features of metaverse healthcare applications significantly (Rafique & Qadir, 2024) (Ali et al., 2023).

Importance of future research to address existing challenges

There are still some open questions regarding the use of blockchain to facilitate metaverse healthcare and further work is needed to tackle these challenges in order to pave the way for the promise of such innovative convergence. The healthcare domain is data-rich but lacks security and privacy solution that could ensure patient information protection from information leakage while ensuring accountability and auditing in the healthcare domain due to its sensitive nature. Finally, the scalability bottleneck of blockchain, which usually illustrates the inefficiency of high data volume regulation, causes the adoption of light-weight implementations that could satisfy the requirements of both performance and decentralization. In fact, these substantial computation and energy needs reflect the cost- and energy-efficient and sustainable systems that are required for blockchain to not only be sustainable, but also to be widely utilized. The metaverse is not just one platform or one technology, it is a decentralized network of platforms that must be able to integrate and interact seamlessly to provide for cohesive healthcare service; this is an example of interoperability that is an important quality of any healthcare solution. In addition, the global and distributed nature of blockchain creates significant regulation and ethics issues that require setting up solid frameworks to regulate this new but already massive ecosystem in an accountable way. It also makes a point of providing empowerment to patients and providers: there needs to be research able to assist on how patients and providers can both be able to own and manage their health data in such a way as to suit their needs (this sounds to me as a relation in which patient data is in or related to many systems that make the work of providers easier). In addition, other potential healthcare applications need more specific investigations especially to tackle the technical challenges where novel dimensions such as Artificial Intelligence (AI) and Internet of Medical Things (IoMT) provide significant integration with Blockchain. Closing these research gaps will facilitate the potential for blockchain to become the core of a secure, transparent and efficient healthcare system in the metaverse.

BLOCKCHAIN AS A SECURE INFRASTRUCTURE FOR METAVERSE HEALTHCARE

Data Security and Privacy

The use of blockchain is another promising infrastructure as it can potentially provide the necessary data security and privacy for metaverse healthcare systems. The decentralized, immutable and transparent characteristics of blockchain promises to address a wide range of health information exchange and privacy-based challenges. The metaverse is about making healthcare services available, affordable, accessible, and secure, which will be facilitated by the application of blockchain together with other technologies, such as artificial intelligence and deep learning. The subsequent explain the key aspects of blockchain-powered metaverse healthcare.

Blockchain: the trusted infrastructure

- Decentralization and Immutability: The decentralized nature of blockchain makes copies of medical data tamper-proof and readable only by authorized parties, which reduces the risk of a massive leak of centralized data. This guarantees confidence and visibility in health care ecosystems (Alanazi et al., 2024).
- Control and Ownership of Data: Patients might own and control their own data, including giving and retracting access. This is inevitable in the metaverse setting that involves persistent data generation and exchange (Alanazi et al., 2024) (Ali et al., 2023).
- Smart Contracts: Another Technical Component for this use case will be smart contracts that are a tool used to automate and secure transactions by providing codified rules that guide the sharing and access of data under specific conditions. It reduces unauthorized access and provides data integrity (Xu, 2024).

Improving Security and Privacy of Data

- Advanced encryption techniques, like the Fractional Order Lorenz system and logistic chaotic encryption, are used to protect medical images and other confidential information. These methods guarantee data secrecy and prevent unauthorized access (Alanazi et al., 2024) (Han et al., 2023).
- Anonymous Signatures and Zero-Knowledge Proofs: Cryptographic tools to enable privacy without disclosing sensitive data. This is especially relevant since patient privacy needs to be protected even in a metaverse environment, which makes for an additional challenge.
- Distributed Storage: Distributed storage systems like proof of retrievability in Blockchain will enable secure and efficient storage and retrieval of data in the metaverse. It solves localization issue in decision-making and single point of failure field (Fang et al., 2024).

AI and Deep Learning Integration

- Explainable AI (XAI): XAI and blockchain can be merged to promote transparency and interpretability for disease diagnosis and prediction in the metaverse. These fosters trust between the patients and the health care providers as it gives a rationale to AI-based decisions (Ali et al., 2023).
- Learn with Deep Data Classification: MobileNetv1 and stacked recurrent neural networks can be used to not only classify medical images, enhancing diagnostic capabilities, but also to ensure data security through blockchain (Alanazi et al., 2024).

Challenges and Future Directions

Despite considerable promise of blockchain to serve as a solid foundation for secure and private access and use of data within a Healthcare metaverses, there are ongoing challenges to address. There are issues of scalability, transaction throughput and latency that must be resolved for it to run effectively in a metaverse context (Fang et al., 2024). Moreover, the convergence between blockchain and other emerging technologies necessitates the careful attention to interoperability and standardization to enable the seamless operation across different systems. Thus, the metaverse is a developing on rung of the ladder of technological advancement and further research and development will be required to address these challenges, making healthcare data security and privacy more watertight.

Decentralized Identity (DID)

Metaverse healthcare services potentially secure infrastructure could be built using Decentralized Identity (DID) blockchain technology. The potential of DID in health information lies in its characteristics of immutability, decentralization, etc., which could strengthen data privacy, interoperability, and the ability of individuals to manage their health information. This allows to scale and adopt changing requirements for metaverse health care where huge number of sensitive data are being handled accross virtual surrounding. DID combined with blockchain will solve the most pressing issues in metaverse healthcare: data security and privacy and interoperability and seamless, safe engagement of the users.

Improving Security and Privacy

- The Security Characteristics of the Blockchain: Blockchain technology offers a secure and unchangeable ledger for the storage of healthcare data, guaranteeing that sensitive data is remain tamper-proof and available to authorized-parties only. This is important in the metaverse, where there are concerns over data breaches and unauthorized access (Alanazi et al., 2024) (Lax et al., 2024).
- Self-Sovereign Identity (SSI): Use of SSI principles can enable users to manage the digital identity that they share and improve their privacy and security in metaverse health care environments. This allows users to have power over their data: who can and cannot use it, and where it can be used.
- Data Encryption and Access Control: Use of advanced encryption methods, such as those that are implemented using chaotic mapping and attribute-based encryption, can enhance the security of healthcare data by ensuring that only authorized entities can access or modify it (Xu, 2024) (Ali et al., 2023).

Interoperability and User Agency

- Cross-Metaverse Interactions: Did provided secure and interoperable interactions across the myriad of metaverse platforms, ensuring seamless interoperability when accessing healthcare services and related data. This is imperative to consolidate the healthcare ecosystem across the metaverses.
- Individual Health-Centeredness: The metaverse will benefit by supporting individual health-centeredness, with the user able to own his/her own health information data using DID. Patients own their health information and may

allow or deny access to their health information (Alanazi et al., 2024) (Ali et al., 2023).

Challenges and Solutions

- Scalability and Efficiency: Blockchain offers robust security, however, in the metaverse, where users, digital assets, and data rapidly increase, there is a scalability bottleneck associated with blockchain. Furthermore, distributed storage paradigm, efficient data transmission and routing protocols, automated load balancing, and other similar technologies can enhance the performance and scalability of blockchain-enabled healthcare applications (Sun et al., 2024).
- AI and IoT Integration: The integration of AI and IoT into blockchain further enhances metaverse healthcare services by enabling smart data processing and real-time health monitoring. This kind of integration could improve diagnostic accuracy and patient outcomes (Jena et al., 2024) (Ali et al., 2023).

Like all other technologies, the incorporation of DOES blockchain in metaverse healthcare comes with its own pros and cons that need to be surmounted. The data being generated in the metaverse is great, and we need to scale the blockchain systems to overcome such challenges as well as need insights on what more will be needed to successful harness use of other critical emerging technology like AI and IoT to fasten health service delivery. DID is a promising solution for metaverse healthcare, but there are limitations that need addressing, such as lack of regulation and standardization thus, it is imperative to create consistent, reliable standards for data sharing and interoperability to unlock the full potential of DID in metaverse healthcare. Focusing on these issues, DID Blockchain would offer a safe and reliable framework for the subsequent treatment landscape in the metaverse.

Smart Contracts

Using smart contracts and Blockchain technology in the metaverse healthcare infrastructure seems to be a potent solution for improving safety, privacy, and efficiency. By utilizing the blockchain's decentralized and immutable perform it, this solution also addresses data integrity, access control, and interoperability issues faced by traditional healthcare systems. Adding smart contracts in the metaverse allows healthcare workers to automate tasks, guarantee secure data exchanges, and foster trust among patients by providing transparency and accountability in actions taken.

Improvements to Security and Privacy

- Privacy and Security via Cryptographic Proofs and Access Control: In healthcare systems-based smart contracts, medical data processing can be secured by cryptographic proof to avoid any repudiation and ensure accountability. An access control array that allows for secure management of Electronic Health Records (EHRs) on the blockchain (Szczepaniuk & Szczepaniuk, 2023).
- Fine-grained access control: The integration of CP-ABE and blockchain leads to fine-grained access control, which not only improves security in EHR management but also automates key management and encryption processes (Ali et al., 2023).
- Immutably Stored Data: The decentralized ledger of blockchain guarantees that the medical data stored remains tamper-proof and accessible only to authorized parties, thereby minimizing the probability of centralized data breaches and promoting trust in healthcare ecosystems (Alanazi et al., 2024).

Efficiency and Scalability

- Distributed Storage and Data Offloading: Blockchain-based distributed storage systems like proof of retrievability can overcome the issues of centralized decision-making, providing better efficiency in data verifiability and better scalability in metaverse health system (Fang et al., 2024). Moreover, smart contracts enable secure data offloading, thereby enhancing resource allocation and reducing costs (He et al., 2024).
- Cloud Integration: The integration of blockchain with cloud computing increases the scalability and resource management, thus it facilitates the efficient management of EHRs which boosts the response time of the healthcare service delivery (Ali et al., 2023).

Trust and Transparency

- Explainable AI and Blockchain: Some evidence should be provided beside the use of explainable AI models in the metaverse; blockchain is another game-changing technology that used together with explainable AI ensures the transparency and trustworthiness of disease diagnosis and data security. Also, this method offers logical reasoning for disease predictions which adds to patient confidence in the health care system (Ali et al., 2023).
- Governance through Smart Contracts: Smart contracts can also govern user behavior in the metaverse, making for a secure and fair environment by reg-

ulating, monitoring, and managing inappropriate behavior, like hate speech and cyberbullying (Rahaman et al., 2024).

ENHANCING PATIENT-CENTRIC CARE

Personalized Healthcare Services

A new avatar of personalized healthcare delivered through a blockchain powered metaverse With the immersive features of the metaverse and the relieving transparency and security of the blockchain, this state-of-the-art model enhances the process of delivering healthcare services. With technologies like metaverse and blockchain, a virtual environment where patients and healthcare professionals can interact can be created without compromising the security and immutability of the health data. That kind of synergy will transform healthcare in terms of providing secure, personalized and effective services.

Healthcare is widely expected to adopt Metaverse and Blockchain

- Healthcare Immersion: The metaverse enables realistic and immersive experiences like virtual consultations and monitoring patients remotely. Thus, it promotes better interaction between patients and their providers, namely avatars for each user (Chengoden et al., 2023) (Ali et al., 2023).
- Data Privacy Protection: Blockchain interspace can also prove the data security and privacy that will be in large demand for the extremely sensitive patient data within the metaverse. It can actually be an important part of data integrity and trust, as it provides you with a decentralized and tamper-free system to store health records. Moreover, aspects of blockchain such as transparency, traceability, and immutability are called upon to make health data transactions secure (Ali et al., 2023).
- Increasingly, blockchain can provide specific medical services to people so personalized healthcare services will become possible. This nature of blockchain can provide a way to maintain personal health records that can enable secure identity for patients, and in turn clinicians will be able to provide state of-the-art personalised treatment plans, physiotherapy and other nursing care (Chen et al., 2024) (S. Wang et al., 2019).

Challenges and Solutions

- Scalability and Efficiency: The metaverse means ever greater amounts of data to connect, creating problems for the scalability and efficiency of blockchains, leading to performance and latency concerns. Some solutions, e.g., distributed storage systems of proof of retrievability and vector commitment, are proposed to solve these problems to motivate the data verification and boost the system scalability automatically (Fang et al., 2024).
- Ethical and Privacy Concerns: Immersive technologies raise ethical considerations around patient privacy and the risk of dehumanizing patient care. However, it is important to create an ethical framework based on respect for the dignity of the patients that would guide the introduction of metaverse platforms in the healthcare practice (Nadarasa, 2024).
- Interoperability and Data Management: As interoperability across multiple types and sources of health data becomes the norm, ensuring a holistic view of patient health is of utmost importance. Blockchain federations are used to bridge and integrate distributed health data to provide a holistic view (world) of the trajectory of patient health.

Telemedicine and Remote Consultations

One such innovative healthcare solution is the incorporation of telemedicine and remote consultations through blockchain technology in the metaverse healthcare environment. This cutting edge construction harnesses the metaverse's volunteer capacities along with the safety and straightforwardness of blockchain to further develop patient consideration and information the board. The metaverse also provides us with a virtual space where healthcare professionals and patients can meet as avatars, thus offering a much more humane interaction than those offered by telemedicine platforms. It not only enhances the quality of remote consultations but also guarantees the security and privacy of patient data through the use of blockchain technology. The two most important characteristics of the integration are discussed below.

Combining the Metaverse with Telemedicine

- In the metaverse, telemedicine transforms into an immersive experience, where patients and healthcare providers can interact through avatars in a virtual environment. This arrangement provides an enhanced experience to the patients as it imitates real-life consultations and makes them an active part of the processes taken, which in return fosters patient engagement and satisfaction (Ali et al., 2023) (Sestino & D'Angelo, 2023).

- AR and VR technologies can augment remote metaverse-based consultations; such augmented consultations facilitate detailed visualizations and simulations that assist the metaverse-based doctor with diagnosis and treatment planning. For specialities such as cardiology, this has the advantage of a hybrid approach of virtual face-to-face consultations extending to telemedical devices to monitor patients (Skalidis et al., 2022).

Use of Blockchain to Store Data Securely and Trustably

- Blockchain technology One important aspect of the metaverse healthcare model is the blockchain technology that enables secured and private information integrity. It provides a permanent and decentralized protocol for verstiling patient data which enhances trust and transparency between users (Ali et al., 2023) (Fang et al., 2024).
- The use of blockchain in health care metaverse settings could reduce concerns with data leaking and data access without permission, as the use of blockchain provides a secure and traceable record of all interactions and data exchanges (Ali et al., 2023) (Fang et al., 2024).

Applications and Benefits

- The metaverse can provide a range of healthcare use cases: from remote consultations to medical training and patient education It can facilitate mixed reality, such as complete immersive simulations for emergency response training and anatomy learning (Qiu et al., 2022).
- State that Patients may find access to health-related information and resources through the metaverse in ways that empower them to take care of their health and make informed decisions (Ullah et al., 2023).

Challenges and Considerations

- Although it allows novel technological solutions, its combination in the metaverse (i.e. integration of the physical and digital worlds into a single space) has its own challenges in facing high latency and blocked transaction throughput throughput of present day blockchain systems that may act as a bottleneck of data retrieval and storage (Fang et al., 2024).
- Lastly, the digital divide will need to be addressed, given that the metaverse environment may not be accessible to everyone, especially poorer or less

technology-savvy populations, which could increase health inequality (Qiu et al., 2022).

While blockchain plus telemedicine in the metaverse integration offers some actual positive developments in healthcare delivery, without careful consideration of the implications, it can never be real long-term success. We need to be mindful of the digital divide and where technology does not enable great access and cost-effectiveness. Furthermore, we must continue the innovation to refine these technologies and facilitate their transformative ability to disrupt healthcare systems.

Patient Empowerment

How we can use blockchain in the metaverse for empowering the patient. Combining the fully immersive possibilities of the metaverse with blockchain's inherent security and transparency makes for a patient-controlled healthcare ecosystem. This can greatly empower patients by giving them more control over their health information as well as their interactions with healthcare providers, as secure data exchange fosters trust. In the following sections we will discuss how both elements are intertwined and what this means for the empowering of patients.

Integrating Blockchain & Metaverse into Healthcare

- Secure Data Management: Blockchain technology allows to secure, private, and unchangeable patient data in the metaverse. This is vital for ensuring trust between patients because the interactions and exchanges of data are documented on the blockchain, so that no individual can use the data that does not belong to him and at the same time protects against data breaches (Ali et al., 2023) (Hylock & Zeng, 2019).
- She overhauls the main topics into a significant scale and inquires of interest for coliseum fairs. This enables patients to choose who can see their health information and in what circumstances (Zhuang et al., 2023).
- Enhanced Interoperability and Data Exchange: Blockchain enables the secure and efficient exchange of health data between disparate healthcare systems, allowing patients to benefit from more complete and current medical record histories. Interoperability is important for patient empowerment, as it allows patients to make educated decisions regarding their health based on comprehensive health data (Hylock & Zeng, 2019).

Empower Patients With Blockchain

- Autonomy and Control: Blockchain technology encourages patient empowerment through autonomy over their health data. Patients can control access to their data, and can participate in their healthcare decisions instead of being passive subjects, increasing their sense of control and involvement (Aujoulat et al., 2012).
- Improved Communication and Decision-Making: Digital resources like Empowering Providers to Empower Patients (EPEP) show the promise of enhancing the exchanges between patients and providers. Blockchain can enhance this further by making sure that all the information that is shared is accurate and secure, thus, promoting better shared decision making.
- Building Trust and Transparency: Blockchain transactions based on transparency and traceability enhance trust between patient and healthcare provider. Patients demonstrate improved engagement with healthcare systems when they trust their data is in safe and transparent hands (Ali et al., 2023) (Dewangan & Chandrakar, 2023).

NTEGRATION WITH EMERGING TECHNOLOGIES

Artificial Intelligence (AI) and Machine Learning (ML)

One of these types even extends to a new metaverse landscape to prove its ability to enable accurate diagnosis and predictions through the blockchain contribution to AI model. It is an exciting new metaverse that integrates the processing capabilities of AI with the protective mechanisms of blockchain to advance healthcare. The combined utilization of these technologies aims to provide a secure, efficient, and transparent healthcare ecosystem capable of meeting the challenges posed by the technical and ethical facets of digital health environments. In this blog, we discuss various details of this integration and how it can benefit.

Use of Blockchain and AI in Metaverse Healthcare

- Security & Privacy of Patient Data: Blockchain technology using decentralized and immutable ledger secures the patient data. It keeps data secure and minimizes the risks of hacking and breaches so that rigorously protects customers and healthcare providers trust each other (Ali et al., 2023) (Alanazi et al., 2024).

- AI-Driven Diagnosis and Predictions: AI models, especially deep learning ones, are used for complex medical data analysis and real-time disease prediction. The real-world data generated in the metaverse enriches these models, making them more accurate and reliable (Rahal et al., 2024).
- Explainable AI (XAI): The application of explainable AI models like GradCAM & LIME adds transparency & trust to AI-driven diagnoses by reasoning the prediction. Tuning AI systems is vital in order to gain patient and clinician trust (Ali et al., 2023).

Reasons for Benefits of Blockchain-Enabled AI in healthcare

- Better Diagnostic Accuracy: The Improved Diagnostic Accuracy from Portable AI Models Using Multiple Data Sources It utilizes model assembling and federated learning, two processes that enable the use of different datasets without compromising data privacy (Rahal et al., 2024).
- Decentralization and Data Sharing: While blockchain allows secure data to be shared across sectors in health care, creating composite datasets for robust machine-learning models. This distributed approach decreases the risk of centralized data storage (S. Wang et al., 2019).
- User Control: Patients have the ability to grant or revoke access to their data. The ethical use of data and patient autonomy are upheld as paramount principles; hence this is key.

Challenges and ethical considerations

- Data Bias and Discrimination: AI models can mirror biases in the training data, causing biased outcomes. To avoid these pitfalls, a diverse, representative dataset is critical (Curtis & Brolan, 2023).
- Issues of Regulation and Governance: The use of both blockchain and AI in healthcare will need strong governance frameworks to manage issues of privacy, security and ethics. In their absence, the potential remains for misuse of data and violations of privacy (Curtis & Brolan, 2023).
- Technical Limitations While blockchain and AI provide substantial advantages, there are also technical limitations, such as high-demand computational power and challenges in integrating these technologies into current healthcare systems (C. Wang et al., 2024).

Blockchain-Enabled AI Metaverse Models For Healthcare Come with Unique Challenges These technologies' full promise will be realized only if issues related to data bias, privacy, and governance can be tackled. The fourth, fifth, sixth and seventh hurdles: The Future of the Metaverse in Healthcare Although the integration of the metaverse in healthcare holds great promise, there also exist some challenges that will need to be addressed in order for the concept to succeed in the long run.

Internet of Medical Things (IoMT)

The Internet of Medical Things (IoMT), along with the metadata and cyber-layers as part of the metaverse healthcare ecosystem, presents significant security concerns that are key to the success of using blockchain technology. These concerns can be efficiently stored using Blockchain which gave it one of the best places to store data. Blockchain is one of the most significant enabling technologies of the Fourth Industrial Revolution; IoMT devices can create security vulnerabilities where sensitive health information could be exposed; Blockchain integration can allow to enhance security by immutability, decentralize control, and secured authentication mechanisms. In this answer, we take a closer look at the important elements associated with securing IoMT devices in metaverse healthcare ecosystems using blockchain.

Role Based Access and Authentication

- As a result, we could develop a role-based access framework employed over a blockchain to validate various participants of a healthcare ecosystem to provide role-based access to health data. This alternative reduces the burden on administrators but also raises the security through avoiding access to the non-authorized data sets. Dynamic access rights enable flexibility and security to the owner in this system (Aslam et al., 2024).
- This can greatly broaden the security offered by quantum secure authentication approaches embedded into the blockchain avoiding the requirement of third-party agency and/or the later exploitation of user functions by clinicians. It is resilient to all the attacks encountered by which it is security against communication security attacks in IoMT networks(Prajapat et al., 2024).

Data Integrity and Intrusion Detection

- In one of the research, they proposed an Integration of Blockchain with Intrusion Detection Systems (IDS) to safeguard IoMT networks. This coalition utilizing cryptographic hashes and decentralized peer-to-peer networks for data secrecy and integrity. It is proved to be resistant against DoS, impersonation and MITM attacks, having a very high accuracy at the threat detection process.

- Use of Blockchain in IoMT system also helps overcome data privacy challenges by sharing private information safely. Techniques such as encrypted K-means clustering and elliptic curve-based authentication protocols help in enhancing data privacy and protection against internal and external attacks (Lin, 2023).

Corroborated Communications and Information Shielding

- Certificateless aggregate signcryption schemes under blockchain enables data confidentiality and authentication in IoMT systems. In these schemes, fog computing is implemented to sign/unsigncrypt the data stating that we obtain a less resource-intensive secure communication channel (Tomar & Tripathi, 2023).
- Unlike traditional authentication processes, the smart contract-based schemes use the decentralization provided by blockchain with protection against the distributed denial service attack and are guaranteed integrity of information. They are providing secure firmware update and anti-counterfeiting, which ameliorate overall IoMT security.

Limitations and Future Work

- Nevertheless, data storage, architecture, standardization, security, and high computing power requirements are barriers to the integration of IoMT with blockchain in healthcare. Dealing with these issues requires innovative strategies that can facilitate security while maintaining practicality (Ahmed et al., 2024) (Lin, 2023).
- Designing and Developing Lightweight Blockchains in IoMT Devices: Future studies can focus on formulating solutions for lightweight blockchains that can be used in IoMT devices with lower computational power. Abstract Blockchain is a game-changing technology and when considered with some of the recent technologies like quantum computing, it could be a possible solution for securing metaverse healthcare ecosystem.

When metaverse is integrated into the healthcare ecosystem, possible solutions of Blockchain can secure IoMT, yet providers face limitations and challenges. IoMT devices have limited computational and storage capabilities, and hence, the requirements of the blockchain can become a burden for them. Therefore research and development still runs in the background so that new and good blockchain solutions can land where they can and should be best fitted.

Non-Fungible Tokens (NFTs)

The potential use cases for NFTs in health care are numerous, promising to solve some of the longest-standing issues facing the industry. NFTs or non-fungible tokens are unique digital assets and can help in securing, increasing the transparency and efficiency of the healthcare sector based on blockchain technology. Which means they can be used in different fields such as tracking medical records, certificates, and personalized treatment plans, among others. This response explains these possible applications and supports with new research insight.

Medical Records Management

- This means that for instance, you can integrate NFTs as a different perspective, and it allows you to access data through secured, trustworthy, and decentralized methods. As data is encrypted through this and stored in decentralized networks, cohesive and immutable proof of ownership, strengthens data security and decreasing the threat of manipulation or theft (Bendayan et al., 2024).
- When they share it, with whom they share it, and allowing them to maintain the high ground on their own health data, allowing a more democratic and transparent health information exchange (Kostick-Quenet et al., 2022).

Certification and Traceability

- NFTs can help provide authenticity and traceability certifications of medical devices, particularly for refurbished MDDs. We can use NFTs to ensure the safety and quality of these devices while also reducing the risk of counterfeiting and fraud by creating a secure, reliable and verifiable record of the refurbishment process.
- NFTs can be applied in the pharmaceutical industry for asset ownership and trading, creating a transparent and efficient system for tracking cases of provenance and authenticity of medical products (Srinivas & Pradhan, 2024).

Unique Treatment Plans

- This layer of NFT technology can then allow doctors to aggregate patient data across hospitals, clinics, and mHealth devices to then determine the best patient-specific treatment. Such a wealth of data allows for more accurate diagnosis, and a more tailored treatment pathway to be developed (Bendayan et al., 2024).

- Patients move from passive subjects to active entities that monitor and record their own health; patients guarantee, mediated by NFTs, access to care in the physical and digital dimensions (Bendayan et al., 2024).

Supply Chain Management

- Domestic energy crisis, protests in Haiti, NFTs for HC supply chain By using smart contracts ownership can also be ensured, enabling trade and delivery of healthcare products that can be traced, audited and verified by all.

Despite the broad application of NFTs in healthcare, it is important to examine the challenges and the constraints in utilizing them. Immediate considerations regarding ethical, technical and moral protection (eg, data, technological and transaction needs), all of which will be raised and interrogated in greater detail as medical technology matures (Bendayan et al., 2024) (Ali et al., 2023), will need to be overcome to help NFT release its untapped potentials in healthcare. In addition, incorporating non-fungible tokens (NFTs) into existing healthcare infrastructures will require careful consideration of interoperability and standardization to facilitate seamless implementation and operation.

SCALABILITY AND COST CHALLENGES

Deployment of metaverse healthcare is mostly limited by scalability and cost implications of integration of blockchain systems into the solution in question. The metaverse is an environment that immerses you in it, which means that it needs to store and process big datasets as fast as possible. On the one hand, blockchain can bring great advantages thanks to its decentralized and secure nature, but on the other hand, limitations exist that make blockchain scalability and cost-effective. This trust has serious implications for the efficiency & sustenance of usability of blockchain for metaverse healthcare applications. The sections below highlight these challenges, but we cover them in detail.

Scalability Challenges

- Data Volume and Transactional Throughput: Volumes of data produced in the metaverse need high transaction throughput and low latency. Existing blockchain systems including Ethereum and Filecoin cannot satisfy these requirements due to the insufficient throughput, which can degrade the performance of healthcare applications in metaverse (Fang et al., 2024) (Mazlan et al., 2020).

- Network Requirements: The immersive nature of the metaverse requires high bandwidth and low latency in transferring real-time healthcare. However, the existing architecture of blockchain could also be less suitable for meeting the demands of these networks, consequently leading to possible data communication and processing bottlenecks (Q. Wang et al., 2023).
- IoMT Combination: The Internet of Medical Things (IoMT) combines verticals to add yet a different set of scalability challenges. The high number of IoMT devices increases the complexity of the blockchain network, so there is a need for tailored scalable solutions to help with the high flows of data and transactions (Adavoudi Jolfaei et al., 2021).

Cost Challenges

- High Resource Consumption: The majority of the blockchains are high computational power and energy consuming blockchains. The metaverse is composed of data being processed 24/7 across vast landscapes and the result is high operational costs.
- Building Infrastructure — As the metaverse healthcare value grows, integrating blockchain could require substantial infrastructure expenditure. In a decentralized architecture, the hardware and software capabilities of healthcare providers play a significant role in determining whether privacy protocols can be established, and this does come with a price to pay for healthcare providers.
- Cloud Integration: While there is always the possibility for greater scalability and efficiency, the price of cloud computing and association is a drawback. It should combine the cost advantages of existing cloud services with the safety and privacy benefits of blockchain, by means of the natural fusion of systems (Ismail et al., 2021).

Possible Solutions and Things to Contemplate

- Storage Optimization and Redesign– Storage optimization and blockchain redesign, as some solutions, can fix scalability problems. Improvements in blockchain scalability are examples of these, such as off-chain storage and consensus mechanisms (Mazlan et al., 2020).
- Multipath Transmission: Research on multipath transmission architectures can provide benefits in terms of data flow optimization, latency reduction,

and also meeting the scalability requirements for metaverse healthcare applications (Q. Wang et al., 2023).

- Cloud Computing with Blockchain Integration (BcC):BcC is a solution that offers great promise to circumvent scalability and cost issues. It merges the advantages of both technologies, which allow to become the use of this tech as a health data management solution large-scale and economical(Ismail et al., 2021).

Though promising, the key strength of blockchain as a secure and decentralized method for data management in metaverse healthcare may be quenched by inherent scalability and cost challenges of blockchain. Much of these are perhaps challenges we need to address but the hybrid models and optimizing the current blockchain architectures can lead us forward. However, the full promise of blockchain will require that scalability, security, and cost trade-offs be managed to put these tools to use in metaverse healthcare systems.

REGULATORY AND ETHICAL CONSIDERATIONS

However, harnessing blockchain systems in the metaverse to provide healthcare services also involves the following unique, wider regulatory and ethical issues. In this context, the metaverse emerges as a potentially valuable platform for healthcare delivery with expected advantages in data security, patient empowerment, and access to quality healthcare. On the other hand, these innovations also introduce issues that must be dealt with to guarantee ethical and regulatory conformance. These considerations are examined in the sections that follow.

Regulatory Considerations

- Data Security and Privacy: Blockchain technology plays a crucial role in ensuring the security of medical data in the metaverse through privacy and integrity via decentralized data storage and cryptographic techniques such as zero-knowledge proofs and secure multi-party computation (Divyashree, 2024) (George & Kizhakkethottam, 2024). However, regulatory frameworks need to be developed that will allow for the innovation, scaling, and future-proofing of these technologies against forthcoming threats such as quantum computing (George & Kizhakkethottam, 2024).
- Regulatory Compliance: The compliance with healthcare regulations in place is also a requirement for metaverse healthcare solutions, which are often challenging to assure due to the borderless nature of virtual environments (Aditya

Shastry & Mohan, 2025). Policymakers must also work internationally to create comprehensive regulations that meet the complexities of metaverse healthcare.

- Interoperability and Integration: Integrating blockchain with existing healthcare systems necessitates substantial infrastructure investments and regulatory oversight to ensure interoperability and seamless data exchange (Aditya Shastry & Mohan, 2025).

Ethical Considerations

- Blockchain enables more control of data for patients, which would contribute to a more patient centric approach in the metaverse (Divyashree, 2024) (George & Kizhakkethottam, 2024). Ethical frameworks should guarantee respectful treatment of patients' autonomy regarding informed consent about use and sharing of their data.
- These principles include the following: Bioethical Principles: The employment of metaverse technology in healthcare should be guided by bioethical principles such as beneficence, nonmaleficence, autonomy, and justice (Gaur et al., 2023). These principles ensure reduced risks of negative consequences and equitable access to a health service.
- The immersive nature of the metaverse heightens the ethical challenges of access who is granted access to whom, fairness the degree to which the metaverse's content and experience represents an equitable and just perspective, discrimination and privacy. This complexity makes a careful re-examination of the ethical frameworks that currently underpin much of executed digital medicine necessary to meet these challenges.

Here is the one-liner:Regulations and ethical concerns must be addressed to harness the true features of blockchain systems in metaverse healthcare. Navigating these challenges, however, will require the establishment of new laws specifically governing the metaverse, along with an ethical framework to draw upon as a guidepost in the development of new healthcare networks.

FUTURE USE CASES IN METAVERSE HEALTHCARE

The metaverse, a cutting-edge immersive virtual space system, is set to transform healthcare because it provides solutions in many areas. The combination of XR with advanced technologies, such as virtual reality (VR), augmented reality (AR), artificial intelligence (AI), and blockchain, provides many possible future applications in healthcare. Applications may include improving medical education, providing psychosocial support, or aiding patient care. While these are exciting possibilities, the metaverse offers many challenges and the adoption of such a technology will require significant thinking through.

Medical Education and Training

- The metaverse can be used to create an immersive, engaging virtual implementation of real world medical education where students as well as professionals can have a realistic simulation experience and even a way to train themselves to dynamically solve problems with the help of dynamic scenarios without any geographical limitations.
- These technologies can simulate elaborate complex surgeries — providing a safe and controlled environment to practice (Morgan, 2024).
- Digital twins in the metaverse can be used to device personalized treatment plans and increase diagnostic accuracy (Morgan, 2024).

Psychosocial Support

- It provides a well-suited platform to provide psychosocial support for patients, especially those with rare diseases or those patients undergoing extended treatment. For example, avatar-mediated experiences for paediatric and adolescent cancer patients have shown to mitigate stigma and provide emotional relief (Hasei et al., 2024).
- For chronic patients who rely on community, virtual support communities within the metaverse can help significantly, as it enables patients to connect with peers, share experiences, and gain emotional support from fellow patients, thus, helping them form a sense of community and fostering a sense of belonging (Hasei et al., 2024).

Patient Care and Management

- In healthcare, the metaverse and AI can increase patient care via some integrated AI avatars for telemedicine, advanced patient monitoring, and remote patient management (Morgan, 2024).
- Some examples of the application of the metaverse can be, in fertility clinics offering virtual tours & simulations for patients to understand the procedures better (Morgan, 2024).

- Wearables in the Metaverse can assist in remote management and therapeutic treatment of patients, enhancing the ability to provide quality care and improve patient outcomes.

Mental Health Applications

- VR and AR interventions in the metaverse can help treat and diagnose mental health disorders like phobias, anxiety, and PTSD.
- Virtual mental health clinics and group therapy sessions in the metaverse can deliver real-time, on-demand support and therapy (8) expanding access to mental health services in new innovative and effective ways.

The metaverse can offer promising solutions to the way healthcare centres operate, but it also poses unique challenges involving data privacy, security and ethical concerns. Patient trust: The technologies of the metaverse need to be woven together carefully to address these issues to permit safe delivery to the patient. In addition, it is essential to work toward closing the digital divide and addressing technological gaps to ensure equitable access to metaverse-based health care solutions for everyone, no matter the socioeconomic standing or national borders. The evolution of the metaverse throughout these, as well as the continued alignment with industry stakeholders, will be paramount to realize this potential for health.

RECENT TECHNIQUES IN BLOCKCHAIN-ENABLED METAVERSE HEALTHCARE

The above ash note reflects how far we have come in healthcare technology in the last couple of years with regards to the degree of integration of blockchain in metaverse to enhance patient care, data management and delivery of care. However, the metaverse experience requires a high degree of data security and security due to the inherent sensitivity of health information, information that is best protected using a decentralized, unchangeable blockchain ledger system. Automation: Transparency and Trust: Tech like smart contracts provide rule-based access control tht enables automated and secured transaction, leading to increased trust between stakeholders in the healthcare value chain. In addition, decentralized identity (DID), self-sovereign identity (SSI approaches provide patients complete ownership and control of their health data, enabling secure and seamless interoperability between multiple metaverse platforms. Further data confidentiality is available through advanced encryption techniques like Zero-Knowledge proofs and chaotic encryption. Simultaneously, the intersection of both tracks yields blockchain-powered explainable Ai models for real-time accurate diagnostics, and implenting multi-layer IoMT fortified by the blockchain for real-time monitoring of health parameters. Emerging use cases in the form of non-fungible tokens (NFTs) are also being developed for medical record management, device certifications, and customized treatment plans. Although such initiatives represent key steps forward, however, there remain considerable barriers to the adoption and effective use of blockchain in metaverse healthcare. While existing high transaction volume and data in real-time healthcare applications require high throughput and low latency, scalability continues to be a challenge; these are two areas that challenge much existing blockchain frameworks. Inadequate protocol encryption or systems that are not integrated can lead to complications with interoperability which can prevent efficient data transfer across many platforms. 2) Resource constraints: Deploying a blockchain requires expensive computational power and infrastructure to get started with Access, a potential roadblock in favour of developing regions. And there are ethical and privacy issues such as the possibility of dehumanizing treatment and worsening the digital divide that will require careful consideration. Regulatory compliance presents another hard problem, as old laws for healthcare and data governance may be unable to keep up with metaverse realities resulting in unfettered movement across borders. Additionally, the high energy consumption and operating costs of the blockchain technology pose doubts on sustainability in the long run.

The Intended goals to overcome these challenges includes building scalable and metaverse-based clinical blockchain architectures for healthcare applications with high privacy, security, and patient autonomy. A core aim is to enhance person-centered care, which regulation will help facilitate through individualized treatment plans existing alongside decentralization of digital identities allowing individual citizens agency over their data. The emergence of federated blockchain networks and standardized protocols will increase interoperability and will be crucial to achieving effective healthy ecosystems across multiple metaverse platforms. This framework to securely mix or link AI and IoMT aims to increase diagnostic accuracy, and enable continuous patient monitoring. And ethical regulatory frameworks around the governance of data must ensure patient rights, promote equity of access, and guide the governance of data. Moreover, off-chain storage wrapper like hybridization will help to optimize blockchain working (e.g. blockchain-cloud integration) will increase & cost benefits (these hybridization-based techs are easier and more achievable to tons of healthcare providers to adapt real-world-wise. The performance fronts on which the existing metaverse healthcare models enabled by blockchain are largely evaluated include data security, system scalability, interoperability, patient empowerment and operational efficiency. Cryptographic guarantees for high confidentiality and integrity, distributed storage and consensus optimization for high throughput but low latency. Features that put the patient at the centre such as decentralized identity management enhance transparency and trust, resulting in better engagement with healthcare providers and shared decision-making. Also addressed are cost-effective solutions, with architectural innovations that will allow lower computation overhead, and better utilization of cloud resources that will lower energy and infrastructure costs. The combined use of explainable AI models under the blockchain umbrella improves diagnostic reliability through a transparent rationale which is a prerequisite for clinical deployment and patient trust.

By contrast, healthcare data systems today are notorious for centralized models that fail on numerous fronts, from security to transparency to patient control–all of which can be enabled with blockchain-based metaverse models. While existing blockchain solution face challenges due to the lack of solution scalability and interoperability, the proposed approaches integrating decentralized identity and hybrid storage mechanisms in this context indicates remarkable progress on how to seamlessly gain access to large scale and highly efficient healthcare data storage through the unique health data identifier. In addition, other existing systems are not able to combine several limited features for practical realization, unlike the proposed one, where blockchain integration with AI and IoMT emphasizes high diagnostic potential and real-time monitoring. Furthermore, the proposed model emphasizes comprehensive governance frameworks and further demonstrates how previous approaches often miss ethical and regulatory considerations necessary for an ethical and fair delivery of healthcare in the metaverse.

Table 1. Comparative Analysis with Existing Techniques

Aspect	Existing Techniques	Proposed Model Highlights	Advantage / Improvement
Data Security	Centralized databases prone to breaches	Decentralized, immutable blockchain ledger	Higher trust, tamper-proof data storage
Scalability	Limited throughput in blockchain	Distributed storage, blockchain-cloud hybrid	Improved scalability, lower latency
Patient Control	Limited patient data ownership	Decentralized Identity, Self-Sovereign Identity	Empowered patients with data ownership
Interoperability	Fragmented healthcare systems	Blockchain federations and standardized DID	Seamless cross-platform data exchange
AI Integration	AI with limited transparency	Explainable AI integrated with blockchain	Increased trust and explainability
Cost Efficiency	High infrastructure and operational cost	Off-chain storage and cloud integration	Reduced computational and storage costs
Ethical Considerations	Under-addressed in traditional models	Frameworks emphasizing patient autonomy and equity	Responsible and fair healthcare delivery

CONCLUSION AND RESEARCH ROADMAP

This combination of blockchain technology with metaverse healthcare can open up new avenues to transform the way we deliver care, manage data, and streamline operations. Utilizing the inherent strengths of blockchain in areas such as security, transparency, and decentralization, metaverse health care has the potential to overcome significant challenges like data privacy, interoperability, and trust among stakeholders. If this ecosystem develops, research will need to work towards sustainable best practices that provide scalability, cost-effectiveness, and accessibility while still engaging in equitable and ethical practices. Next-generation technologies such as AI, IoMT, and NFTs to extend the capabilities of Blockchain create way for Customization in care, secure connectivity of devices, and transformative use cases in medical applications. To make these advancements a reality, however, we will first have to jump some hurdles namely regulatory complexities and energy consumption, as well as educating the public about these technologies. So, the future of healthcare in the metaverse with blockchain will depend on experts from various fields of technology, health care, politics and ethics getting together. Collectively, they can create strong frameworks that enables seamless incorporation of blockchain within healthcare ecosystems that are inclusive, resilient, and able to withstand Realtime future disruptions. Leveraging the clarity of a well-defined research roadmap and tackling the mentioned challenges, this amalgamation of technologies can bring about a paradigm shift in healthcare, making it patient-centric, process-oriented, as well as creating a global, connected, and secure health ecosystem.

REFERENCES

Adavoudi Jolfaei, A., Aghili, S. F., & Singelee, D. (2021). A Survey on Blockchain-Based IoMT Systems: Towards Scalability. *IEEE Access : Practical Innovations, Open Solutions*, *9*, 148948–148975. DOI: 10.1109/ACCESS.2021.3117662

Aditya Shastry, K., & Mohan, S. G. (2025). The Metaverse in Healthcare: Emerging Technologies, Challenges, and Research Directions. In Chhabra, G., & Kaushik, K. (Eds.), *Understanding the Metaverse* (pp. 113–135). Springer Nature Singapore., DOI: 10.1007/978-981-97-2278-5_6

Ahmed, S. F., & Alam, Md. S. B., Afrin, S., Rafa, S. J., Rafa, N., & Gandomi, A. H. (2024). Insights into Internet of Medical Things (IoMT): Data fusion, security issues and potential solutions. *Information Fusion*, *102*, 102060. DOI: 10.1016/j.inffus.2023.102060

Alanazi, A. A., Karim, F. K., Ghorashi, S. A., Amoudi, G., & Hamza, S. H. A. (2024). Blockchain with optimal deep learning assisted secure data sharing and classification on future healthcare systems. *Alexandria Engineering Journal*, *99*, 168–179. DOI: 10.1016/j.aej.2024.05.023

Ali, S., Abdullah, Armand, T. P. T., Athar, A., Hussain, A., Ali, M., Yaseen, M., Joo, M.-I., & Kim, H.-C. (2023). Metaverse in Healthcare Integrated with Explainable AI and Blockchain: Enabling Immersiveness, Ensuring Trust, and Providing Patient Data Security. *Sensors (Basel)*, *23*(2), 565. DOI: 10.3390/s23020565 PMID: 36679361

Aslam, M. S., Altaf, A., Iqbal, F., Nigar, N., Galán, J. C., Aray, D. G., Díez, I. D. L. T., & Ashraf, I. (2024). Novel model to authenticate role-based medical users for blockchain-based IoMT devices. *PLoS One*, *19*(7), e0304774. DOI: 10.1371/journal.pone.0304774 PMID: 38985779

Aujoulat, I., Young, B., & Salmon, P. (2012). The psychological processes involved in patient empowerment. *Orphanet Journal of Rare Diseases*, *7*(Suppl 2), A31. DOI: 10.1186/1750-1172-7-S2-A31

Bak, O., Braganza, A., & Chen, W. (2023). Exploring blockchain implementation challenges in the context of healthcare supply chain (HCSC). *International Journal of Production Research*, •••, 1–16. DOI: 10.1080/00207543.2023.2286491

Bendayan, S., Cohen, Y., Bendayan, J., Windisch, S., & Afilalo, J. (2024). Nonfungible Tokens in Cardiovascular Medicine. *The Canadian Journal of Cardiology*, *40*(10), 1959–1964. DOI: 10.1016/j.cjca.2024.07.010 PMID: 39032555

Chen, X., He, G., & Li, Q. (2024). Can Fintech development improve the financial inclusion of village and township banks? Evidence from China. *Pacific-Basin Finance Journal*, *85*, 102324. DOI: 10.1016/j.pacfin.2024.102324

Chengoden, R., Victor, N., Huynh-The, T., Yenduri, G., Jhaveri, R. H., Alazab, M., Bhattacharya, S., Hegde, P., Maddikunta, P. K. R., & Gadekallu, T. R. (2023). Metaverse for Healthcare: A Survey on Potential Applications, Challenges and Future Directions. *IEEE Access : Practical Innovations, Open Solutions*, *11*, 12765–12795. DOI: 10.1109/ACCESS.2023.3241628

Curtis, C., & Brolan, C. E. (2023). Health care in the metaverse. *The Medical Journal of Australia*, *218*(1), 46–46. DOI: 10.5694/mja2.51793 PMID: 36437589

Dewangan, N. K., & Chandrakar, P. (2023). Patient-Centric Token-Based Healthcare Blockchain Implementation Using Secure Internet of Medical Things. *IEEE Transactions on Computational Social Systems*, *10*(6), 3109–3119. DOI: 10.1109/TCSS.2022.3194872

Divyashree, K. S. (2024). Blockchain Application on Healthcare Services in Metaverse. In Hiran, K. K., Doshi, R., & Patel, M. (Eds.), *Advances in Medical Education, Research, and Ethics* (pp. 141–158). IGI Global., DOI: 10.4018/979-8-3693-5493-3.ch009

Fang, G., Sun, Y., Almutiq, M., Zhou, W., Zhao, Y., & Ren, Y. (2024). Distributed Medical Data Storage Mechanism Based on Proof of Retrievability and Vector Commitment for Metaverse Services. *IEEE Journal of Biomedical and Health Informatics*, *28*(11), 6298–6307. DOI: 10.1109/JBHI.2023.3272021 PMID: 37126619

Gaur, L., Gaur, D., & Afaq, A. (2023). Ethical Considerations in the Use of the Metaverse for Healthcare. In Gaur, L., & Jhanjhi, N. Z. (Eds.), (pp. 248–273). Advances in Medical Technologies and Clinical Practice. IGI Global., DOI: 10.4018/978-1-6684-9823-1.ch008

George, L., & Kizhakkethottam, J. J. (2024). Unleashing the Future of Healthcare in the Metaverse: The Pivotal Role of Blockchain in Data Privacy. In Nijalingappa, P., Gururaj, T., Goyal, S. B., Shukla, V., & Bruno, A. (Eds.), (pp. 77–102). Advances in Medical Technologies and Clinical Practice. IGI Global., DOI: 10.4018/979-8-3693-1515-6.ch004

Han, D., Yu, D., & Qiu, J. (2023). Assessing coupling interactions in a safe and just operating space for regional sustainability. *Nature Communications*, *14*(1), 1369. DOI: 10.1038/s41467-023-37073-z PMID: 36914668

Hasei, J., Ishida, H., Katayama, H., Maeda, N., Nagano, A., Ochi, M., Okamura, M., Iwata, S., Ikuta, K., Yoshida, S., Fujiwara, T., Nakata, E., Nakahara, R., Kunisada, T., & Ozaki, T. (2024). Utilizing the Metaverse to Provide Innovative Psychosocial Support for Pediatric, Adolescent, and Young Adult Patients with Rare Cancer. *Cancers (Basel)*, *16*(15), 2617. DOI: 10.3390/cancers16152617 PMID: 39123345

He, Q., Feng, Z., Fang, H., Wang, X., Zhao, L., Yao, Y., & Yu, K. (2024). A Blockchain-Based Scheme for Secure Data Offloading in Healthcare With Deep Reinforcement Learning. *IEEE/ACM Transactions on Networking*, *32*(1), 65–80. DOI: 10.1109/TNET.2023.3274631

Hylock, R. H., & Zeng, X. (2019). A Blockchain Framework for Patient-Centered Health Records and Exchange (HealthChain): Evaluation and Proof-of-Concept Study. *Journal of Medical Internet Research*, *21*(8), e13592. DOI: 10.2196/13592 PMID: 31471959

Ismail, L., Materwala, H., & Hennebelle, A. (2021). A Scoping Review of Integrated Blockchain-Cloud (BcC) Architecture for Healthcare: Applications, Challenges and Solutions. *Sensors (Basel)*, *21*(11), 3753. DOI: 10.3390/s21113753 PMID: 34071449

Jena, S. K., Barik, R. C., & Priyadarshini, R. (2024). A systematic state-of-art review on digital identity challenges with solutions using conjugation of IOT and blockchain in healthcare. *Internet of Things : Engineering Cyber Physical Human Systems*, *25*, 101111. DOI: 10.1016/j.iot.2024.101111

Kostick-Quenet, K., Mandl, K. D., Minssen, T., Cohen, I. G., Gasser, U., Kohane, I., & McGuire, A. L. (2022). How NFTs could transform health information exchange. *Science*, *375*(6580), 500–502. DOI: 10.1126/science.abm2004 PMID: 35113709

Lax, G., Nardone, R., & Russo, A. (2024). Enabling secure health information sharing among healthcare organizations by public blockchain. *Multimedia Tools and Applications*, *83*(24), 64795–64811. DOI: 10.1007/s11042-024-18181-4

Lin, J. (2023). Study on Brand Management of Fashion Brands. *Advances in Economics. Management and Political Sciences*, *55*(1), 24–29. DOI: 10.54254/2754-1169/55/20230955

Liu, S., Liu, C., & Lang, C. (2024). Consumer Engagement in Fashion Circularity in China: Exploring Consumer Online Fashion Resale through the Lens of Social Practice Theory. *Sustainability*, *16*(11), 4733. DOI: 10.3390/su16114733

Mazlan, A. A., Mohd Daud, S., Mohd Sam, S., Abas, H., Abdul Rasid, S. Z., & Yusof, M. F. (2020). Scalability Challenges in Healthcare Blockchain System—A Systematic Review. *IEEE Access : Practical Innovations, Open Solutions, 8*, 23663–23673. DOI: 10.1109/ACCESS.2020.2969230

McCourt, C. (2024). Exploring the intersection of the medical metaverse and healthcare ethics: Future considerations and caveats. *Global Health Journal (Amsterdam, Netherlands), 8*(1), 36–40. DOI: 10.1016/j.glohj.2024.02.005

Morgan, J. (2024). P-462 Exploring the potential of fertility clinics in the metaverse: Opportunities, challenges, and ethical implications. *Human Reproduction, 39*(Supplement_1), deae108.292. https://doi.org/DOI: 10.1093/humrep/deae108.292

Nadarasa, A. (2024). Social prescribing in the metaverse: A new frontier for primary care practice. *Global Health Journal (Amsterdam, Netherlands), 8*(1), 32–35. DOI: 10.1016/j.glohj.2024.02.006

Prajapat, S., Kumar, P., Kumar, D., Kumar Das, A., Shamim Hossain, M., & Rodrigues, J. J. P. C. (2024). Quantum Secure Authentication Scheme for Internet of Medical Things Using Blockchain. *IEEE Internet of Things Journal, 11*(23), 38496–38507. DOI: 10.1109/JIOT.2024.3448212

Qiu, C. S., Majeed, A., Khan, S., & Watson, M. (2022). Transforming health through the metaverse. *Journal of the Royal Society of Medicine, 115*(12), 484–486. DOI: 10.1177/01410768221144763 PMID: 36480946

Rafique, W., & Qadir, J. (2024). Internet of everything meets the metaverse: Bridging physical and virtual worlds with blockchain. *Computer Science Review, 54*, 100678. DOI: 10.1016/j.cosrev.2024.100678

Rahal, H. R., Slatnia, S., Kazar, O., Barka, E., & Harous, S. (2024). Blockchain-based multi-diagnosis deep learning application for various diseases classification. *International Journal of Information Security, 23*(1), 15–30. DOI: 10.1007/s10207-023-00733-8

Rahaman, Md. T., Pranta, A. D., Repon, Md. R., Ahmed, Md. S., & Islam, T. (2024). Green production and consumption of textiles and apparel: Importance, fabrication, challenges and future prospects. *Journal of Open Innovation, 10*(2), 100280. DOI: 10.1016/j.joitmc.2024.100280

Sestino, A., & D'Angelo, A. (2023). My doctor is an avatar! The effect of anthropomorphism and emotional receptivity on individuals' intention to use digital-based healthcare services. *Technological Forecasting and Social Change, 191*, 122505. DOI: 10.1016/j.techfore.2023.122505

Skalidis, I., Maurizi, N., Kaldasch, M., El Idrissi, B., Briante, N., Fournier, S., Muller, O., & Skalidis, E. (2022). Feasibility of clinical and electrocardiographic follow-up of prinzmetal angina using the metaverse. *European Heart Journal - Digital Health, 3*(4), ztac076.2817. https://doi.org/DOI: 10.1093/ehjdh/ztac076.2817

Srinivas, O., & Pradhan, N. R. (2024). A Novel NFT Framework for Pharmaceutical Asset Ownership and Trading: TokenPharma. *IEEE Access : Practical Innovations, Open Solutions, 12*, 171418–171433. DOI: 10.1109/ACCESS.2024.3500092

Sun, N., Cao, B., & Mu, X. (2024). Research on the Future Trends of the Integration of Artificial Intelligence and Fashion Design of Clothing. *Applied Mathematics and Nonlinear Sciences, 9*(1), 20242181. DOI: 10.2478/amns-2024-2181

Szczepaniuk, H., & Szczepaniuk, E. K. (2023). Cryptographic evidence-based cybersecurity for smart healthcare systems. *Information Sciences, 649*, 119633. DOI: 10.1016/j.ins.2023.119633

Tomar, A., & Tripathi, S. (2023). BCSoM: Blockchain-based certificateless aggregate signcryption scheme for Internet of Medical Things. *Computer Communications, 212*, 48–62. DOI: 10.1016/j.comcom.2023.09.027

Ullah, H., Manickam, S., Obaidat, M., Laghari, S. U. A., & Uddin, M. (2023). Exploring the Potential of Metaverse Technology in Healthcare: Applications, Challenges, and Future Directions. *IEEE Access : Practical Innovations, Open Solutions, 11*, 69686–69707. DOI: 10.1109/ACCESS.2023.3286696

Wang, C., Wang, L., Zhao, S., Yang, C., & Albitar, K. (2024). The impact of Fintech on corporate carbon emissions: Towards green and sustainable development. *Business Strategy and the Environment, 33*(6), 5776–5796. DOI: 10.1002/bse.3778

Wang, Q., Liu, C., & Lan, S. (2023). Digital literacy and financial market participation of middle-aged and elderly adults in China. *Economic and Political Studies, 11*(4), 441–468. DOI: 10.1080/20954816.2022.2115191

Wang, S., Zhang, D., & Zhang, Y. (2019). Blockchain-Based Personal Health Records Sharing Scheme With Data Integrity Verifiable. *IEEE Access : Practical Innovations, Open Solutions, 7*, 102887–102901. DOI: 10.1109/ACCESS.2019.2931531

Xu, S. (2024). Research on financial innovation and Risk Management in the digital Economy Era. *Applied Mathematics and Nonlinear Sciences, 9*(1), 20242488. DOI: 10.2478/amns-2024-2488

Zhuang, Y., Shyu, C.-R., Hong, S., Li, P., & Zhang, L. (2023). Self-sovereign identity empowered non-fungible patient tokenization for health information exchange using blockchain technology. *Computers in Biology and Medicine*, *157*, 106778. DOI: 10.1016/j.compbiomed.2023.106778 PMID: 36934533

Chapter 9

Navigating the Ethico-Legal Landscape of Blockchain in Healthcare: A Critical Analysis

Ananya Pandey
https://orcid.org/0000-0002-2419-6314
Christ University, India

ABSTRACT

Blockchain technology offers improved data security, interoperability, and patient empowerment, which could revolutionize the healthcare industry. Its incorporation, however, calls for thorough evaluation of the complicated legal and ethical issues. The global pandemic has exposed the current healthcare system's lack of interoperability and the requirement for reliable clinical data that can be efficiently and securely disseminated to healthcare providers on a large scale. This analysis explores important issues such as algorithmic bias, informed consent, data privacy and ownership, and legal barriers. It looks at current regulatory frameworks and new best practices for using blockchain responsibly in the healthcare industry, highlighting the necessity of stakeholder collaboration to guarantee safe, reliable, and equitable healthcare systems. In light of the above perspective, this chapter explores the ethical and legal implications of blockchain in the healthcare sector. It critically overviews the current laws and regulations in force to implement blockchain in healthcare.

DOI: 10.4018/979-8-3373-1225-5.ch009

INTRODUCTION

Blockchain technology records data in a way that makes it difficult or impossible for the system to be altered, compromised, or manipulated. It is a distributed ledger that replicates transactions among the participating computers in the network (Srivastava, 2019). Blockchain technology is a system that keeps public transactional records, or blocks, in several databases, or the "chain," in a network that is connected by peer-to-peer nodes. This type of storage is commonly known as a "digital ledger" (Collomb & Sok, 2016). The digital signature of the owner authenticates each transaction in this ledger and prevents manipulation through authorization. Because of this, the data in the digital ledger is extremely safe. With the use of this technology, transactions cannot be changed or removed once they have been recorded without the consent of all network users. Three essential features—decentralization, immutability, and transparency—are at the center of blockchain's core ideas (Kumar et al., 2023). Blockchain technology has become a potent instrument for improving accountability and transparency in corporate governance, especially in transaction tracking and financial reporting. Organizations can guarantee that financial data is more dependable, verifiable, and accessible by utilizing its special qualities (Paik et al., 2019).

Blockchain is an innovative technology that is being used to develop creative solutions in a number of industries, including healthcare. The healthcare system uses a blockchain network to store and share patient data amongst doctors, diagnostic labs, pharmacies, and hospitals. In the medical area, blockchain applications can precisely detect serious errors, even those that are harmful (Haleem et al., 2021). As a result, it can enhance the efficiency, safety, and openness of medical data exchange throughout the healthcare system. Medical institutions can improve the analysis of medical records and obtain new insights with the help of this technology. Blockchain is essential in combating clinical trial fraud; in this case, the technology has the ability to increase healthcare data efficiency. It offers a distinct data storage pattern at the highest level of security and can help allay concerns about data manipulation in the healthcare industry. It offers adaptability, connectivity, responsibility, and data access authentication. Health records need to be kept private and secure for various reasons. Blockchain prevents some dangers and aids in the decentralized safeguarding of healthcare data (Andrew et al., 2023). However, concerns like data ownership and control over data processing and storage are relevant in blockchains and pose an ethical conundrum. It is also necessary to address concerns about data subjects' rights to access, confirm, and request correction of their personal data. In light of the above perspective, this chapter explores the substantial advantages of blockchain technology in the medical field. It also critically examines the associated difficulties, moral dilemmas, and legal issues.

BLOCKCHAIN IN HEALTHCARE: AN OVERVIEW

Blockchain technology aids marketers in keeping track of medical product usage. Blockchain technologies will help the pharmaceutical and health industries eradicate fake drugs and make it possible to track down all of these products (Uddin et al., 2021). It aids in identifying the root reason of false information. Patient records can be kept private because of blockchain technology; once a medical history is created, it can be stored on the blockchain and cannot be altered. The hospital's commodity hardware is all connected to this decentralized network (Haleem et al., 2021).

Core Principles

It is essential to comprehend the fundamentals, workings, and benefits of blockchain technology in order to promote its adoption in a variety of sectors, including digital health, retail, advertising and marketing, and financial services.

Decentralization

A decentralized blockchain network eliminates the need for people to know or trust one another. Every individual within the network possesses a duplicate of the identical data in the form of a distributed ledger (Tripathi et al., 2023). The majority of network members will reject a member's ledger if it is changed or corrupted in any way. Businesses have recognized the opportunity for innovation and adaptation in response to the decentralization trend. In addition to being in line with consumer values of autonomy and democratic justice, embracing decentralization offers companies the chance to enter new markets, create cutting-edge goods and services, and apply decentralized governance models inside their own companies (Darvishmotevali, 2019).

Immutability

Ideally, one would want to maintain a precise record of occurrences and ensure that it doesn't deteriorate over time as a result of fraud, human mistake, or natural disasters. Digital information can be updated regularly to stop deterioration, but physical objects can alter over time. Maintaining a digital history that doesn't change over time is the goal of implementing an immutable blockchain (Peppet, 2011). Businesses find this particularly helpful when determining who owns an asset, determining its legitimacy, or verifying one or more transactions. An unchangeable record of transactions is essential for legal and corporate regulation purposes because it streamlines these procedures and can save time and money. Hashing techniques are used to encode data in a well-designed blockchain. This guarantees that a transaction can only be verified by those who possess adequate knowledge (Ma et al., 2018).

Transparency

Consensus and governance systems must function transparently for businesses to generate the intended audience engagement for blockchain, as well as eventual mainstream acceptance and success. In order to determine what can be saved and potentially shared on-chain, users must be aware of who has access to what data (Hussein et al., 2023). Users agree to share their data under these contractual terms. Consumers might be forced to exercise the right for their data to be destroyed, which normally is a capability offered via auxiliary, 'off-chain' databases (Pandey and Joseph, 2025). On the other hand, only hashed data—which is essentially meaningless—is kept on-chain indefinitely (Andrew et al., 2023). Another essential quality that users and customers rightfully look for is trust, in addition to openness. Since systems must also be trusted, trust must extend beyond the individuals involved (Kuo et al., 2019).

Applications of Blockchain in Healthcare

With the patient at the core of the healthcare ecosystem and improved security, privacy, and interoperability of health data, blockchain technology has the potential to revolutionize the medical field. By improving the efficiency, disintermediation, and security of electronic medical data, this technology may offer a new paradigm for health information exchanges. Some of the potent applications of blockchain technology in healthcare are classified below.

Maintaining Electronic Health Records

Accessing health care services across several hospitals or clinics for diagnosis and treatment has become increasingly widespread because of the rising specialization of health care services and high levels of patient mobility, especially for patients with chronic conditions (Starfield et al., 2005). The blockchain network's synchronous nodes are able to detect data changes instantly and forbid data manipulation. The blockchain-based health data storage system is a key telemedicine trend that will be essential to maintaining patient privacy and legitimacy (Ghosh et al., 2023; Pandey & Joseph, 2025b). In order to better patient diagnosis and treatment globally, hospitals and other key stakeholders in the healthcare sector can exchange medical information about patients using Electronic Health Record (EHR) systems, which are a useful and efficient tool. An important turning point in healthcare technology, EHR systems have drastically changed how patient health information is maintained and made available (Velmurugun et al., 2024). Large amounts of patient data, including prescriptions, treatment plans, medical histories, and diagnoses, are digitized and consolidated by these systems. EHRs improve provider-to-provider communication, streamline workflows, and enhance patient care by providing rapid access to critical data (Ratwani, 2017). They make it easier for patients to access their medical records, encourage data-driven decision-making to provide individualized treatment, and enable the safe exchange of information.

Medical Data Exchange for Patients

An "isolated island of information" exists in the medical profession as a result of traditional medical records being kept in the central databases of different hospitals (Mackey et al., 2019; Xie et al., 2021). Blockchain gives patients access to their medical records and gives them the freedom to give third parties access to their EHRs as they see fit. Regardless of when and where medical services are rendered, health care practitioners have simple access to all patient medical data (Fan et al., 2018). The healthcare system uses a blockchain network to store and share patient data amongst doctors, diagnostic labs, pharmacies, and hospitals. In the medical area, blockchain applications can precisely detect serious errors, even those that are harmful (Haleem et al., 2021).

Analyzing the effect of procedure on a patient

Verified access to patient data allows researchers to analyze any given procedure on a sizable portion of the patient population. This yields noteworthy outcomes that improve the way certain patient groups are managed (Khatoon, 2020). Pharmaceutical companies will collect data in real-time with the Blockchain infrastructure in order to provide patients with a variety of precisely tailored prescription medications or services (Vaishya et al., 2021). Because blockchain contains all the data on top of it, it makes pharmacies' jobs easier. Based on these findings, they will effectively advise patients on how to take the prescription. Using wearable data collected in real-time, it will notify clinicians of any emergencies and provide them with an update on the patient's current status (Haleem et al., 2021).

Information Display

To guarantee high quality and that the maker of the authorized drug is supplying it, the Blockchain system will show details about the medication's origins. When utilized properly, blockchain offers more protection for private information than before (Haleem et al., 2021). The Blockchain app trend has been used by a number of industries, including finance, retail, and immobilization, and it offers numerous advantages for information display. It is also believed that healthcare is complex and multifaceted (Zarour et al., 2020). There will be serious disagreements about this proclamation. Due to its intricacy, the industry has experienced significant advancements in a number of areas, including the adoption of cloud computing, clinical trials, pharmaceuticals, vaccines, and medical products (Khujamatov et al., 2020).

Supply Chain Tracking for Pharmaceuticals

There are numerous advantages to using a blockchain-powered supply chain. It provides a comprehensive description of the complete process from beginning to end. The entire supply chain can be managed by a single piece of software (Akram et al., 2024). With consent, it also improves communication between parties. Another significant advantage of blockchain is the increased security and traceability it provides. Products may be tracked, traced, and recalled via a blockchain system. Transactions involving pharmaceutical drugs may be tracked from suppliers of raw materials to final customers because of blockchain-based pharmaceutical supply chain management (Ahmed & MacCarthy, 2023). Because of its transparency, immutability, and auditability, the pharmaceutical blockchain has promise for improving the supply chain's security, integrity, data provenance, and functioning (Longo et al., 2019).

BENEFITS AND CHALLENGES OF BLOCKCHAIN IN HEALTHCARE

Blockchain technology offers transformative potential in healthcare by enhancing data security, interoperability, and transparency. Its decentralized structure allows secure, tamper-proof sharing of patient records among authorized stakeholders, improving care coordination and reducing administrative burdens. Smart contracts automate processes such as insurance claims and consent management, increasing efficiency and reducing costs. Blockchain also bolsters data integrity in clinical trials, supply chain traceability for pharmaceuticals, and real-time health monitoring.

However, several challenges hinder its widespread adoption. Technical issues such as scalability, energy consumption, and integration with legacy systems limit practical deployment. Data privacy regulations like HIPAA and GDPR pose compliance hurdles due to the immutable nature of blockchain records. Additionally, the lack of standardized frameworks and industry-wide collaboration complicates interoperability. High implementation costs and the need for specialized knowledge further discourage adoption, especially in resource-limited settings. Moreover, ethical concerns regarding patient consent and data ownership remain unresolved. Despite these challenges, with the right regulatory support and technological advancements, blockchain holds promise to revolutionize healthcare delivery by making it more secure, transparent, and patient-centric.

Potential Benefits

Better data security, transparency, and effective claims processing are just a few of the many advantages that blockchain provides the healthcare sector.

Cost Savings

By improving interoperability, expediting data interchange, and simplifying administrative duties, blockchain technology can drastically lower operating costs in the healthcare industry. Healthcare providers can save money by using blockchain technology to automate a number of manual and paper-based procedures, including claims processing, medication supply chain management, and medical record exchange (Fatoum et al., 2021). Additionally, blockchain can offer real-time tracking of the movements of pharmaceuticals and medical supplies. By lowering the likelihood that fake goods may infiltrate the supply chain system, this awareness improves efficiency and stops losses brought on by counterfeit goods (Zakari et al., 2022).

Data Security

Millions of individuals worldwide are impacted by healthcare data breaches, which are a serious problem. In the first half of 2023 alone, more than 39 million people were affected by healthcare data breaches, according to research on health IT security (McKeon, 2023). By offering a decentralized and secure platform for storing and exchanging patient data and payment information, blockchain technology can improve data security in the healthcare industry. Furthermore, the blockchain's consensus process lowers the possibility of fraudulent entries by requiring network participants to agree before making any changes or adding new data (Taherdoost, 2023).

Efficiency

By establishing a safe ledger of patient data, blockchain enables seamless information exchange between various healthcare providers while preserving patient ownership and permission. This increases the speed and efficiency of the healthcare system and lessens the need for patients to share their medical details on a regular basis (Ghadi et al., 2024). By tracking the flow of medications, medical equipment, and other healthcare supplies via the supply chain, blockchain integration for the healthcare sector also reduces the possibility of fake medications and improves supply chain management. Additionally, blockchain's smart contract technology automates tracking procedures, cutting down on paperwork and increasing productivity (Nanda et al., 2023).

Barriers and Challenges

With its numerous benefits in the healthcare sector, blockchain has some of the barriers as well. Since blockchain is a relatively new technology, the healthcare industry faces numerous obstacles.

Interoperability

The lack of a single standard for creating blockchain-based healthcare applications is the root cause of the interoperability issue; for instance, apps created by various platforms or manufacturers might not work together (Ali et al., 2021). The development of protocols that guarantee blockchain network interoperability and enable consistent medical record preservation and smooth platform-to-platform transfer is therefore necessary (Habib et al., 2022). Presently, the necessity for interoperability is given less consideration in favor of creating prototypes and proofs-of-concept. Distinct blockchain-based healthcare platforms with differing degrees of smart contract capabilities, transaction mechanisms, and consensus models are the end products (Adere, 2022).

Security and Privacy

It is clear that no single system is completely secure in terms of security. Therefore, even if the blockchain uses cutting-edge encryption techniques, there is still a chance that security flaws could be exploited to compromise the data stored there (Guo & Yu, 2022). The 51% attack, which occurs when the number of malicious nodes in a blockchain network exceeds that of honest nodes, is a well-known security risk in blockchain technology (Aponte-Novoa et al., 2021). In such a scenario, the distributed consensus mechanism may be compromised, allowing the malicious nodes to alter the data on the blockchain and negating the immutability feature of the blockchain. The blockchain's use of private keys for information access presents another security risk because these keys are vulnerable to hacking (Nasir et al., 2024). The saved health data could be accessed without authorization if these private keys are stolen, however the data cannot be accessed if the keys are misplaced. Concerns have also been raised about the possibility that emerging technologies, such quantum computing, would be able to crack the encryption systems currently in use, which form the foundation of the blockchain (Agbo & Mahmoud, 2020).

ETHICAL AND LEGAL CONSIDERATIONS IN BLOCKCHAIN

Traditional business and service models have been upended by the rapid advancements in network technologies and blockchain technology. The healthcare industry is one such application. However, because of the delicate nature and complexity of the field, blockchain-enabled e-healthcare is necessary to guarantee utilitarianism while appropriately resolving the related ethical issues (Srivastava et al., 2021). Different methods and standards for blockchain ethics have developed, depending on the use case. Some of them are as follows.

Accountability

Accountability is a crucial ethical tenet. From the standpoint of responsibility, accountability necessitates that someone take responsibility for their acts and explain what transpired. Accountability helps assign blame when something goes wrong and promotes positive behavior from both individuals and organizations (Srivastava et al., 2021). Even in cases when harm has not resulted from intentional or direct action, accountability also entails responsibility, which aids in determining who should provide compensation if held accountable for an action (Katuwal et al., 2018). This guarantees that extra care is taken at the organizational level to assess which systems are susceptible to loss and who will be held responsible for it. This allows for the development and management of appropriate planning and mitigation methods. Since it shows that companies prioritize ethical work of the highest caliber, accountability becomes a crucial criterion of ethical behavior in the context of technology applications (Tang et al., 2020). Accountability aids in determining who is responsible for any harm or damages brought on by technology. Accountability frameworks assist companies in establishing guidelines for making fair and just decisions about punishment or compensation (Moukalled & Elhaj, 2021).

Patient Privacy and Data Security

The transparency of blockchain technology is a great advantage for data privacy. Every member of a blockchain network has access to the same transaction history, which fosters accountability and trust (Tatineni, 2019). People have more control and transparency over their information since they can see how their data is being used and whether it is accessed properly. GDPR compliance depends on this transparency. Although blockchain has enormous potential to improve data privacy, it is important to understand that putting blockchain-based solutions into practice calls for careful thought (Arabsorkhi & Khazaei, 2024). It can be difficult to strike the correct balance between data privacy and transparency, particularly in public blockchains. Anonymization and pseudonymization are two privacy-enhancing strategies that are frequently required to guarantee GDPR compliance and safeguard sensitive data. Blockchain technology has a strong chance to transform data privacy as it develops further, making it more resilient, transparent, and safe in a society that is becoming more and more reliant on data (de Haro-Olmo et al., 2020).

Regulatory Compliance

In the rapidly evolving field of blockchain technology, legal compliance is not only necessary but also a crucial pillar supporting the validity, dependability, and confidence that are necessary for the technology's adoption and mainstream incorporation (Han et al., 2023). Building legitimacy and trust is a key component in bringing blockchain technology into compliance with legal requirements. Respect for accepted legal standards turns blockchain from a purely technological advancement into a trustworthy and valid platform (de Filippi et al., 2020). Such conformance gives stakeholders confidence that the technology operates in accordance with laws and social standards, which is necessary for its broad adoption. This alignment is essential for integrating blockchain technology into different industries, presenting it as a dependable, well-received solution rather than a disruptive force (Tripathi et al., 2023).

Smart Contracts and Liability

Any transaction in which the parties' rights and responsibilities are encoded in a code is known as a smart contract. Such a contract, which is the outcome of the use of Blockchain technology, suggests that the parties to the contract must have faith in one another (Levy, 2017). The question of accountability for fulfilling contractual obligations is brought up by Blockchain (smart contract) technology as a legal phenomenon. In addition to making contract execution easier, smart contracts can reduce some contract risks (Pandey, 2025). They take effect right away, negating the need for any additional communication between the parties (ALqodsi & Arenova, 2024). Digitally verified data and the automatic execution of legally pertinent activities based on digitally received and processed information are the fundamental elements of smart contracts. Every issue highlighted is crucial to comprehending the accountability of Blockchain actors. Since at least the industrial revolution, the question of whether humans are accountable for the functioning of machines has been discussed in legal discourse (Taherdoost, 2023). The answer to this question has been the same in every jurisdiction: new situations and inventions that are suitably tailored to the new circumstances will be covered by and subject to the law. However, ideas about liability did not keep up with technological advancements (Pandey and Joseph, 2025a). As the use of automated systems increased, the closest human operators were held accountable for the mishaps and flaws in the supposedly "foolproof" technology (Kavanagh, 2022). Attributions of responsibility and the actual distribution of physical control over the system across a complex system and various actors in time and location were significantly out of sync.

Intellectual Property and Ownership

Since blockchain technology can provide proof of their conception, use, qualification requirements (like originality and the country in which articles made to the design were first marketed), and status, it can also be useful in the context of unregistered intellectual property rights like copyright, which is not a registrable IP right in many jurisdictions and according to the Berne Convention for the Protection of Literary and Artistic Works (Clark & McKenzie, 2018). A time-stamped record and reliable proof of these issues can be produced by uploading an original design or piece of work, together with the designer's or creator's data, to a blockchain. Numerous blockchain start-ups are already working on distributed ledger technology-based repositories for unregistered intellectual property rights, which may be an intriguing and feasible way to handle digital rights management and copyright protection (Quinn & Connolly, 2021).

Equity and Access

Although blockchain technology has the potential to be revolutionary, there are serious ethical issues with guaranteeing fair access. Existing disparities may be made worse by digital divisions in literacy and access to technology (Heeks, 2022). Some blockchains are energy-intensive, which causes environmental issues and disproportionately affects underserved communities. Furthermore, privacy may be jeopardized by blockchain technology's inherent transparency, especially for those who are weak or reside in oppressive countries (Garcia et al., 2024). To maximize blockchain's advantages while reducing its hazards and guaranteeing fair access for everyone, developers and legislators must place a high priority on inclusivity, sustainability, and privacy protection (Lv, 2023).

LEGAL FRAMEWORK AND POLICY IMPLICATIONS

Blockchain requires more than just technology to be implemented widely. It necessitates frameworks that, among other things, identify electronic documents and signatures and make clear the legal standing of blockchain transactions.

Health Insurance Portability and Accountability Act (HIPAA)

Although blockchain technology has the potential to revolutionize healthcare, any integration must comply with the HIPAA regulations. HIPAA requires that sensitive patient data be protected, which is consistent with blockchain's built-in security measures (Khatri et al., 2021). By spreading records across several nodes, blockchain's decentralized architecture improves data security by lowering the possibility of single-point failures and illegal access. Because of its immutability, data integrity is guaranteed, tampering is avoided, and an auditable record of changes is kept (Fatoum et al., 2021). Additionally, blockchain can help authorized entities share data securely, enhancing care coordination while protecting patient privacy. But there are still difficulties. Despite their transparency, public blockchains have the potential to jeopardize patient privacy. Private or permissioned blockchains provide more control over data access to help counteract this (Attaran, 2022). Encryption and strong access restrictions are essential for limiting data visibility to authorized parties. Furthermore, constant adaptability is required due to the changing regulatory environment. Healthcare companies need to keep up with the latest changes to HIPAA regulations that apply to blockchain applications (Lee et al., 2021).

General Data Protection Regulation (GDPR)

The fundamental premise of the GDPR is that, with regard to each piece of personal data, there exists at least one natural or legal entity known as the data controller, to whom data subjects may submit requests in order to exercise their rights under European Union (EU) data protection law (Barati & Rana, 2020). However, blockchains sometimes aim for decentralization by substituting numerous actors for a single unitary actor. This makes distributing accountability and duty difficult, especially given the regulation's ambiguous definition of (joint)-controllership (Teperdijan, 2020). A further complicating aspect in this regard is that determining whether businesses qualify as (joint-)controllers can be difficult due to a lack of legal certainty in light of recent case law developments. GDPR is predicated on the idea that data can be changed or deleted as needed to adhere to legal requirements like GDPR Articles 16 and 17 (Dutta et al., 2020). However, in order to maintain data integrity and boost network trust, blockchains make such data changes intentionally difficult. Once more, the uncertainty that already exists in EU data protection law exacerbates the issues related to this area of data protection legislation (Custers et al., 2019).

CONCLUSION

The need for development in the healthcare industry is growing at ever-increasing rates. High-quality medical facilities backed by more recent and sophisticated technologies are needed today. In this case, blockchain would be essential to changing the healthcare industry. Furthermore, the health system is shifting toward a patient-centered approach that emphasizes two key elements: always available healthcare resources and easily accessible services. The Blockchain helps healthcare organizations deliver high-quality medical facilities and appropriate patient care. Another laborious and repetitive procedure that raises the costs of the health sector is health information exchange, which may be swiftly resolved with the use of this technology. Blockchain technology allows citizens to participate in health research initiatives. Furthermore, improved studies and data on public health will improve care for various populations. There is no denying blockchain's revolutionary potential in the healthcare industry. By using the capabilities of blockchain, healthcare businesses may protect sensitive medical data, aid speedier data interchange, streamline processes, and provide better healthcare services to patients. Blockchain technology can potentially help patients and healthcare professionals save a lot of time and money. eHealth includes remote medical consultation, doctor and patient access to medical data and reports, information-gathering kiosks, and mobile applications that offer information instantly. Appointment scheduling, automated reminders, report collection and storage, and online consultations have all been made simpler by these services. E-health extends beyond services for patients and customers to include services from the viewpoint of other stakeholders, such as physicians and other healthcare service providers. Electronic medical records, drug and clinical trials, gamification, medical supply chain, and other applications are also included in these services. However, the necessity to comprehend the possible repercussions of the technology as well as its moral and ethical issues arises as blockchains are used in more and more fields and domains. It's crucial to keep in mind the ethical implications of its implementation. Strong frameworks that balance innovation, personal privacy, security, and moral principles that are consistent with societal norms must be put in place in order to lessen these ethical ramifications. By doing this, one can optimize blockchain's advantages while reducing any possible hazards and guaranteeing a beneficial social impact.

REFERENCES

Adere, E. M. (2022). Blockchain in healthcare and IoT: A systematic literature review. *Array (New York, N.Y.)*, *14*, 100139.

Agbo, C. C., & Mahmoud, Q. H. (2020). Blockchain in healthcare: Opportunities, challenges, and possible solutions. [IJHISI]. *International Journal of Healthcare Information Systems and Informatics*, *15*(3), 82–97.

Ahmed, W. A., & MacCarthy, B. L. (2023). Blockchain-enabled supply chain traceability–How wide? How deep? *International Journal of Production Economics*, *263*, 108963.

Akram, W., Joshi, R., Haider, T., Sharma, P., Jain, V., Garud, N., & Narwaria, N. S. (2024). Blockchain technology: A potential tool for the management of the pharma supply chain. *Research in Social & Administrative Pharmacy*. PMID: 38423927

Ali, O., Jaradat, A., Kulakli, A., & Abuhalimeh, A. (2021). A comparative study: Blockchain technology utilization benefits, challenges and functionalities. *IEEE Access : Practical Innovations, Open Solutions*, *9*, 12730–12749.

ALqodsi, E. M., & Arenova, L. (2024). Smart Contracts in Contract Law as an Auxiliary Tool or a Promising Substitute for Traditional Contracts. *Journal of Legal Affairs and Dispute Resolution in Engineering and Construction*, *16*(3), 06524004.

Andrew, J., Isravel, D. P., Sagayam, K. M., Bhushan, B., Sei, Y., & Eunice, J. (2023). Blockchain for healthcare systems: Architecture, security challenges, trends and future directions. *Journal of Network and Computer Applications*, *215*, 103633.

Aponte-Novoa, F. A., Orozco, A. L. S., Villanueva-Polanco, R., & Wightman, P. (2021). The 51% attack on blockchains: A mining behavior study. *IEEE Access : Practical Innovations, Open Solutions*, *9*, 140549–140564.

Arabsorkhi, A., & Khazaei, E. (2024). Blockchain technology and GDPR compliance: A comprehensive applicability model. *International Journal of Web Research*, *7*(2), 49–63.

Attaran, M. (2022). Blockchain technology in healthcare: Challenges and opportunities. *International Journal of Healthcare Management*, *15*(1), 70–83.

Barati, M., & Rana, O. (2020). Enhancing user privacy in IoT: Integration of GDPR and blockchain. In *Blockchain and Trustworthy Systems: First International Conference, BlockSys 2019, Guangzhou, China, December 7–8, 2019* [Springer Singapore.]. *Proceedings*, *1*, 322–335.

Clark, B., & McKenzie, B. (2018). Blockchain and IP law: a match made in crypto heaven. *online], WIPO Magazine, published Feb.*

Collomb, A., & Sok, K. (2016). Blockchain/distributed ledger technology (DLT): What impact on the financial sector?. *Digiworld Economic Journal*, (103).

Custers, B., Sears, A. M., Dechesne, F., Georgieva, I., Tani, T., & Van der Hof, S. (2019). *EU personal data protection in policy and practice* (Vol. 29). TMC Asser Press.

Darvishmotevali, M. (2019). Decentralization and innovative behavior: The moderating role of supervisor support. *International Journal of Organizational Leadership*, *8*, 31–45.

De Filippi, P., Mannan, M., & Reijers, W. (2020). Blockchain as a confidence machine: The problem of trust & challenges of governance. *Technology in Society*, *62*, 101284.

de Haro-Olmo, F. J., Varela-Vaca, Á. J., & Álvarez-Bermejo, J. A. (2020). Blockchain from the perspective of privacy and anonymisation: A systematic literature review. *Sensors (Basel)*, *20*(24), 7171. PMID: 33327652

Dutta, R., Das, A., Dey, A., & Bhattacharya, S. (2020). Blockchain vs GDPR in collaborative data governance. In *Cooperative Design, Visualization, and Engineering: 17th International Conference, CDVE 2020, Bangkok, Thailand, October 25–28, 2020* [Springer International Publishing.]. *Proceedings*, *17*, 81–92.

Fan, K., Wang, S., Ren, Y., Li, H., & Yang, Y. (2018). Medblock: Efficient and secure medical data sharing via blockchain. *Journal of Medical Systems*, *42*, 1–11. PMID: 29931655

Fatoum, H., Hanna, S., Halamka, J. D., Sicker, D. C., Spangenberg, P., & Hashmi, S. K. (2021). Blockchain integration with digital technology and the future of healthcare ecosystems: Systematic review. *Journal of Medical Internet Research*, *23*(11), e19846. PMID: 34726603

Garcia, R. D., Ramachandran, G., Dunnett, K., Jurdak, R., Ranieri, C., Krishnamachari, B., & Ueyama, J. (2024). A Survey of Blockchain-Based Privacy Applications: An Analysis of Consent Management and Self-Sovereign Identity Approaches. *arXiv preprint arXiv:2411.16404*.

Ghadi, Y. Y., Mazhar, T., & Shahzad, T., Amir khan, M., Abd-Alrazaq, A., Ahmed, A., & Hamam, H. (2024). The role of blockchain to secure the internet of medical things. *Scientific Reports*, *14*(1), 18422. PMID: 39117650

Ghosh, P. K., Chakraborty, A., Hasan, M., Rashid, K., & Siddique, A. H. (2023). Blockchain application in healthcare systems: A review. *Systems, 11*(1), 38.

Guo, H., & Yu, X. (2022). A survey on blockchain technology and its security. *Blockchain: research and applications, 3*(2), 100067.

Habib, G., Sharma, S., Ibrahim, S., Ahmad, I., Qureshi, S., & Ishfaq, M. (2022). Blockchain technology: Benefits, challenges, applications, and integration of blockchain technology with cloud computing. *Future Internet, 14*(11), 341.

Haleem, A., Javaid, M., Singh, R. P., Suman, R., & Rab, S. (2021). Blockchain technology applications in healthcare: An overview. *International Journal of Intelligent Networks, 2*, 130–139.

Han, H., Shiwakoti, R. K., Jarvis, R., Mordi, C., & Botchie, D. (2023). Accounting and auditing with blockchain technology and artificial Intelligence: A literature review. *International Journal of Accounting Information Systems, 48*, 100598.

Heeks, R. (2022). Digital inequality beyond the digital divide: Conceptualizing adverse digital incorporation in the global South. *Information Technology for Development, 28*(4), 688–704.

Hussein, Z., Salama, M. A., & El-Rahman, S. A. (2023). Evolution of blockchain consensus algorithms: A review on the latest milestones of blockchain consensus algorithms. *Cybersecurity, 6*(1), 30.

Katuwal, G. J., Pandey, S., Hennessey, M., & Lamichhane, B. (2018). Applications of blockchain in healthcare: current landscape & challenges. *arXiv preprint arXiv:1812.02776.*

Kavanagh, C. (2022). *New tech, new threats, and new governance challenges: an opportunity to craft smarter responses?* Carnegie Endowment for International Peace.

Khatoon, A. (2020). A blockchain-based smart contract system for healthcare management. *Electronics (Basel), 9*(1), 94.

Khatri, S., Alzahrani, F. A., Ansari, M. T. J., Agrawal, A., Kumar, R., & Khan, R. A. (2021). A systematic analysis on blockchain integration with healthcare domain: Scope and challenges. *IEEE Access : Practical Innovations, Open Solutions, 9*, 84666–84687.

Khujamatov, K., Reypnazarov, E., Akhmedov, N., & Khasanov, D. (2020, November). Blockchain for 5G Healthcare architecture. In *2020 international conference on information science and communications technologies (ICISCT)* (pp. 1-5). IEEE.

Kumar, A., Bhushan, B., Shristi, S., Chaganti, R., & Soufiene, B. O. (2023). Blockchain-based decentralized management of IoT devices for preserving data integrity. In *Blockchain Technology Solutions for the Security of IoT-Based Healthcare Systems* (pp. 263–286). Academic Press.

Kuo, T. T., Gabriel, R. A., & Ohno-Machado, L. (2019). Fair compute loads enabled by blockchain: Sharing models by alternating client and server roles. *Journal of the American Medical Informatics Association : JAMIA*, *26*(5), 392–403. PMID: 30892656

Lee, T. F., Chang, I. P., & Kung, T. S. (2021). Blockchain-based healthcare information preservation using extended chaotic maps for HIPAA privacy/security regulations. *Applied Sciences (Basel, Switzerland)*, *11*(22), 10576.

Levy, K. E. (2017). Book-smart, not street-smart: Blockchain-based smart contracts and the social workings of law. *Engaging Science, Technology, and Society*, *3*, 1–15.

Longo, F., Nicoletti, L., Padovano, A., d'Atri, G., & Forte, M. (2019). Blockchain-enabled supply chain: An experimental study. *Computers & Industrial Engineering*, *136*, 57–69.

Lv, Y. (2023). Transitioning to sustainable energy: Opportunities, challenges, and the potential of blockchain technology. *Frontiers in Energy Research*, *11*, 1258044.

Ma, Z., Jiang, M., Gao, H., & Wang, Z. (2018). Blockchain for digital rights management. *Future Generation Computer Systems*, *89*, 746–764.

Mackey, T. K., Kuo, T. T., Gummadi, B., Clauson, K. A., Church, G., Grishin, D., & Palombini, M. (2019). 'Fit-for-purpose?'–challenges and opportunities for applications of blockchain technology in the future of healthcare. *BMC Medicine*, *17*, 1–17. PMID: 30914045

McKeon, J. (2023). Biggest healthcare data breaches reported this year, so far. *Health IT Security, 26*.

Moukalled, T., & Elhaj, A. (2021). Patient negligence in healthcare systems: Accountability model formulation. *Health Policy OPEN*, *2*, 100037. PMID: 37383513

Nanda, S. K., Panda, S. K., & Dash, M. (2023). Medical supply chain integrated with blockchain and IoT to track the logistics of medical products. *Multimedia Tools and Applications*, *82*(21), 32917–32939. PMID: 37362711

Nasir, N. M., Hassan, S., & Zaini, K. M. (2024). Securing Permissioned Blockchain-based Systems: An Analysis on the Significance of Consensus Mechanisms. *IEEE Access : Practical Innovations, Open Solutions*.

Paik, H. Y., Xu, X., Bandara, H. D., Lee, S. U., & Lo, S. K. (2019). Analysis of data management in blockchain-based systems: From architecture to governance. *IEEE Access : Practical Innovations, Open Solutions*, *7*, 186091–186107.

Pandey, A. (2025). Blockchain in Industrial Supply Chains: Tracing the Transparency. In *Immersive Technology for the Gig Economy: Transformative Business Practices* (pp. 273-294). IGI Global Scientific Publishing.

Pandey, A., & Joseph, J. (2025). The Convergence of Blockchain and Artificial Intelligence: Transforming Healthcare. In *AI and Blockchain Applications for Privacy and Security in Smart Medical Systems* (pp. 399–416). IGI Global Scientific Publishing.

Pandey, A., & Joseph, J. (2025a). Navigating the HealthTech Ecosystem: Challenges and Roadblocks. In *Synergizing Data Envelopment Analysis and Machine Learning for Performance Optimization in Healthcare* (pp. 31-48). IGI Global Scientific Publishing.

Pandey, A., & Joseph, J. (2025b). Integral Role of Blockchain and Artificial Intelligence in Sustainable Economic Development. In *Driving Socio-Economic Growth With AI and Blockchain* (pp. 271–290). IGI Global Scientific Publishing.

Peppet, S. R. (2011). Unraveling privacy: The personal prospectus and the threat of a full-disclosure future. *Nw. UL Rev.*, *105*, 1153.

Quinn, J., & Connolly, B. (2021). Distributed ledger technology and property registers: Displacement or status quo. *Law, Innovation and Technology*, *13*(2), 377–397.

Ratwani, R. M. (2017). Electronic health records and improved patient care: Opportunities for applied psychology. *Current Directions in Psychological Science*, *26*(4), 359–365. PMID: 28808359

Srivastava, N. (2019). *What is Blockchain Technology, and How Does It Work?*.

Srivastava, V., Mahara, T., & Yadav, P. (2021). An analysis of the ethical challenges of blockchain-enabled E-healthcare applications in 6G networks. *International Journal of Cognitive Computing in Engineering*, *2*, 171–179.

Starfield, B., Shi, L., & Macinko, J. (2005). Contribution of primary care to health systems and health. *The Milbank Quarterly*, *83*(3), 457–502. PMID: 16202000

Taherdoost, H. (2023). Privacy and security of blockchain in healthcare: Applications, challenges, and future perspectives. *Sci*, *5*(4), 41.

Taherdoost, H. (2023). Smart contracts in blockchain technology: A critical review. *Information (Basel)*, *14*(2), 117.

Tang, Y., Xiong, J., Becerril-Arreola, R., & Iyer, L. (2020). Ethics of blockchain: A framework of technology, applications, impacts, and research directions. *Information Technology & People*, *33*(2), 602–632.

Tatineni, S. (2019). Blockchain and Data Science Integration for Secure and Transparent Data Sharing. [IJARET]. *International Journal of Advanced Research in Engineering and Technology*, *10*(3), 470–480.

Tripathi, G., Ahad, M. A., & Casalino, G. (2023). A comprehensive review of blockchain technology: Underlying principles and historical background with future challenges. *Decision Analytics Journal*, 100344.

Uddin, M., Salah, K., Jayaraman, R., Pesic, S., & Ellahham, S. (2021). Blockchain for drug traceability: Architectures and open challenges. *Health Informatics Journal*, *27*(2), 14604582211011228. PMID: 33899576

Vaishya, R., Javaid, M., Khan, I. H., Vaish, A., & Iyengar, K. P. (2021). Significant role of modern technologies for COVID-19 pandemic. *Journal of Industrial Integration and Management*, *6*(02), 147–159.

Xie, Y., Zhang, J., Wang, H., Liu, P., Liu, S., Huo, T., & Ye, Z. (2021). Applications of blockchain in the medical field: Narrative review. *Journal of Medical Internet Research*, *23*(10), e28613. PMID: 34533470

Zakari, N., Al-Razgan, M., Alsaadi, A., Alshareef, H., Alashaikh, L., Alharbi, M., & Alotaibi, S. (2022). Blockchain technology in the pharmaceutical industry: A systematic review. *PeerJ. Computer Science*, *8*, e840. PMID: 35634106

Zarour, M., Ansari, M. T. J., Alenezi, M., Sarkar, A. K., Faizan, M., Agrawal, A., & Khan, R. A. (2020). Evaluating the impact of blockchain models for secure and trustworthy electronic healthcare records. *IEEE Access : Practical Innovations, Open Solutions*, *8*, 157959–157973.

KEY TERMS AND DEFINITIONS

Blockchain: Over the last ten years, blockchain has been one of the major tech narratives. However, amidst the superficial conversation, there is not always a profound and clear comprehension of blockchain—its nature, functionality, or purpose. Even though it has a reputation for being impenetrable, the fundamental concept of blockchain is quite simple. Moreover, it can transform industries from the ground up. In short, blockchain is a technology that allows for the secure sharing of information. As is obvious, a database serves to store data. Transactions are documented in a ledger, which is an account book. A blockchain is a form of distributed database or ledger, implying that the authority to update it is shared among the nodes or participants in a public or private computer network. This is referred to as distributed ledger technology (DLT). To update blockchains, nodes receive digital tokens or currency as a reward.

Data Security: Data privacy refers to the right of individuals and organizations to control how their personal, sensitive, or proprietary information is collected, used, shared, and stored. It involves ensuring that data is handled responsibly, securely, and transparently to protect against unauthorized access, misuse, or breaches. Data privacy laws and policies set standards for consent, purpose limitation, data minimization, and accountability. As digital technologies expand, maintaining data privacy becomes critical to safeguarding trust, autonomy, and security. It applies across sectors, including healthcare, finance, and technology, highlighting the ethical obligation to respect and protect individuals' information in an increasingly interconnected world.

Electronic Medical Records: Electronic Medical Records (EMRs) are digital versions of patients' paper charts maintained by healthcare providers. They contain comprehensive patient information, including medical history, diagnoses, medications, immunization dates, allergies, lab results, and treatment plans. EMRs are designed to streamline clinical workflows, enabling quick access to patient data for better diagnosis and care. They support efficient documentation, enhance communication among healthcare professionals, and reduce medical errors. Unlike Electronic Health Records (EHRs), which are shared across organizations, EMRs typically remain within a single healthcare facility. By improving accuracy and accessibility, EMRs play a crucial role in modernizing healthcare delivery and promoting patient safety.

Equity: Equity refers to fairness, justice, and impartiality within processes, systems, and outcomes. Unlike equality, which treats everyone the same, equity recognizes that individuals have different needs, circumstances, and barriers, and seeks to allocate resources and opportunities accordingly to achieve fair outcomes. In law, equity developed to address the rigidity of common law by focusing on principles of fairness. In social and economic contexts, equity ensures that marginalized or disadvantaged groups receive the support necessary to thrive. It is a fundamental concept in areas like education, healthcare, governance, and business, aiming to create inclusive environments where all individuals can succeed.

Healthcare: Healthcare refers to the organized provision of medical services to maintain or improve individuals' health. It encompasses a broad range of services provided by medical, nursing, and allied health professionals, including prevention, diagnosis, treatment, recovery, and rehabilitation. Healthcare aims to promote well-being, prevent diseases, and manage illnesses through clinical care, public health initiatives, and health education. It operates through various systems like hospitals, clinics, and community health programs and is often supported by government policies and private institutions. Access to quality healthcare is considered a fundamental human right, crucial for enhancing life expectancy, productivity, and overall quality of life.

Intellectual Property Right: Intellectual Property Rights (IPR) refer to the legal protections granted to creators for their inventions, designs, artistic works, and brands. These rights allow creators to control the use of their intellectual efforts and benefit financially from their work. IPR covers categories like copyrights, patents, trademarks, and trade secrets. By securing exclusive rights, IPR encourages innovation, creativity, and investment in new ideas. It also helps in promoting fair competition and economic development. However, IPR must balance protecting creators' interests with public access to knowledge and innovation. Enforcement of IPR varies by jurisdiction and is essential for sustaining creative industries globally.

Smart Contracts: A smart contract is a self-executing digital agreement in which the terms and conditions between parties are directly written into lines of code. It operates on a decentralized blockchain network, ensuring transparency, security, and immutability. Once predefined conditions are met, the contract automatically enforces or executes the agreed-upon actions without the need for intermediaries like banks, lawyers, or notaries. Smart contracts are characterized by their autonomy, accuracy, speed, and trustworthiness. Because they are coded into a blockchain, they cannot be altered once deployed, minimizing risks of manipulation or fraud. They are widely used in various sectors such as finance (for decentralized finance or DeFi applications), supply chain management, real estate, healthcare, and intellectual property management.

Supply Chain: A supply chain is a network of individuals, organizations, resources, activities, and technologies involved in the creation and delivery of a product or service, from the sourcing of raw materials to the final delivery to consumers. It includes every stage of production, procurement, manufacturing, distribution, and retail. Effective supply chain management ensures the efficient flow of goods, information, and finances across all parties. It aims to maximize customer value, reduce costs, and achieve a competitive advantage. Supply chains can be global or local, and their complexity depends on the nature of the product, industry practices, and consumer demands.

Chapter 10
Integrating Blockchain, Smart Contracts, and AI for Decentralized Healthcare in the Metaverse:
Future Research Directions

R. N. Ravikumar
https://orcid.org/0009-0009-3705-1681
Marwadi University, Rajkot, India

A. Satheesh Kumar
Nandha Engineering College, Erode, India

S. Aarthi
https://orcid.org/0009-0006-9064-2091
Marwadi University, Rajkot, India

Sadridin Eshkaraev
Termez State University, Termez, Uzbekistan

Allayarov Dilshodbek
Mamun University, Khiva, Uzbekistan

Kavitha Bharathi Shanmugam
https://orcid.org/0000-0002-5630-7963
Kongu Engineering College, Erode, India

ABSTRACT

This chapter explores how blockchain-based healthcare management technologies, integrated with metaverse developments, address privacy, interoperability, and security challenges. It highlights the role of decentralized ledgers, cryptographic security, and smart contracts in ensuring global privacy compliance and streamlining administrative tasks like insurance claims and prescription management. The chapter reviews blockchain digital identities and their verification protocols

DOI: 10.4018/979-8-3373-1225-5.ch010

for secure patient data use. It also examines the synergy between blockchain and AI in enhancing personalized medical care and treatment analysis within metaverse environments. Despite scalability and regulatory hurdles, the chapter outlines key research directions for developing blockchain solutions that promote widespread metaverse healthcare adoption. The collaboration between healthcare professionals, researchers, and policymakers is pivotal to unlocking the digital potential of future medical systems.

INTRODUCTION

The integration of blockchain technology into metaverse healthcare systems offers transformative potential by enhancing electronic health records (EHR) management, ensuring robust data protection, and enabling secure information sharing. Traditional healthcare systems grapple with operational inefficiencies, security vulnerabilities, and fragmented data access, often leading to procedural errors and compromised patient privacy. Blockchain addresses these challenges through tamper-proof data storage, decentralized control, and immutable audit trails, thereby fostering trust and transparency in healthcare delivery, (Adeghe, Okolo, & Ojeyinka, 2024). Virtual settings using digital avatars enable medical consultations to occur between patients and doctors as the primary development of metaverse healthcare services.

Patients retain secure permanent data storage through blockchain technology since they can permit selected staff members to view their medical records while their system prevents unauthorized editing attempts. Healthcare professionals gain enhanced medical work processes and stronger collaborative opportunities while digital identifications evolve from blockchain-based protocols that assure identity verification. The adoption challenges of blockchain technology in metaverse healthcare systems arise from regulatory restrictions and network constraints that also affect integration of security systems and overcome scalability problems. Research investigates solutions to address present difficulties because they aim to enhance blockchain technology for protected healthcare delivery through the metaverse. New blockchain systems create a dependable digital healthcare infrastructure that provides benefits to public users, (Agbo, Mahmoud, & Eklund, 2019).

Overview of Blockchain Technology in Metaverse Healthcare

Blockchain's decentralized ledger technology (DLT) provides a secure framework for EHR management, enabling real-time data access for authorized providers while maintaining patient privacy. Because of blockchain, healthcare in the metaverse is now more organized, apparent, and convenient. In the world of the metaverse, healthcare is being transformed into digital services, so now people can get consultations, mental health care, wellness advice, and even have their health monitored online, (Benchoufi, Porcher, & Ravaud, 2018). Through blockchain, records of a patient's medical care are made safe from alterations, follow a trackable history, and can only be checked by the right people.

Whenever data in a patient's health record is changed, it is immediately stored as an unchangeable block to guarantee proper data handling and prevent fraud. Using smart contracts, health-related jobs such as processing claims, verifying prescriptions, and controlling consent are automated to enhance operations while preserving the level of trust and following all rules. Furthermore, using blockchain, healthcare apps and wearable devices can exchange and store patients' health data in the metaverse, (Bidve et al., 2023). Health data of patients is theirs to keep, controlled by DIDs and wallets, so that their privacy is maintained. As a result of blockchain and the metaverse working together, people far from medical centers can use remote care and still receive excellent healthcare. All in all, the reliability and strong security offered by blockchain make it possible for metaverse healthcare to deliver better health outcomes for patients. Key features include:

- Immutability: Ensures data integrity by preventing unauthorized alterations.
- Smart Contracts: Automate consent management and regulatory compliance (e.g., HIPAA, GDPR).
- Cryptographic Security: Protects sensitive data through encryption and zero-knowledge proofs (ZKPs).

Table 1. Blockchain benefits in metaverse healthcare

Feature	Traditional System	Blockchain-enabled Metaverse Healthcare
Data Integrity	Prone to manipulation	Tamper-proof and immutable
Privacy Control	Centralized access	Decentralized with DIDs and wallets
Process Automation	Manual processing	Smart contract-based automation
Security	Susceptible to breaches	Encrypted with ZKPs and distributed access
Data Sharing	Limited interoperability	Cross-platform interoperability enabled

The table 1 summarizes the key advantages of integrating blockchain in metaverse-based healthcare, including data immutability, cryptographic security, smart contracts, and decentralized control. It compares traditional vs. blockchain-enabled systems for functions such as data integrity, automation, and patient privacy.

Figure 1. Core applications of blockchain in metaverse healthcare

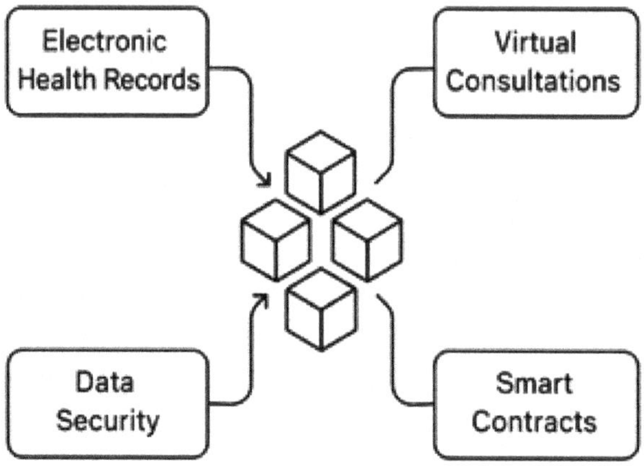

Figure 1 presents the core components enhanced by blockchain. At the center is a cube cluster symbolizing blockchain, with arrows pointing outward to four key applications: Electronic Health Records, Virtual Consultations, Data Security, and Smart Contracts. The layout emphasizes blockchain's central role in enabling secure, decentralized, and efficient healthcare services within the metaverse.

Importance of Secure, Decentralized Healthcare Management

Two major security and patient data protection issues affect the digital health system. During privacy protection, central data systems risk hacker attacks and illegal compromises of patient data. Security vulnerabilities from central administration points are eliminated when blockchain is deployed across several networks, strengthening the healthcare network. Secure points in permissioned blockchain systems allow permitted individuals to access patient record data. Patients may monitor their metaverse data storage locations and maintain safe medical record access rights as healthcare decentralizes, (Chander, 2023). It is very important to have secure and decentralized control over healthcare to protect private data and win the trust of users. Since there are no single points that can be attacked, data breaches and unauthorized entry become unlikely in a decentralized system. By allowing patients to access their health records, the sharing of those records can be made more transparent and with everyone's agreement. Because of these systems, healthcare providers collaborate well and offer efficient care to their patients. What's more, decentralized, secure platforms based on blockchain ensure that vital documents are protected, transparent, and always at hand for effective health care in digital settings, (Dimitrov, 2019).

Key Challenges in Traditional Healthcare Systems

Healthcare systems established in the past suffer from many obstacles that reduce their efficiency and accessibility. When a patient's data has to go across different hospitals or electronic systems, it is difficult for doctors to combine all the information, so medical records might not be complete or similar. This division in healthcare services holds up treatment and also leads to more medical mistakes. Keeping all individuals' health data in a central location exposes it to the dangers of hacking and unauthorized view. Further difficulties come from inefficient management and high costs for health providers, resulting in patients having to wait long and sometimes receive lower-quality care. Lack of healthcare facilities in specific areas results in different degrees of access to healthcare and different health results for people. In addition, problems with transparency in insurance and billing tend to confuse patients and cause them more financial stress. Poor communication between patients and their doctors makes it difficult for decisions to be made as necessary and delays receiving ongoing care. It is becoming more difficult for traditional methods to provide people with modern, immediate, technology-based healthcare services. It is necessary to address these main challenges in healthcare as the system develops, since this will lead to better medical care for everyone in the digital world, (Drosatos & Kaldoudi, 2019).

Table 2. Challenges in traditional healthcare vs blockchain-based solutions

Traditional Challenge	Blockchain-Based Solution
Data Fragmentation	Unified, distributed ledger for consistent records
Centralized Security Risks	Decentralized networks with encrypted nodes
High Operational Costs	Automated processes using smart contracts
Limited Rural Access	Remote care enabled via metaverse consultations
Poor Transparency	Immutable logs and permissioned data access

Table 2 identifies key operational, security, and access-related challenges in traditional systems and maps them to corresponding blockchain-based solutions adopted in metaverse healthcare.

Comparing the Use of Blockchain in Healthcare with Other Sectors

There is significant difference between countries in how blockchain is used in healthcare since this depends on laws, useful digital technologies, and different policy decisions. A comparison of nations offers knowledge about world-wide readiness and main efforts everywhere.

- United States: There have been attempts to use blockchain in healthcare through actions by private companies and associations such as the Synaptic Health Alliance and MedRec in the U.S. However, following HIPAA rules closely and having disconnected healthcare processes make it difficult to integrate patients' information. At the pilot stage, medical credentialing, insurance verification, and exchanging EHRs securely are the main points.
- European Union: One example of the EU using blockchain is MyHealthMyData (MHMD), which puts a main focus on data privacy and following the rules of GDPR. EBSI is also looking into helping health records be exchanged between different countries. While rules and digital IDs have helped innovation, following strict data privacy laws has caused delays in implementing big projects on a large scale.
- India: Blockchain is being introduced in healthcare only at this point in India. The National Digital Health Mission of the government is a basis for using blockchain for ID verification and sharing health-related data. Ensuring the permanence of records and blocking fraud is the main aim of Healthereum and Zebi Health. People still have to overcome the difficulties in understanding technology and wide adaptation.

It is clear from this perspective that cities like Singapore and Zurich are using digital IDs normally, whereas other countries are now following by including blockchain in their healthcare digitization strategies.

Table 3. Comparative overview of blockchain adoption in healthcare by region

Region/ Country	Adoption Stage	Key Initiatives/Projects	Legal & Regulatory Framework	Challenges
USA	Advanced Pilots	Synaptic Health Alliance, MedRec	HIPAA compliance, state-level variations	System fragmentation, high integration cost
European Union	Regulatory & Pilot	MyHealthMyData (MHMD), EBSI	GDPR, EBSI interoperability guidelines	Strict privacy laws, slow multi-state rollout
India	Emerging	National Digital Health Mission (NDHM), Zebi Health	NDHM standards, evolving data privacy laws	Low digital literacy, limited infrastructure
Estonia	Mature	National EHR system using blockchain	National health IT law, strong ID systems	Scalability and integration with new services
UAE	Growing	Dubai Health Authority blockchain record sharing	Blockchain Strategy 2021	Governance and cross-system integration

Table 3 provides a comparative snapshot of blockchain adoption in healthcare across selected regions. It outlines each region's current adoption stage, notable blockchain initiatives, regulatory landscape, and key challenges. This comparison highlights how developed nations like the USA and EU focus on compliance and interoperability, while emerging economies like India are integrating blockchain into national digital health strategies. Estonia stands out as a pioneer with a fully operational blockchain-enabled EHR system, whereas the UAE is rapidly progressing under national blockchain frameworks.

BLOCKCHAIN FOR SECURE PATIENT DATA MANAGEMENT

Data security becomes crucial for healthcare services as they expand into the metaverse. Traditional centralised healthcare databases are vulnerable to cyberattacks, data breaches, and unauthorized users. The implementation of blockchain technology means patients can enjoy medical record data security because it provides tamperproof storage methods that need authorization to access. Secure protection of patient sensitive data becomes possible through distributed ledger procedures that Blockchain offers. Each block-component of the blockchain system timestamps medical history modifications while encrypting complete sections and maintaining a continuous block linkage to safeguard the database from unauthorized modifications. Blockchain technology keeps strict track of every data change to protect complete data security so that it improves visibility while preventing healthcare fraud. A blockchain system enables patients to grant specific permissions for their health records to healthcare providers which builds trust and autonomy between remote medical care services.

The cryptographic core functions of blockchain technology permit safe data exchange between healthcare providers and research teams and medical insurers. The healthcare operations function under GDPR and HIPAA requirements simultaneously, (Hylock & Zeng, 2019). Medical organizations using metaverse healthcare systems rely on blockchain to build superior protective systems for patient data privacy in order to create secure virtual healthcare infrastructure.

Role of Blockchain in Protecting Patient Data Privacy

The highest priority in patient healthcare data protection must be maintained throughout the transfer of medical services from digital health platforms to the metaverse. Public healthcare databases maintain their databases at central locations where they encounter regular security vulnerabilities alongside unauthorized changes and malicious data breaches. The Blockchain technology enables creation of a patient information protection system that implements decentralized security control systems, (Mayer, Costa, & Righi, 2019). The decentralized ledgers in blockchain technology implement secure protection systems that function without any intermediary parties.

Blockchain security provides unrestricted access to health data along with full authority control to medical patients. Blockchain Based digital identity enables permissioned users to both control data sharing permissions and access maintenance privileges for their medical data retrieval process. The system permits external departure from Medicare yet medical providers with administrative access get needed information to enhance security operations. Blocks of data used in healthcare institutions build safe patient data monitoring through blockchain databases which automatically track system access changes and transactions.

The security features of blockchain technology protect healthcare data by stopping unauthorized surveillance practices that endanger AI patient treatment in metaverse healthcare services. Smart contracts enforce regulatory consent measures by implementing a system for the regulation of data sharing activities. The distributed storage model powers blockchain data protection by giving users access to control parts of the database so they cannot possess full database ownership, (Motohashi et al., 2019). The integration of metaverse healthcare systems with blockchain technology protects medical data by setting up privacy standards that create better trust relationships than traditional healthcare practices.

Use of Decentralized Ledgers for Data Security

The implementation of decentralized ledger systems by organizations generates enhanced security capabilities which outstrip central data storage system capabilities. Patient databases stored through conventional methods remain vulnerable to multiple security threats that originate from both hardware system modifications and equipment breakdowns as well as cyber-attacks. Through its distributed architecture blockchains enables doctors to implement distributed patient data storage systems that use several nodes to avoid hardware system breakdowns, (Vazirani et al., 2020).

The decentralized record system functions as an unalterable system which maintains an audit trail of all healthcare transaction information. The encrypted system applies crypto methods for timestamping while multiple nodes store data records to protect integrity. The data backup approach which spreads information across various network nodes provides defense against attacks when one node is compromised. Medical records are managed through Blockchain technology which enables each healthcare body to view all data-modification histories independently from their separately defined data privileges.

The deployment of distributed ledger technology across Metaverse healthcare systems simplifies the distribution of data between medical establishments and insurance companies who execute protected data management protocols as defined by Daniels. Blockchains enable medical staff to create single databases containing patient records which get updated instantly while eliminating duplicate database inputs. Healthcare organizations meet security framework requirements when they use blockchains because the decentralized system allows them to reach compliance. Data security operations in metaverse healthcare platforms depend on Blockchain technology which provides protected access to healthcare patient information. A digital healthcare system needs various essential components from this innovation for implementing safe measures with both observational access and secure implementation.

Cryptographic Techniques for Compliance with Global Regulations

Active data protection platforms based on cryptographic solutions need to serve both HIPAA and GDPR security regulations for healthcare network development. A modern cryptographic model allows Blockchain to build healthcare systems that match privacy standards defined by identity standards, (Wang et al., 2020). Through its primary data encoding cryptographic method Blockchain encrypts medical patient data to defend it from improper access attempts. The double encryption method in Blockchain technology uses decryption keys to determine user identities that can view cryptographic records contained within protected data. ZKPs enable a party to prove data authenticity while safeguarding all information about the data contents from disclosure. Data contents in the metaverse healthcare clinical verification system remain secure because the system implements protective features that stop unauthorized medical record access.

Through the security procedure hash the system transforms patient information into an indestructible special character sequence which functions as a protective measure. Hash values are checked by authorized system personnel who automatically identify data alterations and prevent unauthorized modification from appearing, (Wong, Bhattacharya, & Butte, 2019). Due to their function as surveillance platforms for privacy enforcement smart contracts enhance the regulatory compliance of consent management systems. Healthcare institutions secure patient data storage systems with blockchain cryptographic functions which meet all protective requirement standards. The implementation of blockchain technology by healthcare providers in the metaverse enables security procedures that defend patient trust using international digital health systems standards to prevent data breaches.

Case Study: Blockchain-Based Patient Data Exchange – The Estonia Experience

The country is well-known for its important role in digital governance, mainly thanks to its blockchain-based health record system. Blockchain technology has been used in Estonia's healthcare system since 2012 to make sure data is safe and private. With the system, healthcare providers can securely check and modify patient records, while users can always see who views their records in real time, (Yulianjani, Rosdiana, & Altaufik, 2024). It increases openness and allows patients to keep their data, dealing with a key issue that existed in older systems.

Key Success Factors:

- X-Road lets public services exchange their data securely because of its government-endorsed interoperability technology.
- Through a digital identity, people can confirm their identity and properly enter clinical areas, unlike with traditional IDs.
- Supporting policy: There are strong legal guidelines in Estonia that assist in using blockchain while keeping data safe.

Limitations:

- Scalability: Although things work well on a national scale, linking different countries' healthcare is a tough process.

- Technology dependency: To operate, the model counts on people who are digitally skilled and on regular maintenance of communication infrastructure.
- Initial costs: Setting up the system and maintaining it may not be affordable for countries with few resources.

It has been shown that with the use of blockchain technology, healthcare services can exchange patient information in a safe and easy-to-follow way.

BLOCKCHAIN BASED DIGITAL IDENTITIES IN HEALTHCARE

Through blockchain technology healthcare implements protected decentralized identity systems that enhance security infrastructure by allowing medical staff and patients to control their identities. Current methods of patient verification in healthcare organizations fall short in data protection measures so security problems and steal-thieves continue to perturb medical facilities. Additional trust-based security solutions emerge from blockchain technology implementation because nine problems related to tamper proofness vanish together with cryptographic restrictions, (Garg, 2024).

Virtual visit authentication becomes possible using this platform because it enables digital personifications to safely execute medical data retrieval and insurance process management tasks. The self-sovereign identity capability within the system gives patients control to make decisions about which medical records they wish to show to their health providers. The healthcare field uses autonomous contracts for quick patient authentication yet ensures all exclusive information stays protected from disclosure.

Blockchain digital identifiers ensure the compliance of medical organizations and insurance entities and research establishments with GDPR and HIPAA regulations while protecting data when different systems integrate their functions. By adopting Blockchain technology healthcare organizations defend their operations because it both stops fraud attempts and creates more digital healthcare resources available.

Verification Protocols for Digital Identities

A digital framework needs implementation to achieve secure authentication during all healthcare operations for virtual patient identification management. Identity verification databases feature multiple security points that enable multiple security breaches and unidentified identity theft incidents. The combination of crypto-secure defense that leverage distributed ledger technology lets users verify their identity through blockchain technology. The blockchain enables users to construct digital identity profiles for independent access of their digital assets without needing external authorities. Smart contracts operate automatic verification which makes the retrieval process for medical documents happen seamlessly without interruptions.

The enrolment process for patients at healthcare institutions achieves stronger authentication through Blockchain technology digital verification which provides fraud protection against identity theft and data threats. Healthcare payment processing within the metaverse healthcare system supports remote diagnosis tests and virtual appointment authorizations while providing security and resulting in rapid service delivery and improved trust between patients and providers, (Jusić, 2022).

Data Protection and Patient Identity Management

Block bae Will based digital identities in health systems must protect security information. The centralized healthcare databases containing patient identity information remain at risk of cyber-attacks as well as unauthorized changes. through decentralized identity management Blockchain technology offers a protection system that maintains both data security and complete privacy protection and data integrity.

Cryptographic hashing enables patient identity storage on blockchain so their stored data remains resistant to alterations and unchangeable in permanent form. Ballantine's system grants patients' independent authority over their identity data which lets them determine when to freely give their medical records to doctors or insurance companies or research organizations, (Pokharel et al., 2025). Patients receive protection from data breach risks because the healthcare organization no longer requires external verification systems.

Data privacy regulations including GDPR and HIPAA comply in full manner by using blockchain to enforce strict encryption features along with access controls. Blockchain patient identity management allows healthcare firms to provide metaverse healthcare services for patients and safeguard digital frameworks against fraud.

Enhancing Trust and Security in Virtual Healthcare Interactions

Patients must trust modern diagnostic AI tools and metaverse medical consultancy services with trustworthy security mechanisms to embrace telemedicine systems. Users can trust blockchain technology's tamper-evident features since they can see medical data, identity management, and payment items in their healthcare system. Because Blockchain uses an unmodifiable medical record monitoring system, its authentication process works, (Raasetti, 2024). Distributed ledgers track access activities, verification procedures, and data altering records for transparent accountable systems in every part. Unauthorised modification prevention and secure patient-framework operator connections are possible with the system security architecture. Blockchain security is optimized when smart contracts activate automated authorization processes. Automated contracts authenticate medical staff to secure patient data via permission management and internet intruder avoidance. Blockchain-based cryptographic signatures verify medical prescriptions, lab data, and insurance claims. Blockchain technologies enable healthcare firms to create trust networks that secure patient data and provide improved security frameworks.

Challenges in Digital Identity Verification

Even though blockchain-based digital identity systems make healthcare in the metaverse safer and more private, they present a number of new problems that must be resolved. A major issue is people stealing someone else's identity for their gain. Although the verification of data cannot be changed on blockchain, if anyone uses the user's private keys or credentials, some access may occur without proper protection. As a result, your identity might be taken for unauthorized access to important health records. Managing your cryptocurrencies and recovering your wallet is also a big problem for users. Usually, users of decentralized systems are responsible for saving and managing their digital wallets. If these keys get lost and there is no way to recover them, people may end up losing their health data permanently, something that doesn't happen with centralized storage. Besides, a number of blockchain identity schemes still require trusted third parties to approach and examine any credentials users present. If trust or neutrality is removed from third parties, the problem of blockchain is back, since this dependency can make the blockchain vulnerable again. To deal with these obstacles, the industry should focus on created secure recovery mechanisms, use biometric checks for identification, and increase use of decentralized trust to make sure digital health identities are simple and private.

SMART CONTRACTS FOR HEALTHCARE OPERATIONS

The intelligent contractual framework enhances healthcare operations through its automated execution system which eliminates cumbersome materials regarding official regulations. Personnel can execute blockchain-based self-operating energy transactions through existing contracts while needing no help from outside managers, (Agbo, Mahmoud, & Eklund, 2019). The operation of healthcare facilities depends heavily on smart contracts because they control patient data alongside insurance documents and medical billing functions.

Smart contracts combine to provide users with the highest level of security that links their program systems into synchronization. Computerized systems possessing smart contract functionality allow users to maintain automated consent permissions that both provide access to data exchange between entities while protecting ongoing consent validity. The smart contract functionality allows users to establish access settings that automatically protect patient data privacy while maintaining audit logs on distributed ledger networks, (Aloqaily et al., 2023).

The incorporation of smart contracts helps Mediclaim insurance executives decrease both periods dedicated to processing invalid operations and lowers processing duration. The automated system files claim by itself after all validity requirements are fulfilled so manual checks become unnecessary. Through built-in operational elements the system executes verification of pharmaceutical products and protects supply chains against wrongdoing by preventing unauthorized drugs from reaching distribution routes. Metaverse healthcare operations enabled by smart contracts earn healthcare organizations dual benefits of operating expense reduction and enhanced system safety through increased patient trust, (Arbabi et al., 2023). Medical organizations can now establish decentralized medical service locations that operate directly for patient care.

Automation of Administrative Tasks in Healthcare

Smart contracts enable healthcare administration to transform its operations thus creating higher efficiency because they automate administrative procedures to decrease paperwork. Patients along with healthcare staff need to stay within healthcare facilities because documentation processes for admission along with payment and administrative procedures require significant duration. Healthcare delivery suffers negative impacts from systematic work activities that unite delayed systems with human mistakes and studies of fraudulent behavior to generate operational inefficiencies.

The Blockchain-Based smart contracts within healthcare institutions allow them to define protocols that trigger automated conditional processes according to established protocols. The patient-created digital agreement systems operate without supervision by initiating automatic registrations procedures. The improved data security and complete user system access monitoring comes from healthcare organizations achieving medical regulations through smart contracts, (Atadoga et al., 2024).

Automated systems generate improved healthcare databases without affecting the operational speed between departments. The use of decentralized network communication provides improved operational efficiency and reduced operational costs to medical facilities and governing agencies together with insurers.

Applications in Insurance Claim Processing and Prescription Management

Insurance claims automation and prescription oversight reach high control levels through implementing operational security systems based on transparent procedures which smarter contracts enable. Customers need to provide multiple long documents to insurance companies but face delayed payments when human verification precipitation could result in insurance fraud. Smart contracts employ automatic claim execution through proof of conditions such as policy verification and medical reports. The systematic claim management process boosts operational efficiency because it successfully minimizes both insurance fraud cases alongside claims disputes.

Qualified individuals can use smart contracts to authenticate medical prescription development methods which enhances prescription security systems. The blockchain ledger uses protocol-based systems to offer secure prescription data protection by preventing unauthorized alterations at all times and throughout all regulatory periods, (Attaran, 2020). Drug producers depend on the solution to conduct medical inspections in their entire network infrastructure which prevents the circulation of counterfeit drugs. Smart contracts in healthcare processes enabled profit reductions as well as patient trust growth while delivering precise prescription management to drive system operational improvements.

Table 4. Applications of smart contracts in healthcare

Application Area	Smart Contract Function	Benefit
Insurance Claims	Auto-validate documents and conditions	Fraud reduction, faster reimbursements
Prescription Management	Authenticate and secure prescription data	Prevents tampering, improves patient safety
Billing & Payments	Enforce transparent billing based on pre-set conditions	Eliminates disputes, ensures accuracy
Consent Management	Manage access permissions via logic conditions	Improves compliance with HIPAA/GDPR
Drug Supply Chains	Verify authenticity and traceability	Prevents counterfeit drug distribution

Table 4 outlines the specific applications of smart contracts in metaverse healthcare operations, especially in automating insurance claims, verifying prescriptions, and enhancing data security and efficiency.

Figure 2. Smart contract workflow in healthcare

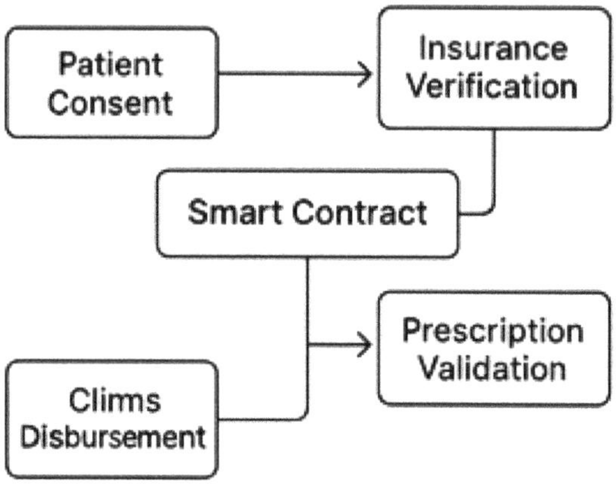

Figure 2 showing the lifecycle of smart contracts managing patient consent, insurance verification, prescription validation, and claims disbursement.

Secure and Transparent Document Sharing Between Healthcare Providers

Healthcare organizations should develop secure document sharing systems in order to enhance team collaboration services for their patient population. Security incidents threaten health data exchange between hospitals due to the creation of possible breaches from different data systems found in healthcare facilities. Healthcare organizations protect their document exchange by using blockchain technology that operates via decentralized protocols which defend against document modifications. The medical documentation system in hospitals becomes protected by blockchain technology which maintains secure access for authorized healthcare staff to medical records. As part of the healthcare industry customers decide how automatic systems determine authorized entities who need access to their health information through authorization arrangements which control both permission beginning and ending points. The system blocks unauthorized access to systems together with improper data handling by preventing these activities from occurring, (Garg et al., 2023). The updating process of blockchain system information streamlines directly to distributed ledgers for change monitoring purposes since blockchain features operate without alterations. Through its protective mechanism the regulatory system makes blockchain technology suitable for health service provider transactions by fulfilling GDPR and HIPAA data safety requirements.

Integration with Legacy Hospital Information Systems

In order for blockchain and smart contracts to help healthcare, they have to connect seamlessly with existing systems used in hospitals. Most hospitals and clinics are still stuck with untouched systems that do not accept decentralized technology. To integrate blockchain with other software, companies should use APIs and middleware systems that help transfer data from the blockchain to regular software. They adjust the data structures, deal with logins, and see to it that communication between the blockchain and HIS/EHRs is always secure. Whenever consent is given by a patient through a smart contract, API relays that and the legacy EHR updates the permissions. It is also possible to use FHIR (Fast Healthcare Interoperability Resources) standards with blockchain so data is transferred in the same structure while remaining standardized. Blockchain-as-a-Service (BaaS) platforms are also being used, providing ready access to various tools that hospitals can integrate instead of having to replace their total IT system. Even though this method is easy to put into action, it introduces new problems like keeping data aligned, dealing with latency, and securing middleware. For these matters to be handled, the design of the architecture must be strong and connect all systems following interoperability standards to ensure data security and connectivity between decentralized and centralized components.

INTEGRATION OF BLOCKCHAIN WITH AI IN THE METAVERSE

The healthcare industry goes through a transformative process because blockchain integration of artificial intelligence into the metaverse develops enhanced security capabilities together with improved treatment systems. Healthcare data protection functions via decentralized blockchain operations that enable AI analysis to produce better medical diagnostic data for better doctor-care improvement, (Jat et al., 2024). Such a trustworthy platform results from the combination of multiple technology components which provide quick and transparent service delivery.

The secure communication protocols enable reliable access to health records stored on blockchain databases where data integrity remains protected against unauthorized edit attempts. Consolidating blockchain technology platforms with medical record analysis and machine learning systems enables healthcare facilities to develop Disease weakness identification services that create personalized treatments and boost distant medical care services. The relationship between automated prescription testing and automated smart contracts delivers superior authorization control to healthcare organizations for both insurance claims and consent authorizations.

Blockchain security technology operates as a united system to build permanent tracking procedures that create secure spaces for AI learning and halt illegal activities and biases. Blockchain systems achieve operational efficiency with the help of artificial intelligence because artificial intelligence generates new consensus protocols accompanied by lower costs and expanded scalability, (Khatib et al., 2023). Blockchain-AI technology integration allows healthcare systems to establish protected virtual healthcare solutions by delivering remote medical services through data distribution systems which effectively track medical records.

AI Powered Blockchain Applications in Virtual Healthcare

Maximum power becomes achievable for health security protection together with blockchain technology when artificial intelligence functions within operational effective parameters for medical services. Doctors can access diagnosis recommendations about their patients through the ongoing patient information monitoring provided by AI systems analyzing medical big data. Basic solutions must be developed for virtual healthcare management to solve two key problems involving data security standards and information protection requirements. Security needs are solved through distributed bookkeeping technology that generates tamper-evident systems for medical record storage.

The blockchain protection system secures medical records using proper storage mechanisms which satisfy regulatory authorization requirements. AI extracts necessary patient data from blockchain databases for physicians because the databases feature security measures that ensure data protection during the retrieval process, (Kumar, Albusaidi, & Halloush, 2023). The smart contract automation framework with network operations provides a safe data exchange environment for healthcare organizations through their insurance checks and consent processing procedures. Hospitals can trust Metaverse virtual healthcare systems to deliver data-driven security features for both patient care processes and treatment procedures through AI blockchain technology.

Figure 3. AI and blockchain integration in the metaverse

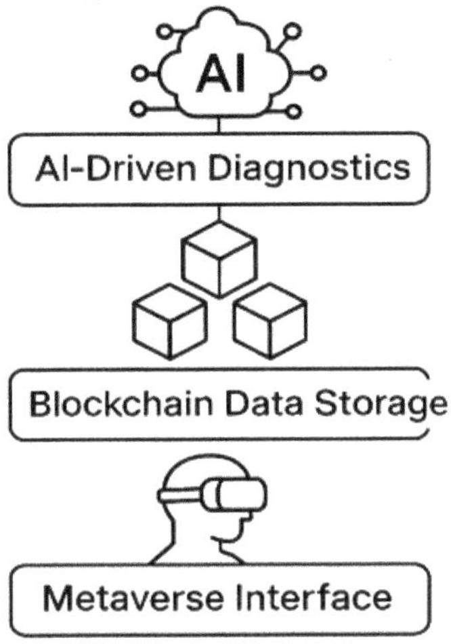

Figure 3 diagram representing the integration of AI diagnostics, blockchain data storage, and the metaverse interface. This illustration demonstrates how intelligent and secure healthcare services are delivered virtually through interconnected technologies.

Personalized Treatment and Predictive Analytics

Healthcare services obtain maximal advantage through integrating AI predictive analytics with Blockchain-powered technology for their clinical work that supports Metaverse patient care. The application of AI models analyzing big patient databases allowed staff members to evaluate genetic test outcomes against clinical documents for disease detection and therapy identification purposes. Core security systems defend health care institutions from threats and simultaneously protect their entire information infrastructure from unauthorized entry. The blockchain recordkeeping system integrates automatic monitoring for instant document edits that users make within its platform, (Mackey et al., 2019).

The blockchain-secured medical patient data processing system uses a verified healthcare recommendation delivery service with untameable verification to serve customers. The authorization features built into smart contracts enable medical service providers to access patient records securely through safety measure systems that protect private health information. Patients who receive equitable health care outcomes now have access to trustworthy AI-generated medical data thanks to healthcare decentralization, (Nguyen et al., 2023). Healthcare providers will establish better preventive care solutions through blockchain integration with AI predictive analytics for delivering affordable wellness protection against diseases to patients.

AI Driven Patient Monitoring and Outcome Assessment

Health monitoring of patients relies on blockchain networks united with AI technology to safeguard patient data from attacks and guarantee safety. AI systems can process disease detection alerts together with significant recovery data and medical guidance through the large patient datasets produced by healthcare systems using wearable IoT devices. The safe protection of patient data along with protecting the integrity of the data represents an essential problem for resolution. Blockchains operating under protection maintain full patient oversight of their healthcare records when they create them, (Yang et al., 2022).

Virtual healthcare services powered by artificial intelligence receive sanctioned access to customized medical care via Blockchain-based medical documentation and provide remote health services to patients. The process of patient data sharing under smart contracts allows safe information exchange between patients and healthcare providers and insurers and physicians while preserving authorized access policies. The performance of treatments and clinical decision improvement and patient care pathway optimization becomes possible through validating AI data models by blockchain systems, (Ahamed, 2024). Medical organizations using monitoring systems enhanced by blockchain technologies deliver safe healthcare services which engage patients deeply to produce better long-term treatment results.

AI Model Bias and Trustworthiness in Healthcare

Since artificial intelligence guides many important medical tasks and choices in metaverse healthcare using blockchain technology, it is essential to ensure that everything is fair, clear, and in line with rules. Even with all its possibilities, AI is susceptible to biased results when the data it uses is not well balanced or representative. Because of these biases, different populations might be given incorrect diagnoses, which could cause discrimination in healthcare. This issue should be dealt with in AI systems used in healthcare by providing bias detection and fixes from development to deployment. Below are practices that must be used: raising data, setting fairness guidelines, and frequently examining the model's results for all demographics. It is also a major issue that models cannot always explain their reasoning. Most modern AI solutions, particularly those based on deep learning, are hard for doctors to explain to their patients because it's unclear how the conclusions were made. When XAI is applied, models share details in a way that is understandable by medical professionals, making everything clearer and more trustworthy in healthcare. Things are moving fast in the creation of AI business regulations for healthcare. Any model used in healthcare clinics needs to be cleared by the FDA, EMA, or similar organizations. Making sure accurate audit and safe storage of patient data with proper verification are required for the security of the blockchain, these things are part of blockchain. Making AI-based blockchain healthcare systems trustworthy requires efforts from multiple fields, regular testing of models, and responsible way of using them.

CHALLENGES AND LIMITATIONS

The implementation of blockchain technology in metaverse healthcare encounters three main challenges because of its scalability problems and regulatory hurdles and organizational obstacles. The general acceptance of blockchain technologies requires solving various obstacles so it can function effectively alongside secure and transparent operations. The healthcare industries in many places deal with difficulties that prevent them from giving services that are efficient, fair, and of good quality. Since health data in many cases is found on different platforms and computers, teams are having a hard time working with each other and accessing all a patient's information. Such separation slows down choices about treatment and also raises the chance of misdiagnoses and medical mistakes. Also, data stored centrally is more likely to be accessed improperly, causing major problems with protecting sensitive medical records.

Administering the country's health system and maintaining older equipment consume a lot of money, making it harder for healthcare providers to offer enough services and adding more stress to patients. In numerous regions, mainly those that are rural or underserved, the access to health services is too limited, which results in different treatment outcomes. Besides, most traditional ways are not sufficiently up-to-date with technology and are unable to provide care that is tailored and immediate, so treatments are not as effective. Following strict rules in the industry may obstruct the use of innovative and advanced solutions. The problems become even worse when people do not embrace technology and patients are not given a chance to take part in making decisions. Dealing with these problems is crucial for creating a health system that cares about patients, performs better, and provides what today's consumers need.

Scalability Concerns in Blockchain Based Healthcare Solutions

Performance issues exist in healthcare systems that implement Blockchain technology because they handle a substantial amount of patient data each day. Traditional blockchains operating at Bitcoin and Ethereum both possess slow operation speeds and high costs that prevent their use for real-time processing of medical records. The digital healthcare models based on Metaverse technology become efficient through high-speed transactions that ensure fast network data access, (Biswas & Singh, 2024).

The implementation of sharding technology in private blockchain networks through Layer2 scaling solutions provides scalability solutions to the system. The system operates by using security protocols with these two components for swift secure transactions. The phaseout of hybrid blockchain systems enables the complete scalability solution since they maintain decentralization by connecting public and private blockchains. Healthcare organizations need appropriate solutions to solve implementation challenges which prevent full system connection deployment success.

Regulatory and Legal Complexities

For successful blockchain technology execution healthcare organizations must adopt international rules which unify HIPAA USA standards with GDPR European standards as well as privacy standards. Blockchains create data security through their protection features which results in challenges for patient data access according to existing governance protocols. Healthcare organizations maintain multiple strict legal requirements that control blockchain applications for standard medical data protection.

Healthcare areas operate with diverse medical regulatory requirements that create multiple operational technical obstacles between them. Different organizations have their own regulatory standards which limit blockchain adoption whereas governments support blockchain when it satisfies their evaluation criteria. Successful implementation of blockchain technology between traditional practices and new methods requires healthcare organizations to standardize their regulatory standards, (Gadicha et al., 2025). Smart contract authority regulations need establishment together with guidelines for AI practices and international data management standards for metaverse healthcare standards.

Organizational and Structural Barriers to Adoption

Healthcare organizations prevent blockchain technology implementation because they need experienced experts and adequate infrastructure to handle employee skill deficits. Blockchain implementation becomes expensive due to the need for integrating systems which fail to meet blockchain requirements. Proper training for both healthcare staff members and IT personnel as well as policymakers is required for the successful operation of blockchain protocol in decentralized healthcare delivery. Several healthcare stakeholders hesitate about implementing Blockchain-Based healthcare solutions because they need to switch away from traditional centralized frameworks. Cloud adoption process progresses slowly since stakeholders maintain concerns about return on investment deductions and implementation security risks together with workflow disturbances, (Jadhav, Sayyed, & Gupta, 2025). Success in blockchain adoption for healthcare demands healthcare institutions and technology providers and policymakers to work together for the development of cost-effective strategies as well as interoperability standards and training programs that support blockchain implementation.

Economic and Environmental Cost of Blockchain in Healthcare

Even though blockchain brings security and creates transparency in the healthcare industry, the process of adopting it has quite a few economic and environmental expenses that should be carefully considered. A main reason for concern is how much energy goes into running the consensus mechanisms. The electricity used to verify transactions in these cryptos contributes a lot to their carbon emission. However, permissioned or private blockchains with PoA or PoS are preferred in healthcare apps, yet wasting less energy is very important for their sustainable operation. Besides, making blockchain work requires buying new hardware, using secure nodes, setting up high-availability servers, and ensuring constant upkeep, which makes everything more costly for users. When there are not enough resources, setting up the necessary infrastructure may be costly for some healthcare organizations. It is very important for a business to calculate its Return on Investment (ROI). Thanks to blockchain, there is less fraud, administration is easier, and costs can be reduced in the long run. However, the results come after many people have adopted the technology and it is connected with other systems. Sustainable and equal introduction of blockchain in healthcare can happen if key players focus on practical solutions, advanced technology, and the use of environmentally friendly systems.

FUTURE RESEARCH DIRECTIONS

The combination of healthcare and metaverse technologies is an important new direction, and there are various important areas that research should focus on for its success. Another main focus is to build blockchain-supported systems for handling health records to make sure the data is secure, available everywhere, and lets patients handle their data themselves. It is very important to study AI-based virtual healthcare solutions, especially for fast diagnostics, custom treatment ideas, and help with mental problems that can be handled through immersive metaverse platforms. Developing digital twins opens new ways for personal healthcare, as they help with simulation and with monitoring patients in real time. In addition, making sure that metaverse platforms, healthcare systems, and wearable devices have the same interoperability standards will allow them to communicate easily. More research should be done on technologies like federated learning and homomorphic encryption to ensure privacy of patients' data during virtual communication. It is also true that using wearable tech along with AR/VR systems can make remote diagnostics, physical rehab, and surgical training much more effective. In the end, researchers must handle issues of ethics and regulations so that digital healthcare within the metaverse is welcoming to all, just, and follows rules worldwide. Ensuring a secure and patient-friendly future in digital health depends greatly on work done in these research areas, (Kashyap, 2024).

Table 5. Future research directions in blockchain-metaverse healthcare

Research Area	Description
Blockchain Interoperability	Cross-platform communication and standard protocols
Privacy-Preserving Techniques	Homomorphic encryption, federated learning, zero-knowledge proofs
Digital Twins for Personalized Care	Real-time simulation and predictive health modelling
Smart Contract Governance	Frameworks for ethical, automated decision-making in healthcare workflows
AR/VR and Wearable Integration	Enhanced remote diagnostics and rehabilitation in immersive environments

Table 5 highlights key future research areas necessary for the advancement of blockchain-enabled metaverse healthcare, including technology, privacy, scalability, and regulatory frameworks.

Enhancing Interoperability Between Blockchain Networks in Healthcare

Further research about blockchain serves a critical purpose because it establishes vital implementation hurdles that drive metaverse healthcare development. Research on blockchain technologies identifies how widely virtual healthcare will spread by establishing standard practices and better solutions for scalable frameworks and privacy protections. To allow medical institutions and digital health platforms to exchange data without issues, it is important for all blockchain networks in healthcare to communicate and work seamlessly. At the moment, healthcare providers have a hard time-sharing patient data in real time because each blockchain system usually operates separately. It requires making standards for how different blockchain platforms receive and send information, ensuring that no one's privacy or data is broken. Movement of medical records and consent authorizations from one blockchain network to another is possible through the help of interoperability bridges and sidechains. The union of universal healthcare standards such as HL7 FHIR and decentralized technology is needed to help with this task. Besides, smart contract interoperability frameworks can handle automated work processes like filing insurance claims and taking part in clinical trials on different blockchains. If medical datasets are interoperable on blockchains, the sharing of information among doctors becomes easier, patients avoid duplicate tests, and they can manage their histories at once. Furthermore, connecting blockchain technology to old EHRs can help gain benefits without interrupting the established systems. For there to be a connected healthcare system put together by patients, it is important to improve how systems interact, (Kavithamani, 2025).

Figure 4. Interoperability across blockchain networks

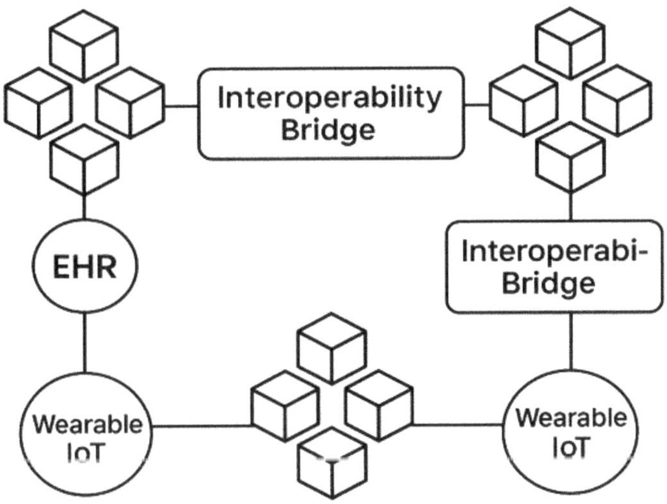

Figure 4 shows multiple blockchain platforms connected via interoperability bridges, with EHR, insurance, and wearable IoT data flowing seamlessly across nodes.

Development of Standardized Frameworks for Blockchain Integration

The implementation rate of blockchain healthcare technology stays low because there is no established protocol for blockchain solution deployment. A prospective research initiative should provide implementation approaches for healthcare blockchain together with solutions to integrate it into medical information technology frameworks that fulfil regulatory needs. Healthcare institutions require standardized protocols that link smart contracts to patient consent systems and data procedures for secure blockchain deployment, (Oduntan et al., 2024). Healthcare industry policies require governmental and healthcare and technology providers to collaborate toward developing blockchain deployment standards that comply with international medical regulations.

Strategies for Improving Blockchain Scalability and Efficiency

Traditional blockchains serve as the main obstacle blocking Blockchain Based healthcare applications from reaching their required speed during transaction processing. People working on innovative scale-up solutions need to conduct thorough research before merging sharding technology with off-chain operations for creating combined blockchain framework designs, (Pathak, Singh, & Roy, 2024). Healthcare organizations choose to avoid blockchain implementation because they lack experienced specialists and appropriate infrastructure required to remediate employee skill shortfalls. The high implementation cost for blockchain relates to system integration efforts when existing systems do not satisfy blockchain standards.

Ethical and Privacy Considerations in Metaverse Healthcare

Healthcare systems powered by blockchain technology must build confidential methods for ethical patient privacy protection since this solution becomes pressing for immediate deployment. Healthcare organizations should move forward with the standardization of blockchain system access at the same time as they work to automate bias reduction through healthcare and develop ethical frameworks for AI research decisions, (Salama & Al-Turjman, 2025). To protect medical records effectively the investigation should examine the combination of zero knowledge proofs (ZKPs) with homomorphic encryption because these methods provide security protection for data. Through decentralization of identity technology patients can manage autonomous health care functions to control their healthcare data access within protected medical record systems. The research frameworks of blockchain systems will establish protected ethical frameworks to support virtual healthcare systems operating in the metaverse.

Research Gaps and Future Technologies

Even though blockchain and healthcare are merging in the metaverse, certain challenges and issues in technology have not yet been resolved, so there is room for more exploration. An important issue is that real-time consensus techniques are not available for healthcare applications. Currently used consensus algorithms, for example Proof of Work (PoW), are not made to cope with the fast and continuous needs of patient monitoring or urgent interventions. It is very important that we find lightweight consensus protocols designed for healthcare applications. It is also true that there are no standard health chain protocols that ensure better coordination and sharing of information among networks, hospitals, and nations globally. Though frameworks like HL7 FHIR work well, no one has managed to fully integrate them with blockchain. Also, the fact that data privacy laws vary from place to place (such as GDPR and HIPAA) can be a hurdle for businesses using blockchain technology. Current methods of encryption might not match up with the changing laws, demanding new privacy protectors. Innovation in quantum blockchain and post-quantum cryptography is expected to solve the network's problems with scalability and security, (Subramani & Manoharan, 2024). It is also an exciting field to research when we combine edge computing, digital twins, and decentralized AI governance. Working on these gaps will help make future healthcare systems more solid, secure, and capable of serving more patients.

CONCLUSION

Healthcare providers must implement blockchain systems to design digital health management tools which will boost system security while offering expedited operations alongside easy access to platforms in their virtual healthcare settings. Blockchain technology resolves simultaneously both healthcare privacy issues and manages complex integration processes through its ability to overcome manager-based system development barriers. The path of blockchain technology development needs obstacle elimination to establish broad market readiness for this technology.

The standalone medical metaverse solution of blockchain maintains secure decentralization of database entries by using built-in cryptographic security features. Medical data breaches along with unauthorized user entries and distributed medical records result in poor patient care and ineffective data management systems. The patient data remains secure through Blockchain since the technology blocks authorized medical staff from viewing files located on mutable information systems. Through security protocols advanced medical data protection becomes possible because HIPAA regulations together with GDPR requirements enable such protection.

Healthcare organizations operating in their districts gain superior benefits by deploying blockchain along with smart contracts to improve operational outcomes in medical settings. Blockchain-Based digital identities perform identity verifications to safeguard patients from theft and protect both their records and identity from unauthorized changes. The implementation of smart contracts in healthcare insurance claim processing leads to fewer medical errors while improving electronic record systems that validate prescriptions. The implementation of Blockchain features acts as a catalyst for medical systems to evolve into metaverse platforms that both improve patient quality of care and strengthen system reliability and safeguard against responses to clients.

The evaluation examines the association between blockchain technology and artificial intelligence which exists during metaverse application development. Information technology systems supported by blockchain enable AI predictive technologies to provide treatment improvements and disease tracking services to patients. The implementation of AI plays an essential role in Blockchain Based healthcare systems because it detects complete patient data relationships in vast healthcare network environments. Better patient success becomes achievable for high-quality medical treatment through remote healthcare applications that utilize these integrated technologies.

To deploy blockchain operations in healthcare settings scientists must first address and resolve the existing implementation barriers. The high resource requirements of blockchain systems prevent proper scalability because of their limited capabilities to handle substantial medical data transfers. The processing requirements of Bitcoin and Ethereum blockchain systems as well as their newer versions demand significant time for completion and significant energy consumption. Scientists need to combine layer2 protocols with sharding methods under network implementation methods to achieve scalability while improving system performance and reducing costs.

Healthcare organizations encounter difficulties when adopting blockchain technology because current healthcare regulations implement operational requirements on their information systems. The regulatory oversight system lacks the capability to monitor blockchain operations because the decentralized approach of blockchain stands in opposite position compared to traditional control mechanisms meant for centralized data. Public authorities must create official operating procedures to protect privacy laws since these procedures establish the methods for applying health information privacy guidelines to technological advancements. should proceed. The implementation of blockchain technology into healthcare demands healthcare institutions to dismantle regulations which impede integration procedures.

The healthcare industry shows comprehensive reluctance to adopt full blockchain implementation because of operational limitations in their current procedures. Medical organizations do not delete current data systems because they need to address rising expenses and difficult operations which result from their insufficient infrastructural capabilities. Healthcare providers must launch education programs for staff and developers need to start academic institution partnerships for filling out the knowledge gap on this technology to deploy blockchain systems.

Research on Blockchain Based metaverse healthcare needs to enhance blockchain network connections together with standardized operational guidelines and privacy security measures and ethical policies. Healthcare institutions achieve unified system success through standard secure data exchange standards that enable them to implement interoperability standards. Healthcare organizations need fewer difficulties in implementing standardized blockchain frameworks because their configured specifications fit existing medical systems. The protection of patient rights and ethical systems that keep AI healthcare decision systems safe from wrongdoings continues through traditional oversight as blockchain develops.

The healthcare industry implements the metaverse through blockchain technology which develops secured patient systems that combine high-level security features with transparent operational views. For successful implementation of this technology institutions must conduct persistent research alongside modern solutions that resolve existing operational problems. Healthcare organizations enhance operational capabilities through blockchain technology because it lets patients maintain secure medical data access during research interactions. Better blockchain technology development will create a worldwide universal medical system within the metaverse healthcare space for patient network connections.

REFERENCES

. Adeghe, E., Okolo, C., & Ojeyinka, O. (2024). Evaluating the impact of blockchain technology in healthcare data management: a review of security, privacy, and patient outcomes. Open Access Research Journal of Science and Technology, 10(2), 013-020. https://doi.org/DOI: 10.53022/oarjst.2024.10.2.0044

Agbo, C., Mahmoud, Q., & Eklund, J. (2019). Blockchain technology in healthcare: A systematic review. *Health Care*, *7*(2), 56. DOI: 10.3390/healthcare7020056

Agbo, C., Mahmoud, Q., & Eklund, J. (2019). Blockchain technology in healthcare: A systematic review. *Health Care*, *7*(2), 56. DOI: 10.3390/healthcare7020056

. Ahamed, M. (2024). Decentralized ai for medical emergency response using blockchain and computer vision. jes, 20(11s), 3479-3490. https://doi.org/DOI: 10.52783/jes.8128

Aloqaily, M., Bouachir, O., Karray, F., Ridhawi, I., & Saddik, A. (2023). Integrating digital twin and advanced intelligent technologies to realize the metaverse. *IEEE Consumer Electronics Magazine*, *12*(6), 47–55. DOI: 10.1109/mce.2022.3212570

Arbabi, M., Lal, C., Veeraragavan, N., Marijan, D., Nygård, J., & Vitenberg, R. (2023). A survey on blockchain for healthcare: Challenges, benefits, and future directions. *IEEE Communications Surveys and Tutorials*, *25*(1), 386–424. DOI: 10.1109/comst.2022.3224644

Atadoga, A., Elufioye, O., Omaghomi, T., Akomolafe, O., Odilibe, I., & Owolabi, O. (2024). Blockchain in healthcare: A comprehensive review of applications and security concerns. *International Journal of Science and Research Archive*, *11*(1), 1605–1613. DOI: 10.30574/ijsra.2024.11.1.0244

Attaran, M. (2020). Blockchain technology in healthcare: Challenges and opportunities. *International Journal of Healthcare Management*, *15*(1), 70–83. DOI: 10.1080/20479700.2020.1843887

Benchoufi, M., Porcher, R., & Ravaud, P. (2018). Blockchain protocols in clinical trials: Transparency and traceability of consent. *F1000 Research*, *6*, 66. DOI: 10.12688/f1000research.10531.5

Bidve, V., Kakakde, K., Sarasu, P., Kediya, S., Tamkhade, P., & Suprakash, S. (2023). Patient data management using blockchain technology. *Indonesian Journal of Electrical Engineering and Computer Science*, *32*(3), 1746. DOI: 10.11591/ijeecs.v32.i3.pp1746-1754

. Biswas, M. and Singh, D. (2024). "application of ai and blockchain in healthcare industry" – a review. jaz. https://doi.org/DOI: 10.53555/jaz.v45i2.3983

Chander, E. (2023). Decentralized healthcare system using blockchain. *Interantional Journal of Scientific Research in Engineering and Management*, *07*(11), 1–11. DOI: 10.55041/ijsrem27214

Dimitrov, D. (2019). Blockchain applications for healthcare data management. *Healthcare Informatics Research*, *25*(1), 51. DOI: 10.4258/hir.2019.25.1.51

Drosatos, G., & Kaldoudi, E. (2019). Blockchain applications in the biomedical domain: A scoping review. *Computational and Structural Biotechnology Journal*, *17*, 229–240. DOI: 10.1016/j.csbj.2019.01.010

. Gadicha, A., Gadicha, V., Burange, M., & Khan, Z. (2025). Leveraging blockchain and ai for sustainable development., 315-338. https://doi.org/DOI: 10.4018/979-8-3693-8664-4.ch014

Garg, A. (2024). Blockchain-based health informatics systems for secure patient data sharing and interoperability. *Seminars in Medical Writing and Education*, *3*, 508. DOI: 10.56294/mw2024508

Garg, S., Kaushal, R., Kumar, N., & Verma, A. (2023). Bibliometric analysis of blockchain in the healthcare domain. *Intelligent and Converged Networks*, *4*(4), 305–312. DOI: 10.23919/icn.2023.0025

Hylock, R., & Zeng, X. (2019). A blockchain framework for patient-centered health records and exchange (healthchain): Evaluation and proof-of-concept study. *Journal of Medical Internet Research*, *21*(8), e13592. DOI: 10.2196/13592

. Jadhav, B., Sayyed, M., & Gupta, S. (2025). Intelligent iot healthcare applications powered by blockchain technology., 1-22. https://doi.org/DOI: 10.2174/9789815305210125010004

Jat, A., Grønli, T., Ghinea, G., & Assres, G. (2024). Evolving software architecture design in telemedicine: A prisma-based systematic review. *Healthcare Informatics Research*, *30*(3), 184–193. DOI: 10.4258/hir.2024.30.3.184

Jusić, A. (2022). Privacy between regulation and technology: gdpr and the blockchain. iuslawjournal, Vol 1(No 1), 47-59. https://doi.org/DOI: 10.21533/iuslawjournal.v1i1.9

Kashyap, G. (2024). Ai in blockchain-enabled healthcare systems. *Interantional Journal of Scientific Research in Engineering and Management*, *08*(12), 1–7. DOI: 10.55041/ijsrem17947

Kavithamani, M. (2025). Blockchain for the next decade: Future trends and predictions in healthcare. *Journal of Information Systems Engineering & Management, 10*(11s), 178–185. DOI: 10.52783/jisem.v10i11s.1510

Khatib, M., Alzoubi, H., Hamidi, S., Alshurideh, M., Baydoun, A., & Al-Nakeeb, A. (2023). Impact of using the internet of medical things on e-healthcare performance: Blockchain assist in improving smart contract. *ClinicoEconomics and Outcomes Research, 15*, 397–411. DOI: 10.2147/ceor.s407778

. Kumar, B., Albusaidi, I., & Halloush, M. (2023). Healthcare information exchange using blockchain and machine learning., 55-69. https://doi.org/DOI: 10.2991/978-94-6463-110-4_6

Mackey, T., Kuo, T., Gummadi, B., Clauson, K., Church, G., Grishin, D., & Palombini, M. (2019). 'fit-for-purpose?' – challenges and opportunities for applications of blockchain technology in the future of healthcare. *BMC Medicine, 17*(1). Advance online publication. DOI: 10.1186/s12916-019-1296-7

Mayer, A., Costa, C., & Righi, R. (2019). Electronic health records in a blockchain: A systematic review. *Health Informatics Journal, 26*(2), 1273–1288. DOI: 10.1177/1460458219866350

Motohashi, T., Hirano, T., Okumura, K., Kashiyama, M., Ichikawa, D., & Ueno, T. (2019). Secure and scalable mhealth data management using blockchain combined with client hashchain: System design and validation. *Journal of Medical Internet Research, 21*(5), e13385. DOI: 10.2196/13385

Nguyen, H., Danh, H., Ma, Q., Měsíček, J., Hajnyš, J., Pagáč, M., & Petrů, J. (2023). A bibliometrics analysis of medical internet of things for modern healthcare. *Electronics (Basel), 12*(22), 4586. DOI: 10.3390/electronics12224586

. Oduntan, O., Bature, H., Wisdom, D., Okechukwu, U., Isaac, S., & Falayi, C. (2024). Artificial intelligence & blockchain technology in modern telehealth systems-a systematic review. kjcs, 1(3), 607-625. https://doi.org/DOI: 10.47514/kjcs/2024.1.3.0015

. Pathak, J., Singh, K., & Roy, S. (2024). Role of artificial intelligence and blockchain on cyber security., 287-320. https://doi.org/DOI: 10.4018/979-8-3693-6537-3.ch013

Pokharel, B., Kshetri, N., Sharma, S., & Paudel, S. (2025). Blockhealthsecure: Integrating blockchain and cybersecurity in post-pandemic healthcare systems. *Information (Basel), 16*(2), 133. DOI: 10.3390/info16020133

. Raasetti, M. (2024). Blockchain technology's role in securing data and preventing cyberattacks: a detailed review. AJSTEME, 4(3), 16-31. https://doi.org/ context. Ccit Journal, 17(1), 10-21. https://doi.org/DOI: 10.69593/ajsteme.v4i03.86re

. Salama, R. and Al-Turjman, F. (2025). Intelligent medical applications blockchain-powered 6g networks. neuaiit, 4(1), 2-15. https://doi.org/DOI: 10.32955/ neuaiit202541922

. Subramani, K. and Manoharan, G. (2024). Ai, iot, and blockchain in healthcare., 161-180. https://doi.org/DOI: 10.4018/979-8-3373-0240-9.ch008

Vazirani, A., O'Donoghue, O., Brindley, D., & Meinert, E. (2020). Blockchain vehicles for efficient medical record management. *NPJ Digital Medicine*, *3*(1). Advance online publication. DOI: 10.1038/s41746-019-0211-0

. Wang, H., Chu, S., Yan, J., Huang, Y., Fang, I., Pan, S., … & Shen, T. (2020). Blockchain-based medical record management with biofeedback information.. https://doi.org/DOI: 10.5772/intechopen.94370

Wong, D., Bhattacharya, S., & Butte, A. (2019). Prototype of running clinical trials in an untrustworthy environment using blockchain. *Nature Communications*, *10*(1). Advance online publication. DOI: 10.1038/s41467-019-08874-y

Yang, Q., Zhao, Y., Huang, H., Xiong, Z., Kang, J., & Zheng, Z. (2022). Fusing blockchain and ai with metaverse: A survey. *IEEE Open Journal of the Computer Society*, *3*, 122–136. DOI: 10.1109/ojcs.2022.3188249

Yulianjani, A., Rosdiana, R., & Altaufik, R. (2024). Analysis of blockchain technology in patient data management system: security, privacy, and efficiency in the digital healthca Feltovic, M. (2024). From theory to practice: the role of cryptography in securing blockchain networks. *Mest Journal*, *12*(2), 93–102. DOI: 10.12709/ mest.12.12.02.12

Chapter 11
Future Research Directions for Blockchain in Metaverse Healthcare

G. Ramya
https://orcid.org/0000-0002-4712-8699
SRM Institute of Science and Technology, India

T. Preethiya
https://orcid.org/0000-0003-3504-1884
College of Engineering and Technology, SRM Institute of Science and Technology, India

R. Nithya Paranthaman
https://orcid.org/0000-0003-2281-1923
College of Engineering and Technology, SRM Institute of Science and Technology, India

S. Ashwini
College of Engineering and Technology, SRM Institute of Science and Technology, India

R. Dhwarithaa
College of Engineering and Technology, SRM Institute of Science and Technology, India

G. Abinaya
College of Engineering and Technology, SRM Institute of Science and Technology, India

ABSTRACT

The inclusion of Blockchain in the Metaverse delivers opportunities for healthcare, contributes to the data security, maintains transparency and decentralization of data. The current Healthcare systems revolve around the immersive data and digitalization of data putting the metaverse as a frontier. This spawned telemedicine, virtual doctor consultations, training people and patient engagement. The integration of Blockchain with the Metaverse healthcare aims to enhance the privacy, security and reliability of data. The key applications of it are patient record management, providing access to valid credentials and decentralized clinical assessments. This

DOI: 10.4018/979-8-3373-1225-5.ch011

chapter tries to provide a comprehensive overview of Blockchain's transformative potential in Metaverse healthcare, highlighting key areas for future research and development. This chapter aims to address several future research directions such as interoperability of devices/data for seamless services, need for privacy-preserving of patient's data, regulatory compliance, ownership of data and other ethical considerations.

INTRODUCTION

The current healthcare sector is digitalizing, and there is a surge for efficient and secure healthcare applications. The Metaverse (Bansal et.al, 2022, Al-Kfairy et.al, 2024), a virtual space where the end users can interact with the computer-generated environment to provide efficient solutions (Bansal et.al, 2022, Al-Kfairy et.al, 2024). Incorporating Blockchain technology in the Metaverse has unleashed a new paradigm in healthcare, deploying plethora of opportunities for patient care, medical training and patient's record management. The Metaverse is emerging as frontier by embracing digitalization and redefining the delivery of medical services. This digital transformation has led to various security challenges in terms of data breaches, low interoperability and ethical concerns. Blockchain, a decentralized architecture aims to provides security in the form of transparency and also plays a vital role in addressing the digital security challenges of Metaverse healthcare (Mozumder, M. A. I et.al, 2023). The integration of these two in healthcare ensures privacy, security, reliability of patients' sensitive data, while fostering innovation in telemedicine, virtual consultations and clinical assessments.

Metaverse in Healthcare – An Overview

From the literature we can see many definitions for Metaverse and few of them are listed here.

Definition 1: It is a virtual ecosystem that effectively combines many aspects of social media applications, gaming, Augmented Reality (AR), Virtual Reality (VR) and cryptocurrencies for interaction of users in the virtual ecosystem (Chengoden et.al, 2023).

Definition 2: It is a network of shared, connected with virtually created ecosystem, where people communicate with each other, connect with each other, play games and do shopping (Chengoden et.al, 2023).

Definition 3: A networked online space that connects environments or creates an ecosystem digitally that people connect, interacts and experiences services virtually, AR, VR, gaming via mobile devices or computers (Chengoden et.al, 2023).

The Metaverse Healthcare is a virtually created ecosystem that comprises Augmented Reality (AR), Virtual Reality (VR), Digital Twinning (DT), Artificial Intelligence (AI) and the Internet of Things (IoT) technologies (Chengoden et.al, 2023, Alghamdi et.al, 2024) to deliver immersive Healthcare applications. The Healthcare system provides service experience that is interactive, immersive and tailors customized applications to meet individual's needs. The application of these technologies offers an experience over new mechanisms of medical treatment in lower cost by enhancing patient experience. It creates the new level experience of virtual medical ecosystem via the Internet by analysing gestures and emotions of human behaviour.

The following are the key applications of Metaverse in Healthcare and is shown in Figure 1.

Figure 1. Key applications of metaverse healthcare

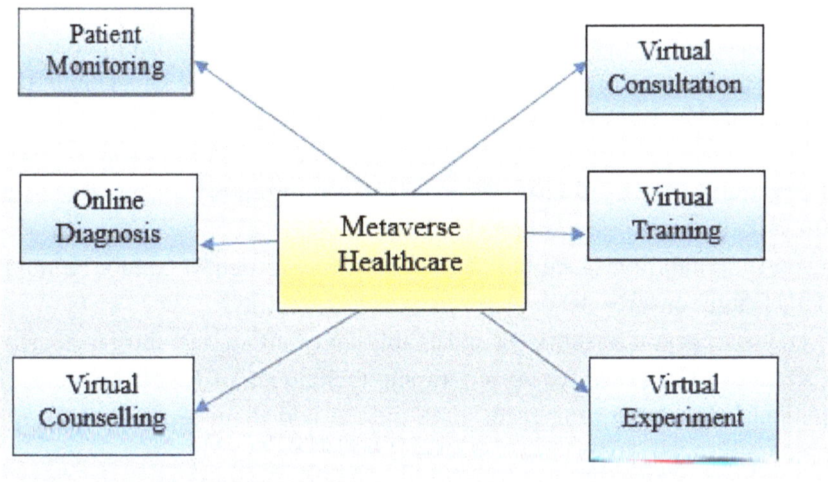

Figure 1.1 Key applications of Metaverse Healthcare

(i) Telemedicine and Virtual Consultations: The Metaverse enables remote connection between patient and doctor for virtual consultations, communication and provide seamless services.

(ii) Training: It facilitates simulations for training the healthcare professional by connecting with the peers in the same healthcare sector to update themselves in the latest technology. This simulation also helps to conduct risk-free ecosystem for learning complex medical procedures in an efficient manner.

(iii) Rehabilitation: This virtual ecosystem facilitates physical and psychological therapies irrespective of the patient location.

Blockchain and its Application in Metaverse

The Metaverse healthcare deals highly sensitive patients' health data which demands highly secured ecosystem. Blockchain is a digital database of transactions that is replicated and distributed over entire Blockchain network (Chengoden et.al, 2023). Each block of it contains several transactions, and any addition of new record is made whenever a new transaction occurs. It is a type of Distributed Ledger Technology (DLT) where the records are immutable and are highly secured by Hash, cryptographic signature. Whenever a block in a chain is modified, it will get notified immediately. If someone wishes to hack the chain, they might have to change every copy of it that are distributed across the entire Blockchain network (Alghamdi et.al, 2024). Blockchain when applied to Metaverse healthcare provides security, data integrity and transparency. The key features of Blockchain that has critical role in Metaverse healthcare ecosystem are as follows.

(i) Decentralization: It eliminates the need for central authorization and also reduces the risk of single point failure.

(ii) Data Immutability: Once the data is entered/recorded, it cannot be modified. This feature ensures data consistency and readability.

(iii) Transparency: It fosters trust and enables only authorized entry to access data.

(iv) Security: The powerful cryptographic techniques of Blockchain safeguards patients' data from tampering, data misuse and illegitimate authorization of data.

The rest of this chapter discusses the current scenario of Blockchain security in Metaverse, challenges and its future research directions. The primary focus aligns to the title by delving into potential benefits of Blockchain in Metaverse healthcare. This chapter outlines a roadmap for future research and development by leveraging Blockchain's potential in reshaping Metaverse healthcare.

LITERATURE SURVEY OF METAVERSE HEALTHCARE

(Mazhar et al., 2025), provided an analysis of the intersection of Generative AI (GenAI), Internet of Things (IoT), and Blockchain in healthcare with a focus on their collaborative value to transform patient-cantered services. The authors emphasized the use of GenAI in generating medical images, making diagnoses automatically, and synthesizing reports with scalable solutions for clinical decision-making and IoT supporting real-time health monitoring via wearable technologies. Blockchain is recognized as a core technology in maintaining data integrity, decentralization, and auditability in electronic health records (EHRs) and access control systems. Nevertheless, these benefits, the authors recognized various challenges such as data privacy issues during AI model training, blockchain scalability problems in high-throughput settings, and interoperability obstacles across heterogeneous healthcare systems. In order to solve these, they suggested a privacy-preserving AI methods like federated learning, scalability enhancements via Directed Acyclic Graphs (DAG) and sharding, along with standardization of IoT protocols and ethical frameworks for AI regulation.

(Bathula et al,2024), present a narrative review presenting the transformative possibility of the trio—Blockchain, Artificial Intelligence (AI), and Healthcare—as one cohesive framework deciding the destiny of medical systems in the future. The authors focus on how blockchain can provide trust in a decentralized manner, offer secure sharing of data, as well as impenetrable audit trails, for healthcare-sensitive data, effectively resolving the eternal issues regarding security and integrity in data. Concurrently, AI is examined for its cross-domain applications across predictive analytics, diagnostic support, targeted medicine, and administrative processes. The essay stresses the symbiotic relationship of blockchain and AI, where blockchain provides trust and transparency in data provenance while AI enables wise insights and decision-making support.

Further this paper addresses integration issues like the absence of standards for interoperability, computational cost, data protection regulations (e.g., compliance with the GDPR), and moral objections to AI bias and impenetrable decision-making. The authors recommend hybrid models like blockchain-enabled federated learning and suggest that future work should aim at scalable, privacy-protecting infrastructure, resilient data governance, and cross-domain collaboration to achieve the maximum potential of this technological combination in healthcare. This review adds to the seminal understanding of how, when positioned strategically, blockchain and AI can support secure, intelligent, and patient-centered digital health ecosystems.

The Metaverse healthcare is fully driven by Blockchain, Digital Twins (DT) and 5G/6G beyond. DT is a visual representation of any physical object, process, system or any entity that is created using real-world data (Bathula et.al, 2024, Okegbile et.al, 2024). These are designed to simulate the ecosystem, monitoring it, and optimizing the real-world applications. The bandwidth offered by 5G and 6G beyond is crucial for any time-sensitive Medicare applications.

Healthify (Healthland, 2022) is a Metaverse wellness program that promotes both mental and physical well-being through personalized health advice, virtual workouts, and guided consultations with wellness specialists. It aimed at preventive care through digital interaction with the users, leverages immersive settings and gamified elements to foster regular user engagement. This promotes healthy living practices and makes resources for easily accessible, especially for the users who are distant from healthcare resources, and it is a scalable digital health tool.

DeHealth (Dehealth, 2022) is a decentralized Metaverse platform aimed to bridge the gap between healthcare practitioners and patients by facilitating immersive virtual consultations. It combines Metaverse and Blockchain to facilitate secure platforms. It uses smart contracts to manage access permission of patient Electronic Health Records (HER), by enabling patients to share the selective health data with professionals. This work introduces a decentralized data storage layer and utilizes Blockchain – based identifiers for preserving patient anonymity and ensure interoperability. It supports various avatars and telepresence using Virtual Reality (VR)/ Augmented Reality (AR).

Bump Galaxy (Bump Galaxy, 2022) adopts a gamified Metaverse architecture to support mental health, in which Blockchain is used to manage user credentials, therapy logs and behaviours. It is built on a modular VR engine integrated with Blockchain – backed mental health journaling. Each and all patients interact via avatars in a decentralized space. This platform emphasizes anonymous peer interaction, certified digital therapeutics and community governance. Blockchain facilitates confidentiality and auditability in a mental health focused Metaverse. AccuVein (AccuVein, 2022), is a vein visualization Metaverse healthcare project, which is used by neurosurgeons and patients. By using this, neurosurgeons can view the blood vessels clearly and treat the patient properly.

HintVR (HealthBlocks, 2022) is an Extended Reality (XR) -based platform for pre and post operative consultation and procedural training. It is integrated with Blockchain for content rights agreement and management, decentralized data access and maintains the provenance of medical simulations. This architecture consists of 3D surgical simulation engine that maps with the patient- specific. It supports privacy-preserving operations using pseudonymized Blockchain identities. It also includes edge computing nodes for local processing, reducing latency in a surgical training environment.

The authors (Gupta, N, 2023) propose HealthBlocks, a Blockchain IoT integrated framework for protecting data from smart devices. It features device-level Blockchain agents to manage data signing, secure channel establishment using elliptic curve cryptography. Each IoT smart device possess a decentralized identifier and fully operated on a federated trust model. It also underpins patient-centric consent mechanisms, by enabling real-time but secure data sharing in the Metaverse Healthcare.

OPEN ISSUES IN METAVERSE HEALTHCARE

The current technology trend in Metaverse healthcare has adapted remote patient monitoring, ensured data privacy and delivered best services.

The following Figure 2 depicts the future research directions in integrated Blockchain Metaverse.

Figure 2. Challenges in blockchain metaverse

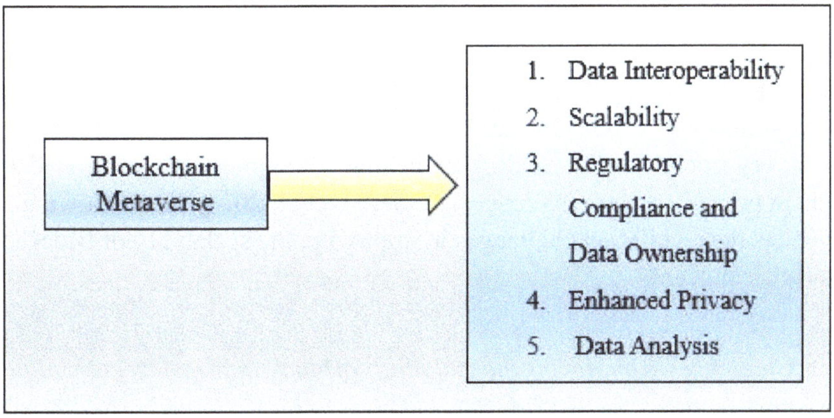

Figure 2.1 Challenges in Blockchain Metaverse

The integration of Blockchain in Metaverse healthcare enables helps in Patient Record Management, Credential Verification, Data Interoperability and Decentralized Clinical Assessments. Despite of the benefits, this integration possesses variety of challenges in terms of Data Interoperability, scalability, Regulatory compliance, Privacy, and Data ownership (Chen, J et.al, 2023).

Data Interoperability

As there are diverse of IoT healthcare devices connected to the Metaverse healthcare poses significant challenge in integration of these devices. The future research should focus on the interoperability of IoT healthcare devices and Blockchain for creating a unified healthcare ecosystem. This challenge can be overcome by applying standardizing protocols cross-chain solutions and implementing API Gateways and Middleware in an efficient manner.

Scalability

As the network scales horizontally, the scalability of Blockchain needs to be addressed. By leveraging the network technologies such as Software Defined Networking (SDN), Network Function Virtualization (NFV) and Fog computing can be applied. Layer 2 solutions can be considered for enhancing the scalability of the Blockchain in Metaverse (Chen, J et.al, 2023).

The healthcare devices collect enormous data which significantly takes time to process at the cloud. Healthcare applications are time-sensitive and the best way to process the data at the edge. The Fog computing lies in the middle of healthcare devices and Cloud reduces the computation time and enhances the performance of the application.

As the number of IoT healthcare devices increases, the network management becomes very complex. The scaling of healthcare applications integrated with Blockchain posses' various challenges (Pervez, F et.al, 2024). The following Figure 3 depicts the significant challenges in improving the scalability of Blockchain Metaverse Healthcare.

Figure 3. Challenges in improving the scalability of blockchain metaverse healthcare

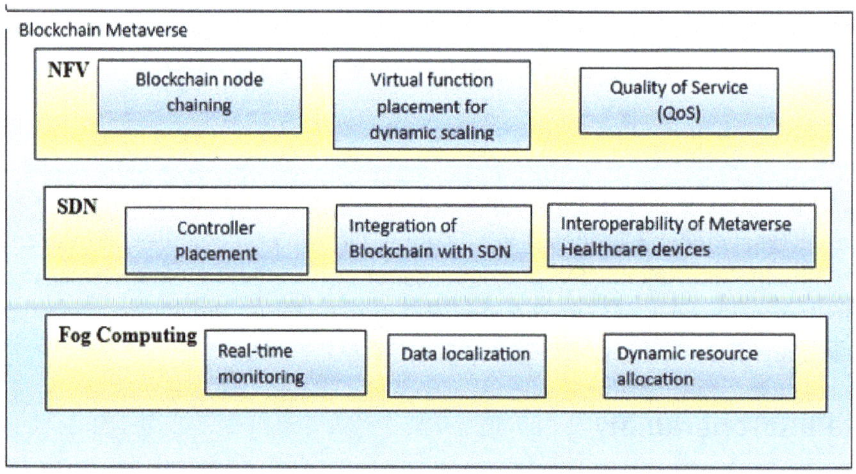

Fig. 2.2 Challenges in improving the scalability of Blockchain Metaverse Healthcare

The application of Software-Define Networking (SDN) to manage the decentralized may results in network traffic optimization, dynamic resource allocation, optimized data flow and enhanced scalability. Further, it also improves the interoperability of devices as there is no proprietary dependency in SDN devices. While the

SDN improves Blockchain node control and data flow, the NFV on the other hand deploys virtualized security functions to enhance security in Metaverse Healthcare. The current research area could be integrating SDN and NFV to improve security. NFV Blockchain node chaining could also be a potential research focus to deploy on-demand scaling of Blockchain nodes and deployment of virtual node functions. Above all, the integration and orchestration of these technologies possess a significant challenge in Metaverse Healthcare.

Regulatory Compliance and Data Ownership

The regulatory compliance is quite essential in everywhere where the data is shared. The Blockchain Metaverse should also incorporate legal framework, Automated Compliance, and Data Sovereignty to ensure data regulations, to enforce standards and to address legal issues related to data breach/transfer. The Blockchain security in Metaverse may define Ownership models to define framework to collect and process the individual data. The research focus could be developing standards to avoid data mishandling and data breaching.

Enhanced Privacy

The Blockchain ensures data security by maintaining the patient privacy in decentralized framework. This needs advanced cryptographic techniques to preserve privacy of patient data. This necessitates Zero-Knowledge Proofs, Multi-party computation and Data anonymization. This emphasis the development of Privacy-Preserving Blockchain Models to be deployed for enhancing security of patient's data.

Summary of Current Challenges in Blockchain Metaverse

The following Table 1 depicts the current challenges in Blockchain Metaverse.

Table 1. Current challenges in blockchain metaverse

Aspect	Current Challenges	Solutions
Data Interoperability	Diverse Healthcare devices	- Development of Standardized protocol - Development of cross- chain platforms-based solution - Implementation of efficient API gateways and Middleware to support Interoperability - Building unified frameworks for Blockchain based IoT Healthcare device interoperability
Scalability	- High volume of data being generated from IoT Healthcare device - Complex network protocols and management - Delay – sensitive environment - Orchestration of new networking technologies	- Usage of Layer 2 Blockchain solutions - Leverage SDN based network infrastructure for efficient network management and traffic optimization - Application of NFV for virtualized security and node functions - Implementation of Fog Computing to achieve low latency
Regulatory Compliance & Data Ownership	- Absence of legal framework in Healthcare Metaverse - Data breaches Lack of standards for ownership and sovereignty.	- Developing legal frameworks for data handling in Metaverse. - Implementation of Automated Compliance mechanisms using smart contracts. - Establishment of data ownership and sovereignty models.
Enhanced Privacy	- As it is sensitive data, enhanced privacy in decentralized health systems - Data exposure risks	- Application of Zero-Trust Authentication (ZTA). – Usage of Multi-Party Computation and anonymization techniques - Designing Privacy-Preserving Blockchain models.

SOCIAL WELFARE AND ETHICAL IMPACT

Blockchain-integrated Metaverse Healthcare refers to the ethical usage of emerging technologies to uplift the society and the overall well-being of it. While Blockchain offers secure, transparent and decentralized control over the data, the metaverse will provide remote healthcare in an efficient manner. The combined effect of them must address the key societal challenges to serve public.

In the perspective of social welfare, it is crucial as well as critical to ensure inclusivity, and data authority. The authorities should have access to these technologies, regardless of their societal status. Blockchain can empower patients by giving them control over their sensitive medical data, by securing them in an effective way. The ethical considerations in the data perspective such as digital literacy, privacy and informed consent needs to be addressed.

Furthermore, Psychological and social impacts of metaverse – based interactions such as virtual consultations or AI driven applications must be carefully designed and chosen to avoid adverse effect of it. The adverse effect may cause mental fatigue, isolation or any other psychological issues of a person or society. Future research must focus on developing affordable solutions, framing global regulatory frameworks and ensure transparency, and privacy of data. The integration of blockchain in metaverse healthcare is not only delivers advance medical technology but also protects patients' data, foster social equity and ensures transparency of data.

FUTURE RESEARCH DIRECTIONS

The following Figure 4 defines the future research directions of Metaverse healthcare. The Metaverse Healthcare is prone to more security threats due to the heterogenous nature of devices involved in monitoring patient health record. The existing Blockchain based secured Metaverse healthcare but the security can be strengthened by applying the Zero-Trust Architecture (ZTA) (Ling, A et.al, 2024, Azad, M et.al, 2024) to enhance context-aware Blockchain access control. It also ensures the continuous verification of nodes in the Blockchain network. This integration opens research challenges such as AI integration, trust management and regulatory compliance.

Figure 4. Dimensions of future research directions in metaverse healthcare

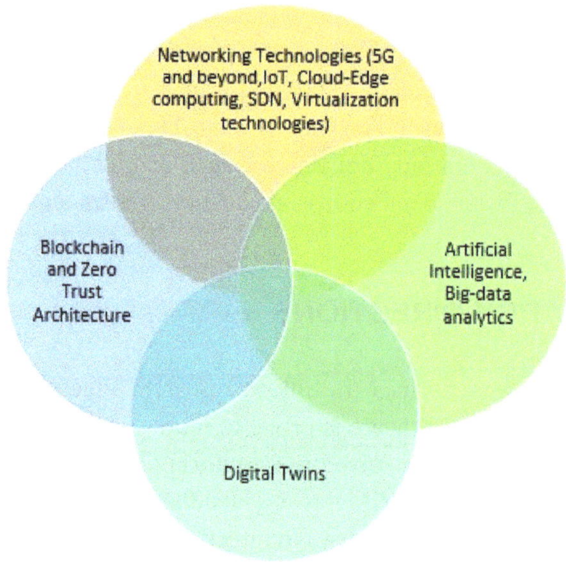

Fig 4.1 Dimensions of future research directions in Metaverse healthcare

The humongous data generated by Metaverse healthcare, needs to be analysed in proper manner using Machine Learning (ML) algorithms to provide enhanced used experience and development of new applications of Metaverse Healthcare. The orchestration of cutting-edge technologies such as SDN, NFV, 5G and beyond, DT needs to be addressed effectively for Qos enhancements. The healthcare devices are resource/energy constrained. Hence an energy efficient metaverse can also be explored to deliver energy-aware healthcare services.

CONCLUSION

The future of Blockchain in Metaverse healthcare is very promising, presenting a multitude of challenges and opportunities to deliver a secure and efficient applications. The challenges include data interoperability, improved security and privacy. By addressing the key challenges and opportunities, the leverage of new technologies helps in delivering efficient applications in Metaverse Healthcare. This chapter addressed the key research challenges and opportunities currently lies in Blockchain Metaverse Healthcare. This chapter also addressed the integration of various technologies to improve overall user experience of Metaverse healthcare users.

REFERENCES

AccuVein. (2022, June). Vein Visualization: The Future of Healthcare is Here. https://www.accuvein.com/why-accuvein/ar/

Al-Kfairy, M., Alomari, A., Al-Bashayreh, M., Alfandi, O., & Tubishat, M. (2024). Unveiling the Metaverse: A survey of user perceptions and the impact of usability, social influence and interoperability. *Heliyon*, *10*, 1–16. PMID: 38826724

Alghamdi, T. A., Khalid, R., & Javaid, N. (2024). A survey of blockchain-based systems: Scalability issues and solutions, applications and future challenges. *IEEE Access : Practical Innovations, Open Solutions*, *12*, 79626–79651.

Azad, M. A., Abdullah, S., Arshad, J., Lallie, H., & Ahmed, Y. H. (2024). Verify and trust: A multidimensional survey of zero-trust security in the age of IoT. *Internet of Things : Engineering Cyber Physical Human Systems*, *27*, 101227.

Bansal, G., Rajgopal, K., Chamola, V., Xiong, Z., & Niyato, D. (2022). Healthcare in metaverse: A survey on current metaverse applications in healthcare. *IEEE Access : Practical Innovations, Open Solutions*, *10*, 119914–119946.

Bathula, A., Gupta, S. K., Merugu, S., Saba, L., Khanna, N. N., Laird, J. R., & Suri, J. S. (2024). Blockchain, artificial intelligence, and healthcare: The tripod of future—a narrative review. *Artificial Intelligence Review*, *57*(9), 238.

Bump Galaxy. (2022, June). Mental Healthcare Metaverse. https://gitcoin.co/grants/2026/bump-galaxy-mental-healthcare-metaverse

Chen, J., Yi, C., Okegbile, S. D., Cai, J., & Shen, X. (2023). Networking architecture and key supporting technologies for human digital twin in personalized healthcare: A comprehensive survey. *IEEE Communications Surveys and Tutorials*, *26*(1), 706–746.

Chengoden, R., Victor, N., Huynh-The, T., Yenduri, G., Jhaveri, R. H., Alazab, M., Bhattacharya, S., Hegde, P., Maddikunta, P. K. R., & Gadekallu, T. R. (2023). Metaverse for healthcare: A survey on potential applications, challenges and future directions. *IEEE Access : Practical Innovations, Open Solutions*, *11*, 12765–12795.

Dehealth. (2022, June). The world's first healthcare metaverse from Dehealth. https://www.dehealth.world/post/the-worlds-first-healthcare-metaverse-from-dehealth

Gupta, N., Bhardwaj, R., & Kumar, A. (2023). Adoption of the Metaverse in the healthcare industry & its impacts on humans: A survey. In *2023 Global Conference on Information Technologies and Communications (GCITC)* (pp. 1–4). IEEE.

HealthBlocks. (2022, June). HealthBlocks Beta. https://www.healthblocks.ai/

Healthland. (2022, June). World's First Sport & Health Metaverse & NFT Store. https://healthland.io/

Ling, A., & Butakov, S. (2024). Trust framework for self-sovereign ID in metaverse health care applications. *Data Science and Management*, *7*, 304–313.

Mazhar, T., Khan, S., Shahzad, T., Khan, M. A., Saeed, M. M., Awotunde, J. B., & Hamam, H. (2025). Generative AI, IoT, and blockchain in healthcare: Application, issues, and solutions. *Discover Internet of Things*, *5*(1), 5. DOI: 10.1007/s43926-024-00059-4

Mozumder, M. A. I., Sumon, R. I., Uddin, S. M. I., Athar, A., & Kim, H.-C. (2023). The metaverse for intelligent healthcare using XAI, blockchain, and immersive technology. In *2023 IEEE International Conference on Metaverse Computing, Networking and Applications (MetaCom)* (pp. 612–616). IEEE.

Okegbile, S. D., Cai, J., & Yi, C. (2024). Concept of Human Digital Twin: An Introduction. In Human Digital Twin: Exploring Connectivity and Security Issues (pp. 3–15). Springer Nature Switzerland.

Pervez, F., Shoukat, M., Usama, M., Sandhu, M., Latif, S., & Qadir, J. (2024). Affective computing and the road to an emotionally intelligent metaverse. *IEEE Open Journal of the Computer Society*, •••, 195–214.

Compilation of References

Abbott, M., & Shaw, P. (2016). *Virtual nursing avatars: Nurse roles and evolving concepts of care*. OJIN Online J. Issues Nurs.

Abu-Elezz I, Hassan A, Nazeemudeen A., Househ M., Abd-Alrazaq A. (2020). The benefits and threats of blockchain technology in healthcare: a scoping review Int. J. Med. Inf. (2020 Aug 14), p. 104246

AccuVein. (2022, June). Vein Visualization: The Future of Healthcare is Here. https://www.accuvein.com/why-accuvein/ar/

Adavoudi Jolfaei, A., Aghili, S. F., & Singelee, D. (2021). A Survey on Blockchain-Based IoMT Systems: Towards Scalability. *IEEE Access : Practical Innovations, Open Solutions*, *9*, 148948–148975. DOI: 10.1109/ACCESS.2021.3117662

Adere, E. M. (2022). Blockchain in healthcare and IoT: A systematic literature review. *Array (New York, N.Y.)*, *14*, 100139.

Aditya Shastry, K., & Mohan, S. G. (2025). The Metaverse in Healthcare: Emerging Technologies, Challenges, and Research Directions. In Chhabra, G., & Kaushik, K. (Eds.), *Understanding the Metaverse* (pp. 113–135). Springer Nature Singapore., DOI: 10.1007/978-981-97-2278-5_6

Agbo, C. C., Mahmoud, Q. H., & Eklund, J. M. (2019). Blockchain technology in healthcare: a systematic review Healthcare, vol. 7, Multidisciplinary Digital Publishing Institute (2019 Jun), p. 562

Agbo, C. C., & Mahmoud, Q. H. (2019, September). Comparison of blockchain frameworks for healthcare applications. *Internet Technology Letters*, *2*(5), e122.

Agbo, C. C., & Mahmoud, Q. H. (2020). Blockchain in healthcare: Opportunities, challenges, and possible solutions. [IJHISI]. *International Journal of Healthcare Information Systems and Informatics*, *15*(3), 82–97.

Agbo, C. C., & Mahmoud, Q. H. (2020, July 1). Blockchain in healthcare: Opportunities, challenges, and possible solutions Int. *J. Healthc. Inf. Syst. Inf.*, *15*(3), 82–97.

Agbo, C. C., Mahmoud, Q. H., & Eklund, J. M. (2019). Blockchain Technology in Healthcare: A Systematic Review. *Health Care*, *7*, 56. PMID: 30987333

Agbo, C., Mahmoud, Q., & Eklund, J. (2019). Blockchain technology in healthcare: A systematic review. *Health Care*, *7*(2), 56. DOI: 10.3390/healthcare7020056

Aggarwal, S., Kumar, N., Alhussein, M., & Muhammad, G. (2021, February 16). Blockchain-based UAV path planning for healthcare 4.0: Current challenges and the way ahead. *IEEE Network*, *35*(1), 20–29.

Ahmad R. W., Salah K., Jayaraman R., Yaqoob I., Ellahham S., Omar M. (2021). The role of blockchain technology in telehealth and telemedicine Int. J. Med. Inf. (2021 Jan 28), p. 104399

Ahmad, M., Bangash, S. A., Shah, S. S., Chemingui, H., & Abubakar, M. (2024). Revolutionizing Healthcare in the Metaverse: The Power of Blockchain. In *Examining the Metaverse in Healthcare: Opportunities, Challenges, and Future Directions* (pp. 51-76). IGI Global.

Ahmed, S. F., & Alam, Md. S. B., Afrin, S., Rafa, S. J., Rafa, N., & Gandomi, A. H. (2024). Insights into Internet of Medical Things (IoMT): Data fusion, security issues and potential solutions. *Information Fusion*, *102*, 102060. DOI: 10.1016/j.inffus.2023.102060

Ahmed, W. A., & MacCarthy, B. L. (2023). Blockchain-enabled supply chain traceability–How wide? How deep? *International Journal of Production Economics*, *263*, 108963.

Ahram, T., Sargolzaei, A., Sargolzaei, S., Daniels, J., & Amaba, B. (2017, June). Blockchain technology innovations. In *2017 IEEE technology & engineering management conference (TEMSCON)* (pp. 137-141). IEEE.

Akram, W., Joshi, R., Haider, T., Sharma, P., Jain, V., Garud, N., & Narwaria, N. S. (2024). Blockchain technology: A potential tool for the management of the pharma supply chain. *Research in Social & Administrative Pharmacy*. PMID: 38423927

Al Omar, A., Rahman, M. S., Basu, A., & Kiyomoto, S. (2017). Medibchain: a Blockchain-based privacy-preserving platform for healthcare data International Conference on Security, Privacy and Anonymity in Computation, Communication and Storage, Springer, Cham (2017 Dec 12), pp. 534-543

Al Omar, A., Bhuiyan, M. Z., Basu, A., Kiyomoto, S., & Rahman, M. S. (2019, June 1). Privacy-friendly platform for healthcare data in cloud-based on blockchain environment Future Generat. *Comput. Syst.*, *95*, 511–521.

Alabdulatif, A., Khalil, I., & Saidur Rahman, M. (2022). Security of blockchain and AI-empowered smart healthcare: Application-based analysis. *Applied Sciences (Basel, Switzerland)*, *12*(21), 11039.

Al-Abdullah, M., Alsmadi, I., AlAbdullah, R., & Farkas, B. (2020). Designing privacy-friendly data repositories: A framework for a blockchain that follows the GDPR. *Digit. Policy Regul. Gov.*, *22*, 389–411.

Alanazi, A. A., Karim, F. K., Ghorashi, S. A., Amoudi, G., & Hamza, S. H. A. (2024). Blockchain with optimal deep learning assisted secure data sharing and classification on future healthcare systems. *Alexandria Engineering Journal*, *99*, 168–179. DOI: 10.1016/j.aej.2024.05.023

Alexis. (2025). Blockchain in Healthcare: Benefits, Challenges, and Future Potential. HealthPoint; healthpoint.com. https://healthpoint.com/technology/blockchain-in-healthcare-benefits-challenges-and-future-potential/ Accessed on: 29/04/2025

AlGhamdi, R., Alassafi, M. O., Alshdadi, A. A., Dessouky, M. M., Ramdan, R. A., & Aboshosha, B. W. (2022). Developing trusted IoT healthcare information-based AI and blockchain. *Processes (Basel, Switzerland)*, *11*(1), 34.

Alghamdi, T. A., Khalid, R., & Javaid, N. (2024). A survey of blockchain-based systems: Scalability issues and solutions, applications and future challenges. *IEEE Access : Practical Innovations, Open Solutions*, *12*, 79626–79651.

Alhadhrami, Z., Alghfeli, S., Alghfeli, M., Abedlla, J. A., & Shuaib, K. (2017, November). Introducing blockchains for healthcare. In *2017 international conference on electrical and computing technologies and applications (ICECTA)* (pp. 1-4). IEEE.

Ali, O., Jaradat, A., Kulakli, A., & Abuhalimeh, A. (2021). A comparative study: Blockchain technology utilization benefits, challenges and functionalities. *IEEE Access : Practical Innovations, Open Solutions*, *9*, 12730–12749.

Ali, S., Abdullah, Armand, T. P. T., Athar, A., Hussain, A., Ali, M., ... & Kim, H. C. (2023). Metaverse in healthcare integrated with explainable AI and blockchain: Enabling immersiveness, ensuring trust, and providing patient data security. *Sensors (Basel)*, *23*(2), 565.

Ali, S., Abdullah, Armand, T. P. T., Athar, A., Hussain, A., Ali, M., Yaseen, M., Joo, M.-I., & Kim, H.-C. (2023). Metaverse in Healthcare Integrated with Explainable AI and Blockchain: Enabling Immersiveness, Ensuring Trust, and Providing Patient Data Security. *Sensors (Basel)*, *23*(2), 565. DOI: 10.3390/s23020565 PMID: 36679361

Al-Kfairy, M., Alomari, A., Al-Bashayreh, M., Alfandi, O., & Tubishat, M. (2024). Unveiling the Metaverse: A survey of user perceptions and the impact of usability, social influence and interoperability. *Heliyon*, *10*, 1–16. PMID: 38826724

Allam, Z., Sharifi, A., Bibri, S. E., Jones, D. S., & Krogstie, J. (2022). The Metaverse as a Virtual Form of Smart Cities: Opportunities and Challenges for Environmental, Economic, and Social Sustainability in Urban Futures. *Smart Cities*, *5*, 771–801.

Aloqaily, M., Bouachir, O., Karray, F., Ridhawi, I., & Saddik, A. (2023). Integrating digital twin and advanced intelligent technologies to realize the metaverse. *IEEE Consumer Electronics Magazine*, *12*(6), 47–55. DOI: 10.1109/mce.2022.3212570

ALqodsi, E. M., & Arenova, L. (2024). Smart Contracts in Contract Law as an Auxiliary Tool or a Promising Substitute for Traditional Contracts. *Journal of Legal Affairs and Dispute Resolution in Engineering and Construction*, *16*(3), 06524004.

Alshehri, F., & Muhammad, G. (2020). A comprehensive survey of the Internet of Things (IoT) and AI-based smart healthcare. *IEEE Access : Practical Innovations, Open Solutions*, *9*, 3660–3678.

Ambhika, C., Gayathri, S., & Sheena, B. G. (2024, August). Enhancing predictive modeling in high dimensional data using hybrid feature selection. In *2024 5th International Conference on Electronics and Sustainable Communication Systems (ICESC)* (pp. 873-879). IEEE.

Andoni, M., Robu, V., Flynn, D., Abram, S., Geach, D., Jenkins, D., McCallum, P., & Peacok, A. (2019). Blockchain technology in the energy sector: A systematic review of challenges and opportunities. *Renewable & Sustainable Energy Reviews*, *100*, 143–174.

Andrew, J., Isravel, D. P., Sagayam, K. M., Bhushan, B., Sei, Y., & Eunice, J. (2023). Blockchain for healthcare systems: Architecture, security challenges, trends and future directions. *Journal of Network and Computer Applications*, *215*, 103633.

Angraal, S., Krumholz, H. M., & Schulz, W. L. (2017). Blockchain technology: Applications in health care. *Circulation: Cardiovascular Quality and Outcomes*, *10*(9), e003800. PMID: 28912202

Angraal, S., Krumholz, H. M., & Schulz, W. L. (2017, September). Blockchain technology: Applications in health care. *Circulation: Cardiovascular Quality and Outcomes, 10*(9), e003800. PMID: 28912202

Anitha, K.; Balasubramani, M.; S, V.P.K. (2023). Smart-fcd: Iot data interoperability using sensor based fuzzy linked rules for cross domain applications. Malays. J. Comput. Sci., sp2023, 54–64.

Aponte-Novoa, F. A., Orozco, A. L. S., Villanueva-Polanco, R., & Wightman, P. (2021). The 51% attack on blockchains: A mining behavior study. *IEEE Access : Practical Innovations, Open Solutions, 9*, 140549–140564.

Arabsorkhi, A., & Khazaei, E. (2024). Blockchain technology and GDPR compliance: A comprehensive applicability model. *International Journal of Web Research, 7*(2), 49–63.

Arbabi, M., Lal, C., Veeraragavan, N., Marijan, D., Nygård, J., & Vitenberg, R. (2023). A survey on blockchain for healthcare: Challenges, benefits, and future directions. *IEEE Communications Surveys and Tutorials, 25*(1), 386–424. DOI: 10.1109/comst.2022.3224644

Ashima, R., Haleem, A., Bahl, S., Javaid, M., Mahla, S. K., & Singh, S. (2021). Automation and manufacturing of smart materials in Additive Manufacturing technologies using Internet of Things towards the adoption of Industry 4.0. *Materials Today: Proceedings*. Advance online publication. DOI: 10.1016/j.matpr.2021.01.583

Aslam, M. S., Altaf, A., Iqbal, F., Nigar, N., Galán, J. C., Aray, D. G., Díez, I. D. L. T., & Ashraf, I. (2024). Novel model to authenticate role-based medical users for blockchain-based IoMT devices. *PLoS One, 19*(7), e0304774. DOI: 10.1371/journal.pone.0304774 PMID: 38985779

Atadoga, A., Elufioye, O., Omaghomi, T., Akomolafe, O., Odilibe, I., & Owolabi, O. (2024). Blockchain in healthcare: A comprehensive review of applications and security concerns. *International Journal of Science and Research Archive, 11*(1), 1605–1613. DOI: 10.30574/ijsra.2024.11.1.0244

Attaran, M. (2022). Blockchain technology in healthcare: Challenges and opportunities. *International Journal of Healthcare Management, 15*(1), 70–83.

Aujoulat, I., Young, B., & Salmon, P. (2012). The psychological processes involved in patient empowerment. *Orphanet Journal of Rare Diseases, 7*(Suppl 2), A31. DOI: 10.1186/1750-1172-7-S2-A31

Azad, M. A., Abdullah, S., Arshad, J., Lallie, H., & Ahmed, Y. H. (2024). Verify and trust: A multidimensional survey of zero-trust security in the age of IoT. *Internet of Things : Engineering Cyber Physical Human Systems*, *27*, 101227.

Bak, O., Braganza, A., & Chen, W. (2023). Exploring blockchain implementation challenges in the context of healthcare supply chain (HCSC). *International Journal of Production Research*, •••, 1–16. DOI: 10.1080/00207543.2023.2286491

Bansal, G., Rajgopal, K., Chamola, V., Xiong, Z., & Niyato, D. (2022). Healthcare in metaverse: A survey on current metaverse applications in healthcare. *IEEE Access : Practical Innovations, Open Solutions*, *10*, 119914–119946.

Barati, M., & Rana, O. (2020). Enhancing user privacy in IoT: Integration of GDPR and blockchain. In *Blockchain and Trustworthy Systems: First International Conference, BlockSys 2019, Guangzhou, China, December 7–8, 2019* [Springer Singapore.]. *Proceedings*, *1*, 322–335.

Bathula, A., Gupta, S. K., Merugu, S., Saba, L., Khanna, N. N., Laird, J. R., & Suri, J. S. (2024). Blockchain, artificial intelligence, and healthcare: The tripod of future—a narrative review. *Artificial Intelligence Review*, *57*(9), 238.

Ben Fekih, R., & Lahami, M. (2020). Application of blockchain technology in healthcare: a comprehensive study. In *The Impact of Digital Technologies on Public Health in Developed and Developing Countries: 18th International Conference, ICOST 2020, Hammamet, Tunisia, June 24–26, 2020* [Springer International Publishing.]. *Proceedings*, *18*, 268–276.

Benaich, R., El Mendili, S., & Gahi, Y. (2023). Advancing Healthcare Security: A Cutting-Edge Zero-Trust Blockchain Solution for Protecting Electronic Health Records. HighTech. *The Innovation Journal*, *4*, 630–652.

Benchoufi, M., Porcher, R., & Ravaud, P. (2018). Blockchain protocols in clinical trials: Transparency and traceability of consent. *F1000 Research*, *6*, 66. DOI: 10.12688/f1000research.10531.5

Bendayan, S., Cohen, Y., Bendayan, J., Windisch, S., & Afilalo, J. (2024). Nonfungible Tokens in Cardiovascular Medicine. *The Canadian Journal of Cardiology*, *40*(10), 1959–1964. DOI: 10.1016/j.cjca.2024.07.010 PMID: 39032555

Berdik, D., Otoum, S., Schmidt, N., Porter, D., & Jararweh, Y. (2021, January 1). A survey on Blockchain for information systems management and security. *Information Processing & Management*, *58*(1), 102397.

Bhattacharya, P., Tanwar, S., Bodke, U., Tyagi, S., & Kumar, N. (2021). Bindaas: Blockchain-based deep-learning as-a-service in healthcare 4.0 applications. *IEEE Transactions on Network Science and Engineering*, *8*(2), 1242–1255.

Bhuvana R., Madhushree L.M., & Aithal P.S. (2020). Blockchain as a disruptive technology in healthcare and financial services-A review-based analysis on current implementations International Journal of Applied Engineering and Management Letters (IJAEML), 4 (1) (2020), pp. 142-155

Bibhu, V., Das, L., Rana, A., Sharma, S., & Salagrama, S. (2023). AI Model for Blockchain Based Industrial Application in Healthcare IoT. In *AI Models for Blockchain-Based Intelligent Networks in IoT Systems: Concepts, Methodologies, Tools, and Applications* (pp. 163–184). Springer International Publishing.

Bidve, V., Kakakde, K., Sarasu, P., Kediya, S., Tamkhade, P., & Suprakash, S. (2023). Patient data management using blockchain technology. *Indonesian Journal of Electrical Engineering and Computer Science*, *32*(3), 1746. DOI: 10.11591/ijeecs.v32.i3.pp1746-1754

Blockchain Consultant. (2025). The Role of Blockchain in Healthcare: Use Cases & Challenges - Chain Consult. https://www.chainconsult.io/the-role-of-blockchain-in-healthcare-use-cases-challenges/ Accessed on: 29/04/2025

Bump Galaxy. (2022, June). Mental Healthcare Metaverse. https://gitcoin.co/grants/2026/bump-galaxy-mental-healthcare-metaverse

Cai, S., Jiao, X., & Song, B. (2022). Open another door to education—Applications, challenges and perspectives of the education metaverse. *Metaverse*, *3*, 11.

Celesti, A., Ruggeri, A., Fazio, M., Galletta, A., Villari, M., & Romano, A. (2020, January). Blockchain-based healthcare workflow for telemedical laboratory in federated hospital IoT clouds. *Sensors (Basel)*, *20*(9), 2590. PMID: 32370129

Chander, E. (2023). Decentralized healthcare system using blockchain. *Interantional Journal of Scientific Research in Engineering and Management*, *07*(11), 1–11. DOI: 10.55041/ijsrem27214

Chelladurai U., Pandian S. (2021). A novel blockchain based electronic health record automation system for healthcare. J. Ambient Intell. Humanized Comput.

Chengoden, R., Victor, N., Huynh-The, T., Yenduri, G., Jhaveri, R. H., Alazab, M., Bhattacharya, S., Hegde, P., Maddikunta, P. K. R., & Gadekallu, T. R. (2023). Metaverse for healthcare: A survey on potential applications, challenges and future directions. *IEEE Access : Practical Innovations, Open Solutions*, *11*, 12765–12795.

Chengoden, R., Victor, N., Huynh-The, T., Yenduri, G., Jhaveri, R. H., Alazab, M., Bhattacharya, S., Hegde, P., Maddikunta, P. K. R., & Gadekallu, T. R. (2023). Metaverse for Healthcare: A Survey on Potential Applications, Challenges and Future Directions. *IEEE Access : Practical Innovations, Open Solutions, 11*, 12765–12795. DOI: 10.1109/ACCESS.2023.3241628

Chen, H. S., Jarrell, J. T., Carpenter, K. A., Cohen, D. S., & Huang, X. (2019). Blockchain in healthcare: A patient-centered model. *Biomedical Journal of Scientific & Technical Research, 20*(3), 15017. PMID: 31565696

Chen, H. S., Jarrell, J. T., Carpenter, K. A., Cohen, D. S., & Huang, X. (2019). Blockchain in healthcare: A patient-centred model. *Biomedical Journal of Scientific & Technical Research, 20*(3), 15017. PMID: 31565696

Chen, J., Yi, C., Okegbile, S. D., Cai, J., & Shen, X. (2023). Networking architecture and key supporting technologies for human digital twin in personalized healthcare: A comprehensive survey. *IEEE Communications Surveys and Tutorials, 26*(1), 706–746.

Chen, X., He, G., & Li, Q. (2024). Can Fintech development improve the financial inclusion of village and township banks? Evidence from China. *Pacific-Basin Finance Journal, 85*, 102324. DOI: 10.1016/j.pacfin.2024.102324

Chowdary, C. D., Chigurupati, S., Surapaneni, P., & Maguluri, L. P. (2024). Blockchain for healthcare management: Enhancing data security and transparency. In community practitioner (Vol. 21, Number 07, pp. 651–665). *Zenodo*. https://doi .org/DOI: 10.5281/zenodo.12704770

Clark, B., & McKenzie, B. (2018). Blockchain and IP law: a match made in crypto heaven. *online], WIPO Magazine, published Feb.*

Coiera, E. (2003). *Guide to health informatics* (2nd ed.). CRC Press., DOI: 10.1201/ b13618

Collomb, A., & Sok, K. (2016). Blockchain/distributed ledger technology (DLT): What impact on the financial sector?. *Digiworld Economic Journal*, (103).

Curbera, F., Dias, D. M., Simonyan, V., Yoon, W. A., & Casella, A. (2019, April 26). Blockchain: An enabler for healthcare and life sciences transformation. *IBM Journal of Research and Development, 63*(2/3), 8–1.

Curtis, C., & Brolan, C. E. (2023). Health care in the metaverse. *The Medical Journal of Australia, 218*(1), 46–46. DOI: 10.5694/mja2.51793 PMID: 36437589

Custers, B., Sears, A. M., Dechesne, F., Georgieva, I., Tani, T., & Van der Hof, S. (2019). *EU personal data protection in policy and practice* (Vol. 29). TMC Asser Press.

Cyran, M. A. (2018, March 23). Blockchain as a foundation for sharing healthcare data. *Blockchain in Healthcare Today*, *1*, 1–6.

Daniel, C., Ouagne, D., Sadou, E., Paris, N., Hussain, S., Jaulent, M.-C., & Kalra, D. (2016). Cross border semantic interoperability for learning health systems: The EHR4CR semantic resources and services. *Learning Health Systems*, *1*, e10014. PMID: 31245551

Darvishmotevali, M. (2019). Decentralization and innovative behavior: The moderating role of supervisor support. *International Journal of Organizational Leadership*, *8*, 31–45.

De Aguiar, E. J., Faiçal, B. S., Krishnamachari, B., & Ueyama, J. (2020, March 13). A survey of blockchain-based strategies for healthcare. *ACM Computing Surveys*, *53*(2), 1–27.

De Filippi, P., Mannan, M., & Reijers, W. (2020). Blockchain as a confidence machine: The problem of trust & challenges of governance. *Technology in Society*, *62*, 101284.

de Haro-Olmo, F. J., Varela-Vaca, Á. J., & Álvarez-Bermejo, J. A. (2020). Blockchain from the perspective of privacy and anonymisation: A systematic literature review. *Sensors (Basel)*, *20*(24), 7171. PMID: 33327652

Dehealth. (2022, June). The world's first healthcare metaverse from Dehealth. https://www.dehealth.world/post/the-worlds-first-healthcare-metaverse-from-dehealth

Dewangan, N. K., & Chandrakar, P. (2023). Patient-Centric Token-Based Healthcare Blockchain Implementation Using Secure Internet of Medical Things. *IEEE Transactions on Computational Social Systems*, *10*(6), 3109–3119. DOI: 10.1109/TCSS.2022.3194872

Dhagarra D., Goswami M., Sarma P. R., & Choudhury A. (2019). Big Data and blockchain supported conceptual model for enhanced healthcare coverage Bus. Process Manag. J. (2019)

Dhinakaran, D., Kumar, N. J., & Ponnuviji, N. P. (2025). Safeguarding confidentiality and privacy in cloud-enabled healthcare systems with spectrasafe encryption and dynamic k-anonymity algorithm. *Expert Systems with Applications*, *279*, 127584.

Dimitrov, D. V. (2019). Blockchain applications for healthcare data management. *Healthcare Informatics Research*, *25*(1), 51–56. PMID: 30788182

Divyashree, K. S. (2024). Blockchain Application on Healthcare Services in Metaverse. In Hiran, K. K., Doshi, R., & Patel, M. (Eds.), *Advances in Medical Education, Research, and Ethics* (pp. 141–158). IGI Global., DOI: 10.4018/979-8-3693-5493-3.ch009

Drosatos, G., & Kaldoudi, E. (2019). Blockchain applications in the biomedical domain: A scoping review. *Computational and Structural Biotechnology Journal*, *17*, 229–240. DOI: 10.1016/j.csbj.2019.01.010

Duan, K., Pang, G., & Lin, Y. (2023). Exploring the current status and future opportunities of blockchain technology adoption and application in supply chain management. *J. Digit. Econ.*, *2*, 244–288.

Dubovitskaya, A., Xu, Z., Ryu, S., Schumacher, M., & Wang, F. (2017). Secure and trustable electronic medical records sharing using blockchain. []. American Medical Informatics Association.]. *AMIA ... Annual Symposium Proceedings - AMIA Symposium. AMIA Symposium*, *2017*, 650. PMID: 29854130

Dutta, R., Das, A., Dey, A., & Bhattacharya, S. (2020). Blockchain vs GDPR in collaborative data governance. In *Cooperative Design, Visualization, and Engineering: 17th International Conference, CDVE 2020, Bangkok, Thailand, October 25–28, 2020* [Springer International Publishing.]. *Proceedings*, *17*, 81–92.

Du, X., Chen, B., Ma, M., & Zhang, Y. (2021, January 12). Research on the application of blockchain in smart healthcare: Constructing a hierarchical framework. *Journal of Healthcare Engineering*, •••, 2021. PMID: 33505644

Ejaz, M., Kumar, T., Kovacevic, I., Ylianttila, M., & Harjula, E. (2021, January). Health-BlockEdge: Blockchain-edge framework for reliable low-latency digital healthcare applications. *Sensors (Basel)*, *21*(7), 2502. PMID: 33916700

Ekblaw, A., Azaria, A., Halamka, J. D., & Lippman, A. (2016). A Case Study for Blockchain in Healthcare: "MedRec" prototype for electronic health records and medical research data In *Proceedings of IEEE Open & Big Data Conference*, vol. 13, p. 13

Ekblaw, A., Azaria, A., Halamka, J. D., & Lippman, A. (2016). A case study for blockchain in healthcare: "MedRec" prototype for electronic health records and medical research data. *Proceedings of IEEE Open & Big Data Conference*, *13*, 13.

Elhoseny, M., Haseeb, K., Shah, A. A., Ahmad, I., Jan, Z., & Alghamdi, M. I. (2021). IoT solution for AI-enabled PRIVACY-PREServing with big data transferring: An application for healthcare using blockchain. *Energies*, *14*(17), 5364.

Engelhardt, M. A. (2017). Hitching healthcare to the chain: An introduction to blockchain technology in the healthcare sector. *Technology Innovation Management Review*, *7*(10).

Fang, G., Sun, Y., Almutiq, M., Zhou, W., Zhao, Y., & Ren, Y. (2024). Distributed Medical Data Storage Mechanism Based on Proof of Retrievability and Vector Commitment for Metaverse Services. *IEEE Journal of Biomedical and Health Informatics*, *28*(11), 6298–6307. DOI: 10.1109/JBHI.2023.3272021 PMID: 37126619

Fan, K., Wang, S., Ren, Y., Li, H., & Yang, Y. (2018). Medblock: Efficient and secure medical data sharing via blockchain. *Journal of Medical Systems*, *42*(8), 136. PMID: 29931655

Fan, K., Wang, S., Ren, Y., Li, H., & Yang, Y. (2018). Medblock: Efficient and secure medical data sharing via blockchain. *Journal of Medical Systems*, *42*, 1–11. PMID: 29931655

Farouk, A., Alahmadi, A., Ghose, S., & Mashatan, A. (2020). Blockchain platform for industrial healthcare: Vision and future opportunities. *Computer Communications*, *154*, 223–235.

Farouk, A., Alahmadi, A., Ghose, S., & Mashatan, A. (2020, March 15). Blockchain platform for industrial healthcare: Vision and future opportunities. *Computer Communications*, *154*, 223–235.

Fatoum, H., Hanna, S., Halamka, J. D., Sicker, D. C., Spangenberg, P., & Hashmi, S. K. (2021). Blockchain integration with digital technology and the future of healthcare ecosystems: Systematic review. *Journal of Medical Internet Research*, *23*(11), e19846. PMID: 34726603

Frank, R. (1957). *The perceptron: A perceiving and recognizing automaton* (Tech. Rep. No. 85-460-1). Cornell Aeronautical Laboratory. McClelland, J. L., Rumelhart, D. E., & the PDP Research Group. (1987). *Parallel distributed processing* (Vol. 2). MIT Press.

Friedman, C. P., Rubin, J. C., & Sullivan, K. J. (2017). Toward an information infrastructure for global health improvement. *Yearbook of Medical Informatics*, *26*(1), 16–23. DOI: 10.15265/IY-2017-004 PMID: 28480469

Fu, J., Wang, N., & Cai, Y. (2020, January). Privacy-preserving in healthcare blockchain systems based on lightweight message sharing. *Sensors (Basel)*, *20*(7), 1898. PMID: 32235389

Games, E. (2017). *Fortnite*. Epic Games.

Ganapathy, K. (2022). Metaverse and healthcare: A clinician's perspective. *Apollo Medicine*, *19*(4), 256–261.

Garavand, A., & Aslani, N. (2022). Metaverse phenomenon and its impact on health: A scoping review. *Informatics in Medicine Unlocked*, *32*, 101029.

Garcia, R. D., Ramachandran, G., Dunnett, K., Jurdak, R., Ranieri, C., Krishnamachari, B., & Ueyama, J. (2024). A Survey of Blockchain-Based Privacy Applications: An Analysis of Consent Management and Self-Sovereign Identity Approaches. *arXiv preprint arXiv:2411.16404*.

Garg, A. (2024). Blockchain-based health informatics systems for secure patient data sharing and interoperability. *Seminars in Medical Writing and Education*, *3*, 508. DOI: 10.56294/mw2024508

Garg, S., Kaushal, R., Kumar, N., & Verma, A. (2023). Bibliometric analysis of blockchain in the healthcare domain. *Intelligent and Converged Networks*, *4*(4), 305–312. DOI: 10.23919/icn.2023.0025

Gaur, L., Gaur, D., & Afaq, A. (2023). Ethical Considerations in the Use of the Metaverse for Healthcare. In Gaur, L., & Jhanjhi, N. Z. (Eds.), (pp. 248–273). Advances in Medical Technologies and Clinical Practice. IGI Global., DOI: 10.4018/978-1-6684-9823-1.ch008

George, L., & Kizhakkethottam, J. J. (2024). Unleashing the Future of Healthcare in the Metaverse: The Pivotal Role of Blockchain in Data Privacy. In Nijalingappa, P., Gururaj, T., Goyal, S. B., Shukla, V., & Bruno, A. (Eds.), (pp. 77–102). Advances in Medical Technologies and Clinical Practice. IGI Global., DOI: 10.4018/979-8-3693-1515-6.ch004

Ghadi, Y. Y., Mazhar, T., & Shahzad, T., Amir khan, M., Abd-Alrazaq, A., Ahmed, A., & Hamam, H. (2024). The role of blockchain to secure the internet of medical things. *Scientific Reports*, *14*(1), 18422. PMID: 39117650

Ghosh, P. K., Chakraborty, A., Hasan, M., Rashid, K., & Siddique, A. H. (2023). Blockchain application in healthcare systems: A review. *Systems*, *11*(1), 38.

Glew, R., Tröger, R., & Schmittner, S. E. (2022). A solution approach for the anonymous sharing of sensitive supply chain traceability data. arXiv preprint arXiv:2204.00317.

Gohar, A. N., Abdelmawgoud, S. A., & Farhan, M. S. (2022). A patient-centric healthcare framework reference architecture for better semantic interoperability based on blockchain, cloud, and IoT. *IEEE Access : Practical Innovations, Open Solutions*, *10*, 92137–92157.

Gökalp, E., Gökalp, M. O., Çoban, S., & Eren, P. E. (2018). Analysing opportunities and challenges of integrated blockchain technologies in healthcare InEurosymposium on Systems Analysis and Design, Springer, Cham (2018 Sep 20), pp. 174-183

Gordon, W. J., & Agrawal, A. (2018). Blockchain Technology for Healthcare: Facilitating the Transition to Patient-Driven Interoperability. *Computational and Structural Biotechnology Journal, 16*, 224–230. PMID: 30069284

Griggs, K. N., Ossipova, O., Kohlios, C. P., Baccarini, A. N., Howson, E. A., & Hayajneh, T. (2018, July). Healthcare blockchain system using smart contracts for secure automated remote patient monitoring. *Journal of Medical Systems, 42*(7), 1–7. PMID: 29876661

Gul, M. J. J., Paul, A., Rho, S., & Kim, M. (2020, December). Blockchain based healthcare system with Artificial Intelligence. In *2020 International Conference on Computational Science and Computational Intelligence (CSCI)* (pp. 740-741). IEEE.

Gul, M. J., Subramanian, B., Paul, A., & Kim, J. (2021, February 1). Blockchain for public health care in smart society. *Microprocessors and Microsystems, 80*, 103524.

Guo, H., & Yu, X. (2022). A survey on blockchain technology and its security. *Blockchain: research and applications, 3*(2), 100067.

Gupta, N., Bhardwaj, R., & Kumar, A. (2023). Adoption of the Metaverse in the healthcare industry & its impacts on humans: A survey. In *2023 Global Conference on Information Technologies and Communications (GCITC)* (pp. 1–4). IEEE.

Gursoy, D., Malodia, S., & Dhir, A. (2022). The metaverse in the hospitality and tourism industry: An overview of current trends and future research directions. *Journal of Hospitality Marketing & Management, 31*, 527–534.

Habib, G., Sharma, S., Ibrahim, S., Ahmad, I., Qureshi, S., & Ishfaq, M. (2022). Blockchain technology: Benefits, challenges, applications, and integration of blockchain technology with cloud computing. *Future Internet, 14*(11), 341.

Haddad, A., Habaebi, M. H., Islam, M. R., Hasbullah, N. F., & Zabidi, S. A. (2022). Systematic review on ai-blockchain based e-healthcare records management systems. *IEEE Access : Practical Innovations, Open Solutions, 10*, 94583–94615.

Haleem, A., Javaid, M., Singh, R. P., Suman, R., & Rab, S. (2021). Blockchain technology applications in healthcare: An overview, International Journal of Intelligent Networks, Volume 2, Pages 130-139, ISSN 2666-6030, https://doi.org/DOI: 10.1016/j.ijin.2021.09.005

Haleem, A., Javaid, M., Singh, R. P., Suman, R., & Rab, S. (2021). Blockchain technology applications in healthcare: An overview. *International Journal of Intelligent Networks*, *2*, 130–139.

Han, D., Yu, D., & Qiu, J. (2023). Assessing coupling interactions in a safe and just operating space for regional sustainability. *Nature Communications*, *14*(1), 1369. DOI: 10.1038/s41467-023-37073-z PMID: 36914668

Han, H., Shiwakoti, R. K., Jarvis, R., Mordi, C., & Botchie, D. (2023). Accounting and auditing with blockchain technology and artificial Intelligence: A literature review. *International Journal of Accounting Information Systems*, *48*, 100598.

Hasei, J., Ishida, H., Katayama, H., Maeda, N., Nagano, A., Ochi, M., Okamura, M., Iwata, S., Ikuta, K., Yoshida, S., Fujiwara, T., Nakata, E., Nakahara, R., Kunisada, T., & Ozaki, T. (2024). Utilizing the Metaverse to Provide Innovative Psychosocial Support for Pediatric, Adolescent, and Young Adult Patients with Rare Cancer. *Cancers (Basel)*, *16*(15), 2617. DOI: 10.3390/cancers16152617 PMID: 39123345

Hasselgren, A., Kralevska, K., Gligoroski, D., Pedersen, S. A., & Faxvaag, A. (2020). Blockchain in healthcare and health sciences—A scoping review. *International Journal of Medical Informatics*, *134*, 104040. PMID: 31865055

Hathaliya, J., Sharma, P., Tanwar, S., & Gupta, R. (2019). Blockchain-based remote patient monitoring in healthcare 4.0 In2019 IEEE 9th International Conference on Advanced Computing (IACC), IEEE (2019 Dec 13), pp. 87-91

HealthBlocks. (2022, June). HealthBlocks Beta. https://www.healthblocks.ai/

Healthland. (2022, June). World's First Sport & Health Metaverse & NFT Store. https://healthland.io/

Heathfield, H. A., & Wyatt, J. (1995). The road to professionalism in medical informatics: A proposal for debate. *Methods of Information in Medicine*, *34*(5), 426–433. DOI: 10.1055/s-0038-1634627 PMID: 8713756

Heeks, R. (2022). Digital inequality beyond the digital divide: Conceptualizing adverse digital incorporation in the global South. *Information Technology for Development*, *28*(4), 688–704.

He, Q., Feng, Z., Fang, H., Wang, X., Zhao, L., Yao, Y., & Yu, K. (2024). A Blockchain-Based Scheme for Secure Data Offloading in Healthcare With Deep Reinforcement Learning. *IEEE/ACM Transactions on Networking*, *32*(1), 65–80. DOI: 10.1109/TNET.2023.3274631

He, W., Zhang, J. Z., Wu, H., Li, W., & Shetty, S. (2022). A Unified Health Information System Framework for Connecting Data, People, Devices, and Systems. *Journal of Global Information Management*, *30*, 2022.

Hirsch, J. A., Leslie-Mazwi, T. M., Nicola, G. N., Barr, R. M., Bello, J. A., Donovan, W. D., & Manchikanti, L. (2015). Current procedural terminology; a primer. *Journal of Neurointerventional Surgery*, *7*(4), 309–312.

Hölbl, M., Kompara, M., Kamišalić, A., & Zlatolas, L. N. (2018). A systematic review of the use of Blockchain in healthcare. *Symmetry*, *10*(10), 470.

Houtan, B.; Hafid, A.S.; Makrakis, D. (2020). A Survey on Blockchain-Based Self-Sovereign Patient Identity in Healthcare. IEEE Access 2020, 8, 90478–90494.

Hubel, D. H., & Wiesel, T. N. (1962). Receptive fields, binocular interaction and functional architecture in the cat's visual cortex. *The Journal of Physiology*, *160*(1), 106–154. PMID: 14449617

Hulsen, T. (2024). Applications of the metaverse in medicine and healthcare. *Advances in Laboratory Medicine/Avances en Medicina De Laboratorio, 5*(2), 159-165.

Hussein, Z., Salama, M. A., & El-Rahman, S. A. (2023). Evolution of blockchain consensus algorithms: A review on the latest milestones of blockchain consensus algorithms. *Cybersecurity*, *6*(1), 30.

Hussien, H. M., Yasin, S. M., Udzir, N. I., Ninggal, M. I., & Salman, S. (2021, June 1). Blockchain technology in the healthcare industry: Trends and opportunities. *Journal of Industrial Information Integration*, *22*, 100217.

Hwang, G.-J., & Chien, S.-Y. (2022). Definition, roles, and potential research issues of the metaverse in education: An artificial intelligence perspective. *Comput. Educ. Artif. Intell.*, *3*, 100082.

Hylock, R. H., & Zeng, X. (2019). A Blockchain Framework for Patient-Centered Health Records and Exchange (HealthChain): Evaluation and Proof-of-Concept Study. *Journal of Medical Internet Research*, *21*(8), e13592. DOI: 10.2196/13592 PMID: 31471959

Ichikawa D., Kashiyama M., Ueno T. (2017). Tamper-resistant mobile health using blockchain technology, Journal of Medical Internet Research, mHealth uHealth 5 (7) (2017) e111.

Imler, T. D., Vreeman, D. J., & Kannry, J. (2016). Healthcare Data Standards and Exchange. In Finnell, J. T., & Dixon, B. E. (Eds.), *Clinical Informatics Study Guide: Text and Review* (pp. 233–253). Springer International Publishing.

Islam, A., & Shin, S. Y. (2020, June 1). A blockchain-based secure healthcare scheme with the assistance of unmanned aerial vehicles in the Internet of Things Comput. *Electrical Engineering*, *84*, 106627.

Islam, N., Faheem, Y., Din, I. U., Talha, M., Guizani, M., & Khalil, M. (2019, November 1). A blockchain-based fog computing framework for activity recognition as an application to e-Healthcare services Future Generat. *Comput. Syst.*, *100*, 569–578.

Ismail, L., Material, H., & Zeadally, S. (2019, October 15). Lightweight blockchain for healthcare. *IEEE Access : Practical Innovations, Open Solutions*, *7*, 149935–149951.

Ismail, L., Materwala, H., & Hennebelle, A. (2021). A Scoping Review of Integrated Blockchain-Cloud (BcC) Architecture for Healthcare: Applications, Challenges and Solutions. *Sensors (Basel)*, *21*(11), 3753. DOI: 10.3390/s21113753 PMID: 34071449

Jabarulla, M. Y., & Lee, H. N. (2021, August). A blockchain and artificial intelligence-based, patient-centric healthcare system for combating the COVID-19 pandemic: Opportunities and applications. [). Mdpi.]. *Health Care*, *9*(8), 1019. PMID: 34442156

Jaleel, A.; Mahmood, T.; Hassan, M.A.; Bano, G.; Khurshid, S.K. (2020). Towards Medical Data Interoperability Through Collaboration of Healthcare Devices. IEEE Access 2020, 8, 132302–132319.

Jat, A., Grønli, T., Ghinea, G., & Assres, G. (2024). Evolving software architecture design in telemedicine: A prisma-based systematic review. *Healthcare Informatics Research*, *30*(3), 184–193. DOI: 10.4258/hir.2024.30.3.184

Javaid, M., & Haleem, A. (2019, May 1). Industry 4.0 applications in medical field: A brief review. *Current Medicine Research and Practice*, *9*(3), 102–109.

Jayabalan, J., & Jeyanthi, N. (2022). Scalable blockchain model using off-chain IPFS storage for healthcare data security and privacy. *Journal of Parallel and Distributed Computing*, *164*, 152–167.

Jena, S. K., Barik, R. C., & Priyadarshini, R. (2024). A systematic state-of-art review on digital identity challenges with solutions using conjugation of IOT and blockchain in healthcare. *Internet of Things : Engineering Cyber Physical Human Systems*, *25*, 101111. DOI: 10.1016/j.iot.2024.101111

Jeong, H., Yi, Y., & Kim, D. (2022). An innovative e-commerce platform incorporating metaverse to live commerce. *International Journal of Innovative Computing, Information, & Control*, *18*, 221–229.

Jiang, S., Cao, J., Wu, H., Yang, Y., Ma, M., & He, J. (2018). Blochie: a blockchain-based platform for healthcare information exchange 2018 IEEE International Conference on Smart Computing (Smart Comp), IEEE (2018 Jun 18), pp. 49-56

Jiang, S., Cao, J., Wu, H., Yang, Y., Ma, M., & He, J. (2018). BlocHIE: a blockchain-based platform for healthcare information exchange, in: IEEE International Conference on Smart Computing (SMARTCOMP), IEEE, 2018, pp. 49–56.

Joshua, J. (2017). Information Bodies: Computational Anxiety in Neal Stephenson's Snow Crash. *Interdisciplinary Literary Studies*, *19*, 17–47.

Jungherr, A., & Schlarb, D. B. (2022). The Extended Reach of Game Engine Companies: How Companies Like Epic Games and Unity Technologies Provide Platforms for Extended Reality Applications and the Metaverse. *Social Media + Society*, *8*, 20563051221107641.

Jusić, A. (2022). Privacy between regulation and technology: gdpr and the blockchain. iuslawjournal, Vol 1(No 1), 47-59. https://doi.org/DOI: 10.21533/iuslawjournal.v1i1.9

Kashyap, G. (2024). Ai in blockchain-enabled healthcare systems. *Interantional Journal of Scientific Research in Engineering and Management*, *08*(12), 1–7. DOI: 10.55041/ijsrem17947

Kassab, M.H., DeFranco j., Malas T., Laplante G.D., & Neto V.V. (2019). Exploring research in Blockchain for healthcare and a roadmap for the future. *IEEE Transactions on Emerging Topics in Computing*.

Kasyapa, M. S. B., & Vanmathi, C. (2024). Blockchain integration in healthcare: A comprehensive investigation of use cases, performance issues, and mitigation strategies. *Frontiers in Digital Health*, *6*, 1359858. DOI: 10.3389/fdgth.2024.1359858 PMID: 38736708

Katuwal, G. J., Pandey, S., Hennessey, M., & Lamichhane, B. (2018). Applications of blockchain in healthcare: current landscape & challenges. *arXiv preprint arXiv:1812.02776*.

Kaur, H., Alam, M. A., Jameel, R., Mourya, A. K., & Chang, V. (2018). A Proposed Solution and Future Direction for Blockchain-Based Heterogeneous Medicare Data in Cloud Environment. *Journal of Medical Systems*, *42*, 156. PMID: 29987560

Kavanagh, C. (2022). *New tech, new threats, and new governance challenges: an opportunity to craft smarter responses?* Carnegie Endowment for International Peace.

Kavithamani, M. (2025). Blockchain for the next decade: Future trends and predictions in healthcare. *Journal of Information Systems Engineering & Management, 10*(11s), 178–185. DOI: 10.52783/jisem.v10i11s.1510

Khansulivong, C., Wicha, S., & Temdee, P. Adaptive of New Technology for Agriculture Online Learning by Metaverse: A Case Study in Faculty of Agriculture, National University of Laos. In Proceedings of the 2022 Joint International Conference on Digital Arts, Media and Technology with ECTI Northern Section Conference on Electrical, Electronics, Computer and Telecommunications Engineering (ECTI DAMT & NCON), Online, 26–28 January 2022; IEEE: Piscataway, NJ, USA, 2022.

Khatib, M., Alzoubi, H., Hamidi, S., Alshurideh, M., Baydoun, A., & Al-Nakeeb, A. (2023). Impact of using the internet of medical things on e-healthcare performance: Blockchain assist in improving smart contract. *ClinicoEconomics and Outcomes Research, 15*, 397–411. DOI: 10.2147/ceor.s407778

Khatoon, A. (2020). A blockchain-based smart contract system for healthcare management. *Electronics (Basel), 9*(1), 94.

Khatoon, A. (2020, January). A blockchain-based innovative contract system for healthcare management. *Electronics (Basel), 9*(1), 94.

Khatri, S., Alzahrani, F. A., Ansari, M. T. J., Agrawal, A., Kumar, R., & Khan, R. A. (2021). A systematic analysis on blockchain integration with healthcare domain: Scope and challenges. *IEEE Access : Practical Innovations, Open Solutions, 9*, 84666–84687.

Khezr, S., Moniruzzaman, M., Yassine, A., & Benlamri, R. (2019). Blockchain technology in healthcare: A comprehensive review and directions for future research. *Applied Sciences (Basel, Switzerland), 9*(9), 1736.

Khujamatov, K., Reypnazarov, E., Akhmedov, N., & Khasanov, D. (2020). Blockchain for 5G healthcare architecture In2020 International Conference on Information Science and Communications Technologies (ICISCT), IEEE (2020 Nov 4), pp. 1-5

Khujamatov, K., Reypnazarov, E., Akhmedov, N., & Khasanov, D. (2020, November). Blockchain for 5G Healthcare architecture. In *2020 international conference on information science and communications technologies (ICISCT)* (pp. 1-5). IEEE.

Khushalani, J., Chandwani, S., Shaikh, A. S., Talreja, B., & Hande, R. Blockchain: The Novel Way to Secure Confidence! In *Proceedings of the International Conference on Electronics and Sustainable Communication Systems (ICESC)*, Coimbatore, India, 2–4 July 2020; IEEE: New York City, NY, USA, 2020; pp. 754–759.

Koo, H. (2021). Training in lung cancer surgery through the metaverse, including extended reality, in the smart operating room of Seoul National University Bundang Hospital, Korea. *Journal of Educational Evaluation for Health Professions, 18*, 33. PMID: 34965648

Koshechkin, K. A., Klimenko, G. S., Ryabkov, I. V., & Kozhin, P. B. (2018, January 1). Scope for the application of blockchain in the public healthcare of the Russian federation. *Procedia Computer Science, 126*, 1323–1328.

Kostick-Quenet, K., Mandl, K. D., Minssen, T., Cohen, I. G., Gasser, U., Kohane, I., & McGuire, A. L. (2022). How NFTs could transform health information exchange. *Science, 375*(6580), 500–502. DOI: 10.1126/science.abm2004 PMID: 35113709

Kouroubali, A., & Katehakis, D. G. (2022). Policy and Strategy for Interoperability of Digital Health in Europe. In *MEDINFO 2021: One World, One Health–Global Partnership for Digital Innovation* (pp. 897–901). IOS Press.

Kraus, S., Kanbach, D. K., Krysta, P. M., Steinhoff, M. M., & Tomini, N. (2022). Facebook and the creation of the metaverse: Radical business model innovation or incremental transformation? *International Journal of Entrepreneurial Behaviour & Research, 28*, 52–77.

Krittanawong, C., Aydar, M., Virk, H. U. H., Kumar, A., Kaplin, S., Guimaraes, L., & Halperin, J. L. (2022). Artificial intelligence-powered blockchains for cardiovascular medicine. *The Canadian Journal of Cardiology, 38*(2), 185–195. PMID: 34856332

Krizhevsky, A., Sutskever, I., & Hinton, G. E. (2012). Imagenet classification with deep convolutional neural networks. In *Advances in Neural Information Processing Systems* (pp. 1097–1105).

Kruse, C. S., Stein, A., Thomas, H., & Kaur, H. (2018). The use of Electronic Health Records to Support Population Health: A Systematic Review of the Literature. *Journal of Medical Systems, 42*, 214. PMID: 30269237

Kumar, P., Kumar, R., Garg, S., Kaur, K., Zhang, Y., & Guizani, M. (2022, December). A secure data dissemination scheme for IoT-based e-health systems using AI and blockchain. In *GLOBECOM 2022-2022 IEEE Global Communications Conference* (pp. 1397-1403). IEEE.

Kumar, T., Ramani, V., Ahmad, I., Braeken, A., Harjula, E., & Ylianttila, M. (2018). Blockchain utilisation in healthcare: key requirements and challenges. In2018 IEEE 20th International Conference on E-Health Networking, Applications and Services (Healthcom), IEEE (2018 Sep 17), pp. 1-7

Kumar, A., Bhushan, B., Shristi, S., Chaganti, R., & Soufiene, B. O. (2023). Blockchain-based decentralized management of IoT devices for preserving data integrity. In *Blockchain Technology Solutions for the Security of IoT-Based Healthcare Systems* (pp. 263–286). Academic Press.

Kumar, A., Singh, A. K., Ahmad, I., & Kumar Singh, P., Anushree, Verma, P. K., ... & Tag-Eldin, E. (2022). A novel decentralized blockchain architecture for the preservation of privacy and data security against cyberattacks in healthcare. *Sensors (Basel)*, *22*(15), 5921. PMID: 35957478

Kuo, T. T., Gabriel, R. A., & Ohno-Machado, L. (2019). Fair compute loads enabled by blockchain: Sharing models by alternating client and server roles. *Journal of the American Medical Informatics Association : JAMIA*, *26*(5), 392–403. PMID: 30892656

Lakumarapu, S., Nithyanandhan, R., Bhargavi, V. S., & TP, A. (2024, August). Machine Learning Approaches for Liver Disease Prediction: A Comparative Analysis. In *2024 5th International Conference on Electronics and Sustainable Communication Systems (ICESC)* (pp. 159-164). IEEE.

Lax, G., Nardone, R., & Russo, A. (2024). Enabling secure health information sharing among healthcare organizations by public blockchain. *Multimedia Tools and Applications*, *83*(24), 64795–64811. DOI: 10.1007/s11042-024-18181-4

Lee, H.-A., Kung, H.-H., Udayasankaran, J. G., Kijsanayotin, B., Marcelo, A. B., Chao, L. R., & Hsu, C.-Y. (2020). An architecture and management platform for blockchain-based personal health record exchange: Development and usability study. *Journal of Medical Internet Research*, *22*, e16748. PMID: 32515743

Leeming, G., Cunningham, J., & Ainsworth, J. (2019, July 24). A ledger of me: Personalising healthcare using blockchain technology. *Frontiers of Medicine*, *6*, 171. PMID: 31396516

Lee, T. F., Chang, I. P., & Kung, T. S. (2021). Blockchain-based healthcare information preservation using extended chaotic maps for HIPAA privacy/security regulations. *Applied Sciences (Basel, Switzerland)*, *11*(22), 10576.

Lehne, M., Sass, J., Essenwanger, A., Schepers, J., & Thun, S. (2019). Why digital medicine depends on interoperability. npj. *Digital Medicine*, *2*, 79. PMID: 31453374

Levy, K. E. (2017). Book-smart, not street-smart: Blockchain-based smart contracts and the social workings of law. *Engaging Science, Technology, and Society*, *3*, 1–15.

Ling, A., & Butakov, S. (2024). Trust framework for self-sovereign ID in metaverse health care applications. *Data Science and Management*, *7*, 304–313.

Lin, J. (2023). Study on Brand Management of Fashion Brands. *Advances in Economics. Management and Political Sciences*, *55*(1), 24–29. DOI: 10.54254/2754-1169/55/20230955

Linn, L. A., & Koo, M. B. (2016, September). Blockchain for health data and its potential use in health it and health care related research. In *ONC/NIST Use of Blockchain for Healthcare and Research Workshop. Gaithersburg, Maryland, United States: ONC/NIST* (pp. 1-10).

Liu, S., Liu, C., & Lang, C. (2024). Consumer Engagement in Fashion Circularity in China: Exploring Consumer Online Fashion Resale through the Lens of Social Practice Theory. *Sustainability*, *16*(11), 4733. DOI: 10.3390/su16114733

Longo, F., Nicoletti, L., Padovano, A., d'Atri, G., & Forte, M. (2019). Blockchain-enabled supply chain: An experimental study. *Computers & Industrial Engineering*, *136*, 57–69.

Lv, Y. (2023). Transitioning to sustainable energy: Opportunities, challenges, and the potential of blockchain technology. *Frontiers in Energy Research*, *11*, 1258044.

Mackey, T. K., Kuo, T. T., Gummadi, B., Clauson, K. A., Church, G., Grishin, D., Obbad, K., Barkovich, R., & Palombini, M. (2019, December). 'Fit-for-purpose?'–challenges and opportunities for applications of blockchain technology in the future of healthcare. *BMC Medicine*, *17*(1), 1–7. PMID: 30914045

Mackey, T. K., Kuo, T. T., Gummadi, B., Clauson, K. A., Church, G., Grishin, D., & Palombini, M. (2019). 'Fit-for-purpose?'–challenges and opportunities for applications of blockchain technology in the future of healthcare. *BMC Medicine*, *17*, 1–17. PMID: 30914045

Mackey, T., Kuo, T., Gummadi, B., Clauson, K., Church, G., Grishin, D., & Palombini, M. (2019). 'fit-for-purpose?' – challenges and opportunities for applications of blockchain technology in the future of healthcare. *BMC Medicine*, *17*(1). Advance online publication. DOI: 10.1186/s12916-019-1296-7

Maithili, K., Ponmalar, A., Yamini, B., Karthikeyan, M., Anish, T. P., Maheswari, B., & Subramanian, R. S. (2024). Advances in AI and Machine Learning for Healthcare Informatics. In *Machine Learning and Generative AI in Smart Healthcare* (pp. 1–22). IGI Global.

Mamoshina, P., Ojomoko, L., Yanovich, Y., Ostrovski, A., Botezatu, A., Prikhodko, P., Izumchenko, E., Aliper, A., Romantsov, K., Zhebrak, A., & Ogu, I. O. (2018, January 19). Converging Blockchain and next-generation artificial intelligence technologies to decentralise and accelerate biomedical research and healthcare. *Oncotarget*, *9*(5), 5665. PMID: 29464026

Mayer, A., Costa, C., & Righi, R. (2019). Electronic health records in a blockchain: A systematic review. *Health Informatics Journal*, *26*(2), 1273–1288. DOI: 10.1177/1460458219866350

Ma, Z., Jiang, M., Gao, H., & Wang, Z. (2018). Blockchain for digital rights management. *Future Generation Computer Systems*, *89*, 746–764.

Mazhar, T., Khan, S., Shahzad, T., Khan, M. A., Saeed, M. M., Awotunde, J. B., & Hamam, H. (2025). Generative AI, IoT, and blockchain in healthcare: Application, issues, and solutions. *Discover Internet of Things*, *5*(1), 5. DOI: 10.1007/s43926-024-00059-4

Mazlan, A. A., Daud, S. M., Sam, S. M., Abas, H., Rasid, S. Z., & Yusof, M. F. (2020, January 24). Scalability challenges in healthcare blockchain system—A systematic review. *IEEE Access : Practical Innovations, Open Solutions*, *8*, 23663–23673.

Mazlan, A. A., Mohd Daud, S., Mohd Sam, S., Abas, H., Abdul Rasid, S. Z., & Yusof, M. F. (2020). Scalability Challenges in Healthcare Blockchain System—A Systematic Review. *IEEE Access : Practical Innovations, Open Solutions*, *8*, 23663–23673. DOI: 10.1109/ACCESS.2020.2969230

McCourt, C. (2024). Exploring the intersection of the medical metaverse and healthcare ethics: Future considerations and caveats. *Global Health Journal (Amsterdam, Netherlands)*, *8*(1), 36–40. DOI: 10.1016/j.glohj.2024.02.005

McGhin, T., Choo, K.-K. R., Liu, C. Z., & He, D. (2019). Blockchain in healthcare applications: Research challenges and opportunities. *Journal of Network and Computer Applications*, *135*, 62–75.

McKeon, J. (2023). Biggest healthcare data breaches reported this year, so far. *Health IT Security, 26.*

McKibbon, K. A., Lokker, C., Handler, S. M., Dolovich, L. R., Holbrook, A. M., O'Reilly, D., Tamblyn, R., Hemens, B. J., Basu, R., & Troyan, S.. (2012). The effectiveness of integrated health information technologies across the phases of medication management: A systematic review of randomized controlled trials. *Journal of the American Medical Informatics Association : JAMIA*, *19*, 22–30. PMID: 21852412

Menachemi, N., & Collum, T. H. (2011). Benefits and drawbacks of electronic health record systems. *Risk Management and Healthcare Policy*, *4*, 47–55. PMID: 22312227

Mertz, L. (2018). (Block) Chain Reaction: A Blockchain Revolution Sweeps into Health Care, Offering the Possibility for a Much-Needed Data Solution. *IEEE Pulse*, *9*, 4–7. PMID: 29757744

Mijwil, M. M., Aljanabi, M., Abotaleb, M., Shukur, B. S., Al Sailawi, A. S. A., Bala, I., Hiran, K. K., Doshi, R., & Dhoska, K. (2025). *Exploring the Impact of Blockchain Revolution on the Healthcare Ecosystem: A Critical Review*. Mesopotamian Journal of CyberSecurity., DOI: 10.58496/MJCS/2025/006

Mistry, C., Thakker, U., Gupta, R., Obaidat, M. S., Tanwar, S., Kumar, N., & Rodrigues, J. J. (2021, June). MedBlock: An AI-enabled and blockchain-driven medical healthcare system for COVID-19. In *ICC 2021-IEEE International Conference on Communications* (pp. 1-6). IEEE.

Mohanasundaram, S., Ramirez-Asis, E., Quispe-Talla, A., Bhatt, M. W., & Shabaz, M. (2022). Experimental replacement of hops by mango in beer: Production and comparison of total phenolics, flavonoids, minerals, carbohydrates, proteins and toxic substances. *International Journal of System Assurance Engineering and Management*, *2022*(13), 132–145.

Moona G., Jewariya M., Sharma R. (2019). Relevance of dimensional metrology in manufacturing industries MAPAN, 34, pp. 97-104, DOI: 10.1007/s12647-018-0291-3

Morar, C. D., & Popescu, D. E. (2024). A Survey of Blockchain Applicability, Challenges, and Key Threats. *Computers*, *13*(9), 223. DOI: 10.3390/computers13090223

Morgan, J. (2024). P-462 Exploring the potential of fertility clinics in the metaverse: Opportunities, challenges, and ethical implications. *Human Reproduction, 39*(Supplement_1), deae108.292. https://doi.org/DOI: 10.1093/humrep/deae108.292

Motohashi, T., Hirano, T., Okumura, K., Kashiyama, M., Ichikawa, D., & Ueno, T. (2019). Secure and scalable mhealth data management using blockchain combined with client hashchain: System design and validation. *Journal of Medical Internet Research*, *21*(5), e13385. DOI: 10.2196/13385

Moukalled, T., & Elhaj, A. (2021). Patient negligence in healthcare systems: Accountability model formulation. *Health Policy OPEN*, *2*, 100037. PMID: 37383513

Mozumder, M. A. I., Sheeraz, M. M., Athar, A., Aich, S., & Kim, H. C. (2022, February). Overview: Technology roadmap of the future trend of metaverse based on IoT, blockchain, AI technique, and medical domain metaverse activity. In *2022 24th International Conference on Advanced Communication Technology (ICACT)* (pp. 256-261). IEEE.

Mozumder, M. A. I., Sumon, R. I., Uddin, S. M. I., Athar, A., & Kim, H.-C. (2023). The metaverse for intelligent healthcare using XAI, blockchain, and immersive technology. In *2023 IEEE International Conference on Metaverse Computing, Networking and Applications (MetaCom)* (pp. 612–616). IEEE.

Munoz, D. J., Constantinescu, D. A., Asenjo, R., & Fuentes, L. (2019). Clinicappchain: a low-cost blockchain hyperledger solution for healthcare International Congress on Blockchain and Applications, Springer, Cham (2019 Jun 26), pp. 36-44

Musamih, A., Yaqoob, I., Salah, K., Jayaraman, R., Al-Hammadi, Y., Omar, M., & Ellahham, S. (2022). Metaverse in healthcare: Applications, challenges, and future directions. *IEEE Consumer Electronics Magazine*, *12*(4), 33–46.

Nadarasa, A. (2024). Social prescribing in the metaverse: A new frontier for primary care practice. *Global Health Journal (Amsterdam, Netherlands)*, *8*(1), 32–35. DOI: 10.1016/j.glohj.2024.02.006

Nanda, A. (2019). Consumers' Intention to use Mobile Wallets. *AIMS Int. J. Manag.*, *13*, 143.

Nanda, S. K., Panda, S. K., & Dash, M. (2023). Medical supply chain integrated with blockchain and IoT to track the logistics of medical products. *Multimedia Tools and Applications*, *82*(21), 32917–32939. PMID: 37362711

Nan, J., & Xu, L.-Q. (2023). Designing Interoperable Health Care Services Based on Fast Healthcare Interoperability Resources: Literature Review. *JMIR Medical Informatics*, *11*, e44842. PMID: 37603388

Nasir, N. M., Hassan, S., & Zaini, K. M. (2024). Securing Permissioned Blockchain-based Systems: An Analysis on the Significance of Consensus Mechanisms. *IEEE Access : Practical Innovations, Open Solutions*.

Natsiavas, P., Mazzeo, G., Faiella, G., Campegiani, P., Dumortier, J., Stan, O., Nalin, M., Martinez, D. M., Theodouli, A., & Moschou, K.. (2021). Developing an infrastructure for secure patient summary exchange in the EU context: Lessons learned from the KONFIDO project. *Health Informatics Journal*, *27*, 14604582211021459. PMID: 34142613

Ngiam, J., Coates, A., Lahiri, A., Prochnow, B., Le, Q. V., & Ng, A. Y. (2011). On optimization methods for deep learning. In *Proceedings of the International Conference on Machine Learning* (pp. 265–272).

Nguyen, D. C., Pathirana, P. N., Ding, M., & Seneviratne, A. (2021). BEdgeHealth: A decentralised architecture for edge-based IoMT networks using blockchain. *IEEE Internet of Things Journal*, *8*(14), 11743–11757.

Nguyen, H., Danh, H., Ma, Q., Měsíček, J., Hajnyš, J., Pagáč, M., & Petrů, J. (2023). A bibliometrics analysis of medical internet of things for modern healthcare. *Electronics (Basel)*, *12*(22), 4586. DOI: 10.3390/electronics12224586

NHS England. (2017). *NHS digital academy*. https://www.england.nhs.uk/digitaltechnology/info-revolution/nhs-digital-academy/

Okegbile, S. D., Cai, J., & Yi, C. (2024). Concept of Human Digital Twin: An Introduction. In Human Digital Twin: Exploring Connectivity and Security Issues (pp. 3–15). Springer Nature Switzerland.

Omodunbi, T., Akindutire, A. S., Awoyelu, T. M., Ikono, R., & Gambo, I. (2023). Integrating Asymmetric Cryptographic Digital Wallet for Online Services in Nigeria. *Int. J. Inf. Eng. Electron. Bus.*, *3*, 29–40.

Onik, M. M., Aich, S., Yang, J., Kim, C. S., & Kim, H. C. (2019). Blockchain in healthcare: challenges and solutions Big Data Analytics for Intelligent Healthcare Management, Academic Press (2019 Jan 1), pp. 197-226

Paik, H. Y., Xu, X., Bandara, H. D., Lee, S. U., & Lo, S. K. (2019). Analysis of data management in blockchain-based systems: From architecture to governance. *IEEE Access : Practical Innovations, Open Solutions*, *7*, 186091–186107.

Pandey, A. (2025). Blockchain in Industrial Supply Chains: Tracing the Transparency. In *Immersive Technology for the Gig Economy: Transformative Business Practices* (pp. 273-294). IGI Global Scientific Publishing.

Pandey, A., & Joseph, J. (2025a). Navigating the HealthTech Ecosystem: Challenges and Roadblocks. In *Synergizing Data Envelopment Analysis and Machine Learning for Performance Optimization in Healthcare* (pp. 31-48). IGI Global Scientific Publishing.

Pandey, A., & Joseph, J. (2025). The Convergence of Blockchain and Artificial Intelligence: Transforming Healthcare. In *AI and Blockchain Applications for Privacy and Security in Smart Medical Systems* (pp. 399–416). IGI Global Scientific Publishing.

Pandey, A., & Joseph, J. (2025b). Integral Role of Blockchain and Artificial Intelligence in Sustainable Economic Development. In *Driving Socio-Economic Growth With AI and Blockchain* (pp. 271–290). IGI Global Scientific Publishing.

Pandey, P., & Litoriya, R. (2020). Implementing healthcare services on a large scale: Challenges and remedies based on blockchain technology. *Health Policy and Technology*, *9*(1), 69–78.

Pandey, P., & Litoriya, R. (2020, March 1). Implementing healthcare services on a large scale: Challenges and remedies based on blockchain technology. *Health Policy and Technology*, *9*(1), 69–78.

Pathak, N., Mukherjee, A., & Misra, S. (2023). SemBox: Semantic Interoperability in a Box for Wearable e-Health Devices. *IEEE Journal of Biomedical and Health Informatics*, *27*, 2306–2313. PMID: 35439151

Peppet, S. R. (2011). Unraveling privacy: The personal prospectus and the threat of a full-disclosure future. *Nw. UL Rev.*, *105*, 1153.

Pervez, F., Shoukat, M., Usama, M., Sandhu, M., Latif, S., & Qadir, J. (2024). Affective computing and the road to an emotionally intelligent metaverse. *IEEE Open Journal of the Computer Society*, •••, 195–214.

Peterson, K., Deeduvanu, R., Kanjamala, P., & Boles, K. (2016). A blockchain-based approach to health information exchange networks InProc. NIST Workshop Blockchain Healthcare, 1 (No. 1) (2016 Sep), pp. 1-10

Pham, H. L., Tran, T. H., & Nakashima, Y. (2018). A secure remote healthcare system for hospital using blockchain smart contract In2018 IEEE Globecom Workshops (GC Wkshps), IEEE (2018 Dec 9), pp. 1-6

Pokharel, B., Kshetri, N., Sharma, S., & Paudel, S. (2025). Blockhealthsecure: Integrating blockchain and cybersecurity in post-pandemic healthcare systems. *Information (Basel)*, *16*(2), 133. DOI: 10.3390/info16020133

Ponnuviji, N. P., Elangovan, G., Sujatha, K., Jambulingam, U., Ganesan, I., & Lalitha, S. D. (2024). IoT-Enabled Assistive Technologies Approach for Personalized Geriatric Health Monitoring and Safety. In *Future of AI in Biomedicine and Biotechnology* (pp. 125–146). IGI Global.

Porras, D. C., Siemonsma, P., Inzelberg, R., Zeilig, G., & Plotnik, M. (2018). Advantages of virtual reality in the rehabilitation of balance and gait: Systematic review. *Neurology*, *90*, 1017–1025. PMID: 29720544

Prajapat, S., Kumar, P., Kumar, D., Kumar Das, A., Shamim Hossain, M., & Rodrigues, J. J. P. C. (2024). Quantum Secure Authentication Scheme for Internet of Medical Things Using Blockchain. *IEEE Internet of Things Journal*, *11*(23), 38496–38507. DOI: 10.1109/JIOT.2024.3448212

Priyadharshini, S. I., Irene, D. S., Beulah, J. R., & Ponnuviji, N. P. (2025). Enhancing real-time health monitoring with hybrid recurrent long short-term tyrannosaurus search for menstrual cups. *Biomedical Signal Processing and Control*, *100*, 107065.

Prybutok, V. R., & Sauser, B. (2022). Theoretical and practical applications of blockchain in healthcare information management. *Information & Management*, *59*(6), 103649.

Qiu, C. S., Majeed, A., Khan, S., & Watson, M. (2022). Transforming health through the metaverse. *Journal of the Royal Society of Medicine*, *115*(12), 484–486. DOI: 10.1177/01410768221144763 PMID: 36480946

Qiu, J., Liang, X., Shetty, S., & Bowden, D. (2018, September). *Towards secure and smart healthcare in smart cities using blockchain. In 2018 IEEE international smart cities conference (ISC2)*. IEEE.

Quinn, J., & Connolly, B. (2021). Distributed ledger technology and property registers: Displacement or status quo. *Law, Innovation and Technology*, *13*(2), 377–397.

Rafique, W., & Qadir, J. (2024). Internet of everything meets the metaverse: Bridging physical and virtual worlds with blockchain. *Computer Science Review*, *54*, 100678. DOI: 10.1016/j.cosrev.2024.100678

Rahal, H. R., Slatnia, S., Kazar, O., Barka, E., & Harous, S. (2024). Blockchain-based multi-diagnosis deep learning application for various diseases classification. *International Journal of Information Security*, *23*(1), 15–30. DOI: 10.1007/s10207-023-00733-8

Rahaman, Md. T., Pranta, A. D., Repon, Md. R., Ahmed, Md. S., & Islam, T. (2024). Green production and consumption of textiles and apparel: Importance, fabrication, challenges and future prospects. *Journal of Open Innovation*, *10*(2), 100280. DOI: 10.1016/j.joitmc.2024.100280

Rajawat, A. S., Bedi, P., Goyal, S. B., Shaw, R. N., Ghosh, A., & Aggarwal, S. (2022). Ai and blockchain for healthcare data security in smart cities. *AI and IoT for Smart City Applications*, 185-198.

Ramani, V., Kumar, T., Bracken, A., Liyanage, M., & Ylianttila, M. (2018). Secure and efficient data accessibility in Blockchain-based healthcare systems In2018 IEEE Global Communications Conference (GLOBECOM), IEEE (2018 Dec 9), pp. 206-212

Ratwani, R. M. (2017). Electronic health records and improved patient care: Opportunities for applied psychology. *Current Directions in Psychological Science*, *26*(4), 359–365. PMID: 28808359

Ray, P. P., Dash, D., Salah, K., & Kumar, N. (2020, January 21). Blockchain for IoT-based healthcare: Background, consensus, platforms, and use cases. *IEEE Systems Journal*, *15*(1), 85–94.

Reegu, F. A., Abas, H., Gulzar, Y., Xin, Q., Alwan, A. A., Jabbari, A., Sonkamble, R. G., & Dziyauddin, R. A. (2023). Blockchain-Based Framework for Interoperable Electronic Health Records for an Improved Healthcare System. *Sustainability*, *15*, 6337.

Ribitzky, R., Clair, J. S., Houlding, D. I., McFarlane, C. T., Ahier, B., Gould, M., Flannery, H. L., Pupo, E., & Clauson, K. A. (2018, March 23). Pragmatic, interdisciplinary perspectives on Blockchain and distributed ledger technology: Paving the future for healthcare. *Blockchain in Healthcare Today*, *1*, 24.

Rosaline, R. A. A., & Ponnuviji, N. P., TC, S. L., & Manisha, G. (2023). Enhancing lifestyle and health monitoring of elderly populations using CSA-TkELM classifier. *Knowledge-Based Systems*, *276*, 110758.

Rouse, W. B., Johns, M. M. E., & Pepe, K. M. (2017). Learning in the health care enterprise. *Learning Health Systems*, *1*(4), e10024. DOI: 10.1002/lrh2.10024 PMID: 31245566

Rumelhart, D. E., Hinton, G. E., & Williams, R. J. (1988). Learning representations by back-propagating errors. In Anderson, J. A., & Rosenfeld, E. (Eds.), *Neurocomputing: Foundations of Research* (pp. 696–699). MIT Press., https://dl.acm.org/citation.cfm?id=65669.104451

Saha, A., Amin, R., Kunal, S., Vollala, S., & Dwivedi, S. K. (2019, September). Review on "Blockchain technology-based medical healthcare system with privacy issues. *Security and Privacy*, *2*(5), e83.

Satamraju, K. P. (2020, January). Proof of concept of scalable integration of internet of things and Blockchain in healthcare. *Sensors (Basel)*, *20*(5), 1389. PMID: 32138380

Schinckus, C. (2022). A Nuanced perspective on blockchain technology and healthcare. Technology in Society, Vol 71, (2022), ISSN 0160-791X, https://doi.org/DOI: 10.1016/j.techsoc.2022.102082

Schinckus, C. (2020). The good, the bad and the ugly: An overview of the sustainability of blockchain technology. *Energy Research & Social Science*, *69*(1), 101614.

Schinckus, C. (2021). Proof-of-work based blockchain technology and Anthropocene: An undermined situation? *Renewable & Sustainable Energy Reviews*, *152*, 111682.

Selvi, D. K., Aswini, J., Balakrishnan, C., Suganya, K., & Sheena, B. G. (2024, May). Revolutionizing cardiovascular care: The role of AI, ML, and DL in early heart disease prediction and treatment. In *2024 International Conference on Electronics, Computing, Communication and Control Technology (ICECCC)* (pp. 1-6). IEEE.

Sestino, A., & D'Angelo, A. (2023). My doctor is an avatar! The effect of anthropomorphism and emotional receptivity on individuals' intention to use digital-based healthcare services. *Technological Forecasting and Social Change*, *191*, 122505. DOI: 10.1016/j.techfore.2023.122505

Sharma, P., Jindal, R., & Borah, M. D. (2021). Healthify: a blockchain-based distributed application for health care. *Applications of blockchain in healthcare*, 171-198.

Shen, B., Guo, J., & Yang, Y. (2019). Med Chain: Efficient healthcare data sharing via Blockchain. *Applied Sciences (Basel, Switzerland)*, *9*(6), 1207.

Shicheng, W., Lin, H., Gan, W., Chen, J., & Yu, P. (2023). The Next Internet Revolution. arXi, arXiv:2304.06111.

Shin, D. (2022). The actualization of meta affordances: Conceptualizing affordance actualization in the metaverse games. *Computers in Human Behavior*, *133*, 107292.

Shinde, R., Patil, S., Kotecha, K., Potdar, V., Selvachandran, G., & Abraham, A. (2024). Securing AI-based healthcare systems using blockchain technology: A state-of-the-art systematic literature review and future research directions. *Transactions on Emerging Telecommunications Technologies*, *35*(1), e4884.

Shiny Irene, D., Ponnuviji, N. P., & Kalaivani, A. (2025). EHECA-HSWS: A Holistic Method for Improving Menstrual Health App User Experience. *Journal of the Institution of Electronics and Telecommunication Engineers*, •••, 1–12.

Shrivastava, U., Song, J., Han, B. T., & Dietzman, D. (2021). Do data security measures, privacy regulations, and communication standards impact the interoperability of patient health information? A cross-country investigation. *International Journal of Medical Informatics*, *148*, 104401. PMID: 33571743

Singh, P., & Singh, N. (2020). Blockchain with IoT and AI: A review of agriculture and healthcare. [IJAEC]. *International Journal of Applied Evolutionary Computation*, *11*(4), 13–27.

Siyal, A. A., Junejo, A. Z., Zawish, M., Ahmed, K., Khalil, A., & Soursou, G. (2019). Applications of blockchain technology in medicine and healthcare: Challenges and future perspectives. *Cryptography*, *3*(1), 3.

Skalidis, I., Maurizi, N., Kaldasch, M., El Idrissi, B., Briante, N., Fournier, S., Muller, O., & Skalidis, E. (2022). Feasibility of clinical and electrocardiographic follow-up of prinzmetal angina using the metaverse. *European Heart Journal - Digital Health, 3*(4), ztac076.2817. https://doi.org/DOI: 10.1093/ehjdh/ztac076.2817

Skalidis, I., Muller, O., & Fournier, S. (2023). CardioVerse: The cardiovascular medicine in the era of Metaverse. *Trends in Cardiovascular Medicine*, *33*(8), 471–476. PMID: 35568263

Smolenskas, A. (2024). Blockchain in healthcare: Benefits, use cases, & challenges. BitDegree. Retrieved from https://www.bitdegree.org/crypto/tutorials/blockchain-in-healthcare#challenges-and-considerations Accessed on 22/04/2025

Soltanisehat, L., Alizadeh, R., Hao, H., & Choo, K. K. (2020). Technical, temporal, and spatial research challenges and opportunities in blockchain-based healthcare: A systematic literature review. *IEEE Transactions on Engineering Management*, •••, 1–16.

Sonkamble, R.G.; Phansalkar, S.P.; Potdar, V.M.; Bongale, A.M. (2021). Survey of Interoperability in Electronic Health Records Management and Proposed Blockchain Based Framework: MyBlockEHR. IEEE Access 2021, 9, 158367–158401.

Sreejith, R., & Senthil, S. (2023). Smart Contract Authentication assisted GraphMap-Based HL7 FHIR architecture for interoperable e-healthcare system. *Heliyon*, *9*, e15180. PMID: 37089400

Sreelakshmi, S., Babu, A. A., Lakshmipriya, C., Gracious, L. A., Nalini, M., & Subramanian, R. S. (2024, October). Enhancing Intrusion Detection Systems with Machine Learning. In 2024 2nd International Conference on Self Sustainable Artificial Intelligence Systems (ICSSAS) (pp. 557-564). IEEE.

Srinivas, O., & Pradhan, N. R. (2024). A Novel NFT Framework for Pharmaceutical Asset Ownership and Trading: TokenPharma. *IEEE Access : Practical Innovations, Open Solutions*, *12*, 171418–171433. DOI: 10.1109/ACCESS.2024.3500092

Sriram, G. (2022). Edge computing vs. Cloud computing: An overview of big data challenges and opportunities for large enterprises. *International Research Journal of Modernization in Engineering Technology and Science*, *2022*(4), 1331–1337.

Srivastava, G., Crichigno, J., & Dhar, S. (2019). A light and secure healthcare blockchain for IoT medical devices In2019 IEEE Canadian Conference of Electrical and Computer Engineering (CCECE), IEEE (2019 May 5), pp. 1-5

Srivastava, N. (2019). *What is Blockchain Technology, and How Does It Work?*.

Srivastava, V., Mahara, T., & Yadav, P. (2021). An analysis of the ethical challenges of blockchain-enabled E-healthcare applications in 6G networks. *International Journal of Cognitive Computing in Engineering*, *2*, 171–179.

Starfield, B., Shi, L., & Macinko, J. (2005). Contribution of primary care to health systems and health. *The Milbank Quarterly*, *83*(3), 457–502. PMID: 16202000

Stearns, M. Q., Price, C., Spackman, K. A., & Wang, A. Y. (2001). SNOMED clinical terms: Overview of the development process and project status. *Proc. AMIA Symp.*, •••, 662–666. PMID: 11825268

Stone, D. (2018). Blockchain: The challenges and opportunities in healthcare. *Divurgent*, *1*, 1–14.

Subha, S., Balakrishnan, C., & Anish, T. P. (2024, August). Optimizing Machine Learning Algorithms for Heart Disease Prediction in Healthcare: A Comparative Study. In *2024 5th International Conference on Electronics and Sustainable Communication Systems (ICESC)* (pp. 866-872). IEEE.

Subramanian, R. S., Ramana, T. V., Ramana, K. V., Prabha, S., & Nivaskumar, V. (2025). Converging Horizons: Synergies of 6G Wireless Communication, Machine Learning, and Embedded Systems for Intelligent Connectivity. *The Intersection of 6G, AI/Machine Learning, and Embedded Systems*, 67-93.

Sudha, K., Nithyanandhan, R., Girija, P., & Nalini, M. (2024, July). Enhancing Healthcare Data Security in the Cloud: Integrating ML-Based Intrusion Detection Systems. In *2024 2nd World Conference on Communication & Computing (WCONF)* (pp. 1-7). IEEE.

Sudha, K., Lakshmipriya, C., Pajila, P. B., Venitha, E., & Anita, M. (2024, January). Enhancing Diabetes Prediction and Management through Machine Learning: A Comparative Study. In *2024 Fourth International Conference on Advances in Electrical, Computing, Communication and Sustainable Technologies (ICAECT)* (pp. 1-6). IEEE.

Sun, Y., Zhang, R., Wang, X., Gao, K., & Liu, L. (2018). A decentralising attribute-based signature for healthcare blockchain In2018 27th International Conference on Computer Communication and Networks (ICCCN), IEEE (2018 Jul 30), pp. 1-9

Sun, N., Cao, B., & Mu, X. (2024). Research on the Future Trends of the Integration of Artificial Intelligence and Fashion Design of Clothing. *Applied Mathematics and Nonlinear Sciences*, *9*(1), 20242181. DOI: 10.2478/amns-2024-2181

Suratkar, S., Shirole, M., & Bhirud, S. Cryptocurrency Wallet: A Review. In Proceedings of the 2020 4th International Conference on Computer, Communication and Signal Processing (ICCCSP), Chennai, India, 28–29 September 2020; pp. 1–7.

Syed, T. A., Alzahrani, A., Jan, S., Siddiqui, M. S., Nadeem, A., & Alghamdi, T. (2019, December 4). A comparative analysis of blockchain architecture and its applications: Problems and recommendations. *IEEE Access : Practical Innovations, Open Solutions*, *7*, 176838–176869.

Szczepaniuk, H., & Szczepaniuk, E. K. (2023). Cryptographic evidence-based cybersecurity for smart healthcare systems. *Information Sciences*, *649*, 119633. DOI: 10.1016/j.ins.2023.119633

Szegedy, C., Liu, W., Jia, Y., Sermanet, P., Reed, S., Anguelov, D., & Rabinovich, A. (2015). Going deeper with convolutions. In *Proceedings of the IEEE Conference on Computer Vision and Pattern Recognition* (pp. 1–9).

Tagde, P., Tagde, S., Bhattacharya, T., Tagde, P., Chopra, H., Akter, R., & Rahman, M. H. (2021). Blockchain and artificial intelligence technology in e-Health. *Environmental Science and Pollution Research International*, *28*, 52810–52831. PMID: 34476701

Taherdoost, H. (2023). Privacy and security of blockchain in healthcare: Applications, challenges, and future perspectives. *Sci*, *5*(4), 41.

Taherdoost, H. (2023). Privacy and Security of Blockchain in Healthcare: Applications, Challenges, and Future Perspectives. *Sci.*, *5*(4), 41. DOI: 10.3390/sci5040041

Taherdoost, H. (2023). Smart contracts in blockchain technology: A critical review. *Information (Basel)*, *14*(2), 117.

Tandon, A., Dhir, A., Islam, A. N., & Mäntymäki, M. (2020). Blockchain in healthcare: A systematic literature review, synthesizing framework and future research agenda. *Computers in Industry*, *122*, 103290.

Tandon, A., Dhir, A., Islam, N., & Mäntymäki, M. (2020, November 1). Blockchain in healthcare: A systematic literature review, synthesising framework and future research agenda. *Computers in Industry*, *122*, 103290.

Tang, Y., Xiong, J., Becerril-Arreola, R., & Iyer, L. (2020). Ethics of blockchain: A framework of technology, applications, impacts, and research directions. *Information Technology & People*, *33*(2), 602–632.

Tan, T. F., Li, Y., Lim, J. S., Gunasekeran, D. V., Teo, Z. L., Ng, W. Y., & Ting, D. S. (2022). Metaverse and Virtual Health Care in Ophthalmology: Opportunities and Challenges. *Asia-Pacific Journal of Ophthalmology*, *11*, 237–246. PMID: 35772084

Tanwar, S., Parekh, K., & Evans, R. (2020, February 1). Blockchain-based electronic healthcare record system for healthcare 4.0 applications. *Journal of Information Security and Applications*, *50*, 102407.

Tatineni, S. (2019). Blockchain and Data Science Integration for Secure and Transparent Data Sharing. [IJARET]. *International Journal of Advanced Research in Engineering and Technology*, *10*(3), 470–480.

Thomason, J. (2022). Metaverse, token economies, and non-communicable diseases. *Global Health Journal (Amsterdam, Netherlands)*, *6*, 164–167.

Tomar, A., & Tripathi, S. (2023). BCSoM: Blockchain-based certificateless aggregate signcryption scheme for Internet of Medical Things. *Computer Communications*, *212*, 48–62. DOI: 10.1016/j.comcom.2023.09.027

Tripathi, G., Ahad, M. A., & Casalino, G. (2023). A comprehensive review of blockchain technology: Underlying principles and historical background with future challenges. *Decision Analytics Journal*, 100344.

Uddin, M., Salah, K., Jayaraman, R., Pesic, S., & Ellahham, S. (2021). Blockchain for drug traceability: Architectures and open challenges. *Health Informatics Journal*, *27*(2), 14604582211011228. PMID: 33899576

Ullah, H. S., Aslam, S., & Arjomand, N. Blockchain in Healthcare and Medicine: A Contemporary Research of Applications, Challenges, and Future Perspectives. arXiv 2020, arXiv:2004.06795.

Ullah, H., Manickam, S., Obaidat, M., Laghari, S. U. A., & Uddin, M. (2023). Exploring the Potential of Metaverse Technology in Healthcare: Applications, Challenges, and Future Directions. *IEEE Access : Practical Innovations, Open Solutions*, *11*, 69686–69707. DOI: 10.1109/ACCESS.2023.3286696

Um, T., Kim, H., Kim, H., Lee, J., Koo, C., & Chung, N. Travel Incheon as a Metaverse: Smart Tourism Cities Development Case in Korea. In Proceedings of the ENTER22 e-Tourism Conference, Tianjin, China, 11–14 January 2022; Springer: Berlin/Heidelberg, Germany, 2022.

Vaishya R., Javaid M., Khan I.H., Vaish A., & Iyengar K.P. (2021). Significant role of modern technologies for COVID-19 pandemic Journal of Industrial Integration and Management (2021 Mar 4), pp. 1-3

Vaishya, R., Haleem, A., Vaish, A., & Javaid, M. (2020, July 1). Emerging technologies to combat the COVID-19 pandemic. *Journal of Clinical and Experimental Hepatology*, *10*(4), 409–411. PMID: 32377057

Vaishya, R., Javaid, M., Khan, I. H., Vaish, A., & Iyengar, K. P. (2021). Significant role of modern technologies for COVID-19 pandemic. *Journal of Industrial Integration and Management*, *6*(02), 147–159.

Vazirani, A., O'Donoghue, O., Brindley, D., & Meinert, E. (2020). Blockchain vehicles for efficient medical record management. *NPJ Digital Medicine*, *3*(1). Advance online publication. DOI: 10.1038/s41746-019-0211-0

Vetrivel, S. C., & Mohanasundaram, T. (2024). Blockchain-empowered metaverse healthcare systems and applications. *Digital Transformation in Healthcare 5.0: Volume 2: Metaverse, Nanorobots and Machine Learning*, 61.

Vorisek, C. N., Lehne, M., Klopfenstein, S. A. I., Mayer, P. J., Bartschke, A., Haese, T., & Thun, S. (2022). Fast Healthcare Interoperability Resources (FHIR) for Interoperability in Health Research: Systematic Review. *JMIR Public Health and Surveillance*, *10*, e35724. PMID: 35852842

Wang, C., Wang, L., Zhao, S., Yang, C., & Albitar, K. (2024). The impact of Fintech on corporate carbon emissions: Towards green and sustainable development. *Business Strategy and the Environment*, *33*(6), 5776–5796. DOI: 10.1002/bse.3778

Wang, Q., Liu, C., & Lan, S. (2023). Digital literacy and financial market participation of middle-aged and elderly adults in China. *Economic and Political Studies*, *11*(4), 441–468. DOI: 10.1080/20954816.2022.2115191

Wang, S., Wang, J., Wang, X., Qiu, T., Yuan, Y., Ouyang, L., Guo, Y., & Wang, F. Y. (2018, August 28). Blockchain-powered parallel healthcare systems based on the ACP approach. *IEEE Transactions on Computational Social Systems*, *5*(4), 942–950.

Wang, S., Zhang, D., & Zhang, Y. (2019). Blockchain-Based Personal Health Records Sharing Scheme With Data Integrity Verifiable. *IEEE Access : Practical Innovations, Open Solutions*, *7*, 102887–102901. DOI: 10.1109/ACCESS.2019.2931531

Wang, Y., Zhu, M., Chen, X., Liu, R., Ge, J., Song, Y., & Yu, G. (2024). The application of metaverse in healthcare. *Frontiers in Public Health*, *12*, 1420367.

Wazid, M., Bera, B., Mitra, A., Das, A. K., & Ali, R. (2020, September). Private blockchain-envisioned security framework for AI-enabled IoT-based drone-aided healthcare services. In *Proceedings of the 2nd ACM MobiCom workshop on drone assisted wireless communications for 5G and beyond* (pp. 37-42).

Wiederhold, B. K. (2022). *Metaverse Games: Game Changer for Healthcare?* Mary Ann Liebert, Inc.

Wong, D., Bhattacharya, S., & Butte, A. (2019). Prototype of running clinical trials in an untrustworthy environment using blockchain. *Nature Communications*, *10*(1). Advance online publication. DOI: 10.1038/s41467-019-08874-y

Wu, T. C., & Ho, C. T. B. (2023). A scoping review of metaverse in emergency medicine. *Australasian Emergency Care (Online)*, *26*(1), 75–83. PMID: 35953392

Xie, Y., Zhang, J., Wang, H., Liu, P., Liu, S., Huo, T., & Ye, Z. (2021). Applications of blockchain in the medical field: Narrative review. *Journal of Medical Internet Research*, *23*(10), e28613. PMID: 34533470

Xu, S. (2024). Research on financial innovation and Risk Management in the digital Economy Era. *Applied Mathematics and Nonlinear Sciences*, *9*(1), 20242488. DOI: 10.2478/amns-2024-2488

Yamini, B., Saraswathi, T., Radhakrishnan, P., Nalini, M., Shanmuganathan, M., & Siva, S. R. (2024). Machine learning algorithms for predicting of chronic kidney disease and its significance in healthcare. *International Journal of Advanced Technology and Engineering Exploration*, *11*(112), 388.

Yang, D.; Zhou, J.; Chen, R.; Song, Y.; Song, Z.; Zhang, X.; Wang, Q.; Wang, K.; Zhou, C.; Sun, J.; et al. Expert consensus on the metaverse in medicine. Clin. eHealth 2022, 5, 1–9.

Yang, Q., Zhao, Y., Huang, H., Xiong, Z., Kang, J., & Zheng, Z. (2022). Fusing blockchain and ai with metaverse: A survey. *IEEE Open Journal of the Computer Society*, *3*, 122–136. DOI: 10.1109/ojcs.2022.3188249

Yang, Y., Zhou, Z., Li, X., Xue, X., Hung, P. C., & Yangui, S. (2023). Metaverse for healthcare: Technologies, challenges, and vision. *International Journal of Crowd Science*, *7*(4), 190–199.

Yaqoob, I., Salah, K., Jayaraman, R., & Al-Hammadi, Y. (2021). Blockchain for healthcare data management: Opportunities, challenges, and future recommendations. *Neural Computing & Applications*, 1–16.

You, Y., & Gui, X. (2020). Self-Diagnosis through AI-Enabled Chatbot-Based Symptom Checkers: User Experiences and Design Considerations. *AMIA ... Annual Symposium Proceedings - AMIA Symposium. AMIA Symposium, 2020*, 1354–1363. PMID: 33936512

Yulianjani, A., Rosdiana, R., & Altaufik, R. (2024). Analysis of blockchain technology in patient data management system: security, privacy, and efficiency in the digital healthca Feltovic, M. (2024). From theory to practice: the role of cryptography in securing blockchain networks. *Mest Journal, 12*(2), 93–102. DOI: 10.12709/mest.12.12.02.12

Zaabar, B., Cheikhrouhou, O., Jamil, F., Ammi, M., & Abid, M. (2021). HealthBlock: A secure blockchain-based healthcare data management system. *Computer Networks, 200*, 108500.

Zakari, N., Al-Razgan, M., Alsaadi, A., Alshareef, H., Alashaikh, L., Alharbi, M., & Alotaibi, S. (2022). Blockchain technology in the pharmaceutical industry: A systematic review. *PeerJ. Computer Science, 8*, e840. PMID: 35634106

Zarour, M., Ansari, M. T. J., Alenezi, M., Sarkar, A. K., Faizan, M., Agrawal, A., & Khan, R. A. (2020). Evaluating the impact of blockchain models for secure and trustworthy electronic healthcare records. *IEEE Access : Practical Innovations, Open Solutions, 8*, 157959–157973.

Zarour, M., Ansari, M. T., Alenezi, M., Sarkar, A. K., Faizan, M., Agrawal, A., Kumar, R., & Khan, R. A. (2020, August 27). Evaluating the impact of blockchain models for secure and trustworthy electronic healthcare records. *IEEE Access : Practical Innovations, Open Solutions, 8*, 157959–157973.

Zeiler, M. D., & Fergus, R. (2014). Visualizing and understanding convolutional networks. In *European Conference on Computer Vision* (pp. 818–833).

Zeng, Y., Zeng, L., Zhang, C., & Cheng, A. S. (2022). The metaverse in cancer care: Applications and challenges. *Asia-Pacific Journal of Oncology Nursing, 9*, 100111. PMID: 36276879

Zhang, P., & Boulos, M. N. (2020). Blockchain solutions for healthcare Precision Medicine for Investigators, Practitioners and Providers, Academic Press (2020 Jan 1), pp. 519-524

Zhang, P., Walker, M. A., White, J., Schmidt, D. C., & Lenz, G. (2017). Metrics for assessing blockchain-based healthcare decentralised apps In2017 IEEE 19th International Conference on E-Health Networking, Applications and Services (Healthcom), IEEE (2017 Oct 12), pp. 1-4

Zhang, P., Schmidt, D. C., White, J., & Lenz, G. (2018). *Blockchain technology use cases in healthcare. Advances in Computers* (Vol. 111). Elsevier.

Zheng, K., Liu, Y., Dai, C., Duan, Y., & Huang, X. (2018). Model checking PBFT consensus mechanism in healthcare blockchain network In2018 9th International Conference on Information Technology in Medicine and Education (ITME), IEEE (2018 Oct 19), pp. 877-881

Zheng, Z., Xie, S., Dai, H. N., Chen, X., & Wang, H. (2018). Blockchain challenges and opportunities: A survey. *International Journal of Web and Grid Services, 2018*(14), 352–3.

Zhuang, Y., Shyu, C.-R., Hong, S., Li, P., & Zhang, L. (2023). Self-sovereign identity empowered non-fungible patient tokenization for health information exchange using blockchain technology. *Computers in Biology and Medicine, 157*, 106778. DOI: 10.1016/j.compbiomed.2023.106778 PMID: 36934533

About the Contributors

Shadab Alam, currently an Associate Professor at Jazan University, KSA, is an accomplished computer science researcher focusing on information security, blockchain, IoT, and smart healthcare. He completed his PhD in Computer Science from Aligarh Muslim University, India, where he also earned his master's and bachelor's degrees. Dr. Shadab Alam has made substantial contributions to the field of computer science, as evidenced by his publication of over 80 research papers in high-impact journals and prominent international conference proceedings. His innovative work has also led to the acquisition of 05 international patents, including those in the US and Australia, and 03 national patents.He was recognized among the World Top 2% Scientists by Stanford University in 2024. Beyond his research, Dr. Alam is actively involved in the professional community as a senior member of IEEE (SMIEEE) and holds memberships in several esteemed organizations, including CSI, CRSI, ACM, IAENG, CSTA, IACSIT, and ICSE, reflecting his wide influence and commitment to the field. Dr. Shadab Alam's editorial achievements include serving as an Academic Editor for several renowned journals: PLOS ONE, Computational and Mathematical Methods in Medicine, Computational and Mathematical Methods, Security and Communication Networks, and Journal of Computational and Cognitive Engineering. These roles are facilitated through collaborations with publishers like Hindawi, John Wiley & Sons, Inc., and BON VIEW PUBLISHING PTE. LTD, Singapore, signifies his expertise and influence in the field.

Mohammed Shuaib is an Assistant Professor at Jazan University, Saudi Arabia, with over 11 years of academic experience. . His international experience includes a visiting research position at INTI International University, Malaysia. Dr. Shuaib's research achievements include 65 peer-reviewed publications in high-impact journals like Elsevier, Springer, and IEEE Access, four patents, and an H-index of 26 with over 1860 citations. He was recognized among the World Top 2% Scientists by Stanford University in 2024. In addition to research, Dr. Shuaib currently serves as an Associate Editor for Sustainable Computing: Informatics and Systems (Elsevier) and the International Journal of Electrical and Computer Engineering (IAES). He also serves as an Academic Editor for PLOS ONE and the International Journal of RF and Microwave Computer-Aided Engineering (Wiley). Moreover, he is on the editorial boards of Mobile Information Systems (Wiley), Discover Internet of Things (Springer), Journal of Economy and Technology (Elsevier), and International Journal of Information Technology and Web Engineering (IGI Global). These journals are indexed in top databases such as ISI, Web of Science, and Scopus.

Rajaram Ayyasamy received the B.E. degree in Electronics and Communication Engineering from the Government College of Technology, Coimbatore, Anna University, Chennai. He received the M.E. degree in Electronics and Communication Engineering (Applied Electronics) from the Government College of Technology, Anna University, Chennai. He received the Full Time Ph.D. degree in Electronics and Communication Engineering from the Anna University of Technology, Coimbatore. He is currently working as a Professor, ECE Department in E.G.S. Pillay Engineering College, Nagapattinam, India. His research interests include Mobile Ad Hoc networks, wireless communication networks (WiFi, WiMax HighSlot GSM), novel VLSI NOC Design approaches to address issues such as low-power, cross-talk, hardware acceleration,Design issues includes OFDM MIMO and noise Suppression in MAI Systems, ASIC design, Control systems, Fuzzy logic and Networks, AI, Sensor Networks. He has published more SCIE indexed journals

***

Usharani Bhimavarapu is an Assistant Professor at Koneru Lakshmaiah Education Foundation in Andhra Pradesh, India, where she teaches Computer Science and Engineering. With a career spanning 17 years, she has become a respected authority in Data Mining, Machine Learning, and Data Structure. Dr. Bhimavarapu's research prowess is evidenced by her publication of over 100 papers and 50 books on programming languages like CPP, Java, Fullstack, Databases, R, Node.js, Python, HTML, and CSS. Ebooks

KarthikA is currently working as an Assistant Professor in the department of Information Technology, Institute of Aeronautical Engineering, Hyderabad. He has completed Ph. D from the Vel Tech Rangarajan Dr. Sagunthala R&D Institute of Science and Technology (Deemed to be University), Chennai on the research work entitled "Enhancing Speech Clarity: An Optimized Approach Using Efficient Convolutional Neural Networks" in 2024. He received M. Tech. in Electronics and Communications Engineering from Malla Reddy Institute of Technology and Sciences, Hyderabad (JNTU Hyderabad) in 2014 and B. Tech from VGSE, Karimnagar (JNTU Hyderabad) in 2012. He has 10 years of teaching experience. He has published 14 international journal papers and 22 international conference papers. His areas of interest include Machine Learning, Signal Processing, Image Processing.

Satheeskumar A is working as the Assistant Professor in the Department of Computer Engineering in Nandha Engineering college, Erode, India

Manjunathan Alagarsamy received the Engineer degree in Electronics and Comunication Engineering from Dr.Navalar Nedunchezhiyan College of Engineering in 2010. He received the Master degree in Embedded System Technologies from Raja College of Engineering and Technology, Madurai, Tamilnadu, India in 2013. He is currently working as an Assistant Professor in the Department of Electronics and Communication Engineering at K.Ramakrishnan College of Technology, Trichy, India. His area of interests includes Embedded Systems, Image processing, Sensors and Interfacing networks and Internet of Things. He has published 72 article in peer reviewed International journals and presented 18 papers in International conferences. He can be contacted at email: manjunathankrct@gmail.com.

Srinivas B V is an Assistant Professor at BMS Institute of Technology & Management, Bengaluru, India. He holds a PhD Degree in Computer and Information Science Engineering with specialization in Cloud Computing from Visvesvaraya Technological University, Belagavi, Karnataka, India. He is UGC-NET qualified, and he has 1year Industry and 12 years of Teaching experience. His main area of research interests are Cloud Computing, Machine Learning and Genetic Algorithms. He has published research articles in renowned SCIE and Scopus indexed journals and is an active reviewer in Scopus indexed journals.He can be contacted at email: srini13986@gmail.com.

Nirmalkumar S. Benni is an Associate Professor at RNS Institute of Technology, Bengaluru, India. He holds a Ph.D. in Electronics and Communication Engineering, specializing in Wireless Communication and Networks, from Visvesvaraya Technological University (VTU), Belagavi. He also earned an M. Tech in Digital Communication & Networking from UBDT, Davangere (affiliated with Kuvempu University, Shimoga), and a B.E. in Electronics and Communication Engineering from Hirasugar Institute of Technology, Nidasoshi (affiliated with VTU, Belagavi). With 18 years of teaching experience, he has taught a wide range of subjects, including Digital Design and Computer Organization, Computer Networks, Principles of Programming Using C, Analog and Digital Electronics, Microcontroller and Embedded Systems, Wireless Communication and Networking, Antenna Theory and Design, Multimedia Communication, and Advanced Computer Networks. His research primarily focuses on Wireless Communication and Networks. He has presented 50+ research papers at national and international conferences and journals. Additionally, he has published 20 patents, copyrights, and books. He is actively involved in academia as a research supervisor, currently guiding a research scholar at RNSIT, Bengaluru. He also serves as a reviewer for several national and international conferences and journals. He is a Senior Member of IEEE (USA) and is affiliated with IEEE Young Professionals, IEEE SIGHT, and IETE.

Ranjeeth KumarC. currently serves as the Dean – Innovation & Entrepreneurship and Professor in the Department of Computer Science and Engineering at G. Pullaiah College of Engineering and Technology, Kurnool. He was awarded a Ph.D. in Information and Communication Engineering by Anna University, Chennai, in 2022. He holds a Master of Engineering in Computer Science and Engineering from Sri Krishna College of Engineering and Technology, Coimbatore (2010), and a Bachelor of Technology in Information Technology from Dr. Mahalingam College of Engineering and Technology, Pollachi (2008). He is also a recognized Research Supervisor under Anna University. With over 15 years of teaching and research experience, his academic interests span Computer Vision, Machine Learning, Deep Learning, and Natural Language Processing. Throughout his career, Dr. Ranjeeth Kumar has actively contributed to industry-focused consultancy and research projects for organizations such as International Aerospace Manufacturing Pvt. Ltd., Bengaluru (a joint venture of Rolls Royce and HAL), Cameron – A Schlumberger Company, GE Healthcare, and L&T Technology Services (LTTS) in the domain of Artificial Intelligence. In recognition of his significant contributions to AI, his former institution, Sri Ramakrishna Engineering College, appointed him as a Co-Founder of the startup Artispec Technologies Pvt. Ltd., incubated at SREC SPARK Incubation Foundation, Coimbatore, with a mission of "Enabling Manufacturing with a Vision." He currently mentors Doctor of Business Administration (DBA) candidates at Golden Gate University, through UpGrad Education Pvt. Ltd., with six learners under his supervision involved in startups, thesis writing, and book publications. Dr. Ranjeeth Kumar was a recipient of the NVIDIA Jetson Nano 2GB Hardware Grant, through which he established an NVIDIA Lab at SREC with 15 kits. He is an NVIDIA Deep Learning Institute (DLI) University Ambassador and a Certified Instructor for courses including Fundamentals of Deep Learning, Computer Vision for Industrial Inspection, and Applications of AI for Predictive Maintenance. Additionally, he has earned IBM badges for Artificial Intelligence Practitioner – Instructor and Enterprise Design Thinking – AI Essentials. He also serves as an Innovation Ambassador (Design Thinking and Innovation) recognized by the Ministry of Education's Innovation Cell (MHRD-IIC) at SREC, Coimbatore.

His contributions have earned him certificates of appreciation from L&T Technology Services for technical evaluation and mentorship (Techgium 6th Edition) and from GE Healthcare for mentorship.He holds one granted patent and has two patents filed in his name. Dr. Ranjeeth Kumar also advises multiple EdTech startups in a part-time capacity. Among his accolades, he was recognized in India's 100 Under 40 (2023) by Fox Story India, awarded in the Elite Category of Top 100 International Distinguished Educators by Green ThinkerZ (2020), named Faculty of the Year (Engineering) by IBAE (2021), and honoured with the Outstanding Faculty Mentor Award by the Novel Research Academy, Puducherry. He has published extensively in reputed international journals, presented papers at national and international conferences (including best paper awards). He has served as a reviewer for many reputed journals that include publishers like Springer, Wiley, Taylor & Francis and Inderscience Publishers. He also mentors students in Hackathons and project contests, and is a life member of professional bodies such as CSI, ISTE, IAENG, and IACSIT.

Raman C J is working as a Professor at St. Joseph's College of Engineering, Chennai, Tamil Nadu, India, in the department of Artificial Intelligence and Machine Learning. He had obtained his PhD in Computer Science and Engineering from Sathyabama Institute of Science and Technology, Tamil Nadu, India. He had obtained his M.E. degree in Computer Science and Engineering from Anna University. He has 18 years of teaching experience. His research interests include Congestion control in Wireless Sensor Networks, Cloud Computing, Network Security, Artificial Intelligence and Machine Learning

Abinaya Gopalakrishnan, currently working as an Assistant Professor in the Department of Networking and Communications at SRM Institute of Science and Technology, holds a PhD in Computer Science from the University of Southern Queensland, Australia, and SRMIST, India. She is a dedicated academic and researcher in Computer Science and Engineering and her research focuses on AI-driven mental health monitoring, Natural Language Processing (NLP), AI driven networks and data analytics. A university rank holder and gold medalist, she has published extensively in reputed journals and conferences. With expertise in machine learning and NLP, she has also contributed as a data analyst and journal reviewer. Passionate about technology-driven solutions, she actively mentors students and collaborates on innovative research projects. She is a life member of ISTE and a member of ACM, reflecting her commitment to academic and professional excellence.

Deepak G. has published extensively in the field of Computer Science and Information Science. His scholarly contributions span a range of high-impact journals, international conferences, patents, and book chapters. His research covers diverse areas within the discipline and has been featured in reputed academic and scientific publications, reflecting his ongoing commitment to advancing knowledge and innovation in the field.

RamyaG. earned her Ph.D. in Computer Science and Engineering from Pondicherry University in 2023. Currently serving as an Assistant Professor in the Department of Networking and Communications at SRM Institute of Science and Technology, she has extensive teaching experience and over six years of research expertise. Dr. Ramya has published extensively in SCIE and Scopus-indexed journals, contributed to international conferences, and actively participates in technical committees and peer-reviewing activities. Her research interests extend to Intelligent Networks, IoT Smart Cities and Machine Learning algorithms. She has been a mentor and trainer in programming and placement preparation. She is been a reviewer in peer-reviewed journal and IEEE International Conferences. She is a life member of ISTE and a member of ACM, reflecting her commitment to academic and professional excellence.

Vibha T G is working as an Assistant Professor in the Department of Electronics and Communication Engineering at Dayananda Sagar College of engineering.

G.C. Jagan, was born in Marthandam on 11th June 1981. He received his Bachelor Degree in Electronics and communication Engineering from Noorul Islam College of Engineering, Kumarakoil, Kanyakumari District, Tamilnadu. India in the year 2002. He received his Master's Degree in Communication Systems from Noorul Islam College of Engineering, Kumarakoil, Kanyakumari District, Tamilnadu. India in the year 2006, and Ph.D degree in Electronics Engineering from Sathyabama Institute of Science and Technology, Chennai, Tamilnadu, India in the year 2023. He is currently working as Assistant Professor in Department of ECE, Jeppiaar Engineering College, Chennai. His research interest includes wireless communication, wireless sensor network, Signal Processing and Image Processing. He has Research publications in SCI, WEB OF SCIENCE and SCOPUS indexed National / International Journals / Conferences.

Subhojit Ghosh is a student pursuing Bachelor of Technology in Computer Science and Engineering in Artificial Intelligence and Machine Learning.

Neha Gupta has done her PhD from Manav Rachna International University and has total of 18+ year of experience in teaching and research. She is currently working as professor at School of Computer Applications, MRIIRS. She has authored and coauthored 85 research papers in SCI/SCOPUS/Peer Reviewed Journals (Scopus indexed) and IEEE/IET Conference proceedings in areas of Web Content Mining, Mobile Computing, and Cloud Computing. She has 9 national and international patents published and 2 national & 4 international patents granted to her credit. She has published books with publishers like Springer, Taylor & Francis, IGI Global & Pacific Book International and has also authored book chapters with Elsevier, Springer, CRC Press and IGI global USA. Six scholars have successfully completed their PhD in her guidance. Her areas of research include Cloud Computing, Network Intrusion Detection, Cryptography and Cyber Physical Systems. She is a technical programme committee (TPC) member in various conferences across globe. She has been conferred with best researcher award by the university as well as best associate award in the year 2024.

ElavarasiJ. is an Assistant Professor in the Department of Artificial Intelligence and Data Science at Vel Tech High Tech Dr. Rangarajan Dr. Sakunthala Engineering College. She specializes in machine learning, deep learning, and intelligent systems. She is dedicated to guiding students in innovative AI-based projects and research initiatives. Her academic involvement includes publishing papers and participating in technical workshops and FDPs. Ms. Elavarasi strives to create an engaging learning environment that nurtures technical excellence and creativity.

SudarvelJ. working as an Assistant Professor of Management at Karpagam Academy of Higher Education. He produced five Ph.D. Scholars and four Ph.D. Scholars are under his guidance. Further, to his credit he published more than five articles in Scopus indexed journals and published more than 50 articles in international journals. He is acting as a Subject Experts in Board of studies of various autonomous colleges.

Deepa K. is affiliated with the Department of Information Technology at Karpagam College of Engineering in Coimbatore, India.

Shashi Raj K received Bachelor of Engineering degree in Electronics & Communication Engineering from Vivekananda Institute of Technology, Bengaluru, M.Tech. degree in VLSI Design & Embedded Systems from Reva Institute of Technology and Management, Bengaluru and obtained his Ph.D. in Wireless Networks from Visvesvaraya Technological University, Belagavi, Karnataka, India. He is currently working as Assistant Professor in the department of Electronics and Communication Engineering, Dayananda Sagar College of Engineering, Bengaluru, Karnataka, India. He has published more than 30 research papers in reputed peer reviewed International Journals and Conferences. His research interests include

Wireless Networks, Network Security, Machine Learning, Medical Imaging, VLSI Design and Embedded system. He can be contacted at email: shashiraj-ece@ dayanandasagar.edu

Vinutha K Obtained her Bachelor's Degree In Engineering from Channabasaveshwara Institute Of Technology, Tumkur, In 2011. Subsequently, She Completed her Master's Degree In Computer Science and Engineering from AMC Engineering College in 2013 and Completed her Doctor of Philosophy (Ph.D.) In CSE from VTU, Belagavi In 2023. With a remarkable Teaching Experience, She is actively involved In Research, specifically focusing on Prediction models using Machine Learning Techniques. She has published more than 15 Publications in reputed International Journals and Conferences and delivered 10 Invited Talks in the area of Machine Learning, RPA etc. Her Keen areas of interest encompass Machine Learning and Data Mining. She is a dedicated Life Member of the "Indian Science Congress Association".

Anto GraciousL. A. is an accomplished academic professional in Information Technology and Computer Science, known for his dedication to education, technology, and research. He holds a B.Tech in IT from C.S.I Institute of Technology (2006), an MBA in Technology Management, and an M.Tech in IT from Francis Xavier Engineering College (2011). He began his career as a Programmer at Software Solutions Integrated Limited, later transitioning to academia in 2011 as an Assistant Professor at Marthandam College of Engineering and Technology. Over eight years, he excelled in teaching, led the Software Development Cell, and earned multiple awards for his contributions. He later served at St. Xavier's Catholic College of Engineering and currently holds a position at R.M.K. College of Engineering and Technology. A prolific researcher, Anto focuses on machine learning, wireless sensor networks, and healthcare technologies. His work is widely published, and he has received accolades such as the Best Paper Award and multiple Best Faculty Awards.

EzhilvendanM. is an Assistant Professor in the Department of Artificial Intelligence and Machine Learning at Panimalar Engineering College, Chennai. He specializes in AI technologies, machine learning algorithms, and data-driven application development. He is actively involved in academic research, student project guidance, and technical training programs.Mr. Ezhilvendan regularly contributes to seminars, workshops, and faculty development initiatives. He is dedicated to fostering innovation, critical thinking, and hands-on learning in the field of AI and ML.

Mehedi Masud (Senior Member, IEEE) is a Professor in the Department of Computer Science at the Taif University, Taif, KSA. Dr. Mehedi Masud received his Ph.D. in Computer Science from the University of Ottawa, Canada. His research interests include machine learning, distributed algorithms, data security, formal methods, and health analytics. He has authored and co-authored around 70 publications, including refereed IEEE/ACM/Springer/Elsevier journals, conference papers, books, and book chapters. He has served as a technical program committee member in different international conferences. He is a recipient of many awards, including the Research in Excellence Award from Taif University. He is on the Associate Editorial Board of IEEE Access, International Journal of Knowledge Society Research (IJKSR), and editorial board member of Journal of Software. He also served as a guest editor of ComSIS Journal and Journal of Universal Computer Science (JUCS). Dr. Mehedi is a Senior Member of IEEE, a member of ACM.

PavithraN. is an Assistant Professor in the Department of Information Technology at Jeppiaar Institute of Technology, Chennai.She has expertise in areas such as programming, database systems, and emerging IT technologies. She is actively involved in student mentoring, academic coordination, and technical training initiatives. Her contributions include participation in faculty development programs, workshops, and academic projects. Ms. Pavithra is dedicated to fostering a learner-centric environment and promoting innovation in IT education.

R. Nagarajan received his B.E. in Electrical and Electronics Engineering from Madurai Kamarajar University, Madurai, India. He received his M.E. in Power Electronics and Drives from Anna University, Chennai, India. He received his Ph.D in Electrical Engineering from Anna University, Chennai, India. He has worked in the industry as an Electrical Engineer. He is currently working as a Professor of Electrical and Electronics Engineering at Gnanamani College of Technology, Namakkal, Tamilnadu, India- 637 018. He has published more than 130 papers in various peer reviewed International Journals and Conferences. He has published more than 80 books and book chapters in various international publications.His research interest includes Power Electronics, Power Systems, Power Converters, PWM Control Techniques, Electrical Engineering, Electrical Drives & Control, Communication Engineering, Network Security, Digital Image Processing, Soft Computing Techniques, Cloud Computing, Big Data Analysis and Renewable Energy Sources.

Ananya Pandey is a Research Scholar in School of Law at Christ University, Bangalore. She has her research interests in the field of Constitutional Law, Environment Law, Human Rights, Food Security, Intellectual Property Law and Jurisprudence.

Kavitha S Patil received B.E. degree in electronics in 2002 from VTU and M.Tech degree in Digital Electronics and Communication from M S Ramaiah Institute of Technology (MSRIT). She completed Ph.D in Network Security from Visvesvaraya Technological University, Belagavi. She is working as an Assistant Professor in Atria Institute of Technology and has an experience of 17 years. Her main area of research interests are Embedded System, IoT, Machine Learning and Network Security. Iam now asociate professor in ISE department of atria and also designated as a program coordinator of CSE(data science) which is an allied branch of ise.and piblished various journals of sci index and scopus indexed . and also attended international and national conferences . My patent got granted in 2022. and also served as institution level NBA coordinator for 2024-25 and attended many workshops on Outcome based education.

Priya is working as an Assistant Professor in the Computer Application Department of Manav Rachna International Institute of Research and Studies, Faridabad. She has completed her BCA from KL Mehta Dayanand College, followed by MCA from Institute of Information Technology & Management institute affiliated to Guru Gobind Singh Indraprastha University, followed by M.Tech from J.C. Bose University of Science and Technology, YMCA. Her research interest includes Data Mining, Botnet Detection, Blockchain, Artificial Intelligences and Machine Learning. She has participated in various workshops and Faculty development programmes. She is actively involved in research activities.

Anand BabuR. is an Associate Professor in the Department of Artificial Intelligence and Machine Learning at Panimalar Engineering College, Chennai. He holds a doctorate in Computer Science and has extensive experience in teaching, research, and academic mentoring. His areas of expertise include machine learning, deep learning, and intelligent systems. Dr. Anand Babu has contributed to numerous research publications and actively participates in conferences and faculty development programs. He is committed to advancing AI education and nurturing innovation among students and researchers.

Bhuvaneswari R. working as an Assistant Professor of English at Dr.Mahalingam College of Engineering and Technology, Pollachi. To her credit she completed 10 NPTEL / SWAYAM and published few articles in Scopus indexed journals.

Dhwarithaa R. is an Assistant Professor at SRM Institute of Science and Technology, Chennai, specializing in Artificial Intelligence and Networking. With prior experience as a lecturer and software trainer, she has taught programming languages, mentored students, and contributed to academic administration. She holds a B.E. and M.E. in Computer Science from Sethu Institute of Technology and is currently pursuing a Ph.D. Her skills include Java, Python, HTML, and CSS.

Nithya Paranthaman R. is an Assistant Professor at SRM Institute of Science and Technology with over 10+ years of academic and research experience in Electronics and Communication Engineering. Specializing in Cybersecurity, IoT, and Digital Image Processing, she holds a Ph.D. from SIMATS University. Her award-winning research on adaptive security for IoT-enabled vision sensors was recognized by the Ministry of Defence and NCSSS. A published author, patent holder, and certified in cloud computing and computer vision, she is passionate about mentoring and technological innovation in secure systems.

Velmurugan R. presently working as an Associate Professor in Commerce, Karpagam Academy of Higher Education, Coimbatore. He started his career as a Project Fellow under UGC Sponsored Major Research Project at NGM College, Pollachi. He has 18 years of teaching experience has 15 years of research experience. To his credit he produced 22 Ph.D. Scholars and 5 M.Phil. Scholars. At present 1 scholar submitter his thesis, 6 Ph.D. Scholars are under his guidance. Moreover, to his credit he published 168 articles in various International Journals, of which 58 articles are published in Scopus Indexed Journals and 15 articles in Web of Science and 76 articles in edited volumes. He also participates and presented 27 papers in various International Seminar / Conference and 54 National Seminar / Conference. He acted as an external examiner for various M.Phil. and Ph.D. Viva voce examinations. He acted as a Vice Chancellor nominee for Doctoral Committee Expert at Bharathiar University, Coimbatore and Periyar University, Salem. He acted as a Chairperson at various National Level Conferences. He also acted as an Expert for Syllabus Scrutiny Committee, Question Paper Scrutiny Committee and Expert members for Board of Studies at various reputed Colleges. Considering his meritorious contribution, he received awards like Best Paper Presenter, Best Research Supervisor and Best Faculty Awards from various research foundations and councils. He too acted as a resource person for 27 Guest Lectures, 30 Workshops and 10 faculty development programmes.

Ravikumar R. Natarajan is an experienced academician with over 12+ years of teaching and research expertise across institutions in India, the UAE, and the Maldives. He currently serves as an Assistant Professor at Marwadi University, Rajkot, specializing in Machine Learning, Recommender Systems, and AI-driven applications in healthcare and security. He holds a Ph.D. in Machine Learning and Recommender Systems from Amity University, Jaipur, a Master of Engineering in CSE from VMRF University, Salem, and a Bachelor of Engineering in CSE from

Anna University. He also has a MiniMBA from the Swiss eLearning Institute. Dr. Ravikumar has authored more than 8+ multiple SCIE/Scopus-indexed journal articles, 25+ IEEE/Springer conference papers, and co-authored a book on Artificial Intelligence. He has also published 9 patents and contributed 10+ book chapters in emerging domains such as Federated Learning, Blockchain, and Digital Twins for IGI Global, Wiley and Springer publisher. He actively mentors students through initiatives like the Research Activities Club (RAC) and Student Research Internship Training (SRIT), promoting innovation and research culture.

Jyoti Rani, Assistant professor, school of fashion design and technology. Research and Academic experience. 2-year experience in academics and research. Research area: fashion, textile, natural dyeing, consumer behavior, AI, merchandising. she has published 28 research paper in referred journal and 5 book chapters.

Ramesh S. is an AI and Machine Learning researcher with over 17 years of experience in academia and industry. Currently the Research Head at Saveetha School of Engineering, Chennai, he specializes in data science, deep learning, and IoT-based intelligent systems. He holds a Ph.D. in Wireless Communication and is an AWS Certified Machine Learning Specialist. Dr. Ramesh has published extensively in SCIE and Scopus-indexed journals and holds multiple international patents. His work focuses on medical imaging, anomaly detection, and cloud-based AI solutions.

Ravindra S (born July 1 1980) is a research scholar. He has done his engineering in the field of Telecommunication engineering and M.Tech in the field of VLSI and embedded systems. He is pursuing his PhD on Qos based D2D Wireless communication in LTE-A networks.

Aarthi S is a dedicated Assistant Professor in Computer Science with over six years of teaching experience. She is currently pursuing her Ph.D. at Marwadi University, Gujarat, and holds an M.Phil. and MCA from Bharathiar University, Tamil Nadu. Throughout her academic career, Aarthi has specialized in programming languages such as C++, Java, and C, and contributed to research in recommender systems and AI-related data privacy. She has published journal articles, contributed to book chapters, and actively participated in technical workshops. Known for her student mentorship and engagement in academic events, Aarthi remains committed to fostering innovation and excellence in computer science education.

Ashwini S. is an Assistant Professor in the Department of Computing Technologies at SRM Institute of Science and Technology, Kattankulathur. She holds a Ph.D. in Computer Science and Engineering from Saveetha Institute of Medical and

Technical Sciences, Chennai, an M.E. in CSE from Rrase College of Engineering under Anna University, and a B.Tech. in Information Technology from Sri Sairam Engineering College. With over 9 years of academic and research experience, her expertise spans Deep Learning, Machine Learning, Artificial Intelligence, Data Mining, Python Programming, Cryptography and Network Security, and Compiler Design. She has taught various subjects including C, Java, Data Structures, Operating Systems, and Statistics with R. Dr. Ashwini has published over 25 research papers in reputed international journals and conferences, with research interests focused on Deep Learning applications in medical imaging, cybersecurity, and IoT. She has also contributed a book chapter on deep learning in cancer research. Actively involved in academic development, she has organized workshops, webinars, and coding contests, and participated in numerous faculty development programs. She is a member of professional bodies such as IAENG, IRED, IFERP, and NCSSS, and has handled academic roles in project evaluation, exam coordination, and accreditation processes. Her dedication and commitment to continuous learning mark her as a sincere and hardworking academician.

Kavitha Bharathi Shanmugam is working as Associate Professor in Computer Technology, Kongu Engineering College, and Perundurai. She has industrial experience and 20 years of experience in Teaching. She completed her UG degree in Computer Science, MCA from Vellalar College for Women, M.phil degree from Bharathiar University, Coimbatore and Ph.D from Anna University, Chennai. Her area of interest in Mobile Grid Computing and Internet of Things. She has published more than 30 papers in National and International Journals, presented more than 15 papers in national and International conferences, completed two Projects for academics and organized various funded programs, Seminars and Workshops, Published 2 books. Guided more than 100 UG, PG projects in various emerging trends in technology such as Internet of Things, Mobile Application Development, Augmented and Virtual Reality.

Senthilkumar S., currently working as Assistant Professor in Finance and Management, Skyline University, Nigeria. His qualifications are MBA, M.Com, M.Phil, MS, and PhD. He has rich experience in teaching and academic of 18.2 years. He had published 58 papers Publications in National and International Journals and Proceedings. He Authored 4 books in Research Methodology, Corporate Finance, Principles of Accounting and Business Policy & Strategic management. Participated and presented 62 papers in National & International Seminars and Conferences. He acted as resource person and Guest lecture around 25 Programmemes. He guided 225 projects in M.B.A., 36 M.Phil, and 9 PhD. He got Authorized Guide ship for PhD & M.Phil from Indian Universities such as Anna University, Karpagam University,

Bharathiar University, Periyar Manimai University and AMIET University and Vinayaka Mission University and Bahir Dar University, Ethiopia. He performed as Foreign examiner for evaluating PhD Thesis around 18 Thesis of Indian universities such as Bharathiar University, Visvesvaraya Technological University, University of Mumbai, MS University and Bharathidasan university.

Manas Saha has completed his Bachelor's Degree (B.Tech) from MSIT (Techno India) with First Class. After that he has completed his Master's Degree (M.Tech) from Jadavpur University, Kolkata with First Class. In this while, he has worked as "Trainee Software Engineer" from Dec, 2022- July, 2023. Currently he is working as "Assistant Professor" in the Department of Computer Science and Engineering-AI, Brainware University from Aug 1, 2023.

Ahmad Tasnim Siddiqui is working as Faculty at the School of Computing, Horizon University College (Formerly, Skyline University College), UAE. He is Ph.D. in Computer Science. He also holds a Master of Computer Applications, and an M. Phil (Computer Science) from Madurai Kamaraj University, Madurai, India. He has many publications in reputed journals indexed at SCI, SCIE, and SCOPUS. He has also published book chapters in EMERALD insight, Taylors & Francis, SPRINGER, and IGI Global publications. His research interest includes e-commerce, e-learning, active learning, web mining, IoT, ICT, e-health, and cloud computing. He has a total of 15+ years of experience including 4.7 years of software industry experience. His favorite subjects are E-commerce and web Technologies using .net.

Siva Subramanian is an faculty member in the Department of Computer Science and Engineering at SRM Institute of Science and Technology. He is engaged in academic research and teaching in the field of computer science. His interests include programming, data science, and emerging technologies.

KannadadhasanSuriyan is working as an Associate Professor and HoD in the department of Electronics and Communication Engineering at Study World College of Engineering, Coimbatore, Tamil Nadu, India. He completed his Ph.D. in the field of smart antennas at Anna University in 2022. He has thirteen years of teaching and research experience. He obtained his B.E. in ECE from Sethu Institute of Technology, Kariapatti, in 2009 and his M.E. in Communication Systems from Velammal College of Engineering and Technology, Madurai, in 2013. He obtained his M.B.A. in Human Resources Management from Tamil Nadu Open University, Chennai. He has published around 110 papers in the reputed international journals indexed by SCI, Scopus, Web of Science, and Major Indexing, and more than 250 papers have been presented or published in national and international journals and conferences. Besides, he has also contributed a book chapter. He also serves as a board member, reviewer, speaker, session chair, and member of the advisory and technical committees of various colleges and conferences.

VenketbabuT. is an Assistant Professor (Senior Grade) in the Department of Computer Science and Engineering, School of Computing at Vel Tech Rangarajan Dr. Sagunthala R&D Institute of Science and Technology, Chennai. He specializes in advanced computing technologies, with research interests spanning artificial intelligence, data analytics, and software engineering. Dr. Venketbabu has published research papers in reputed journals and actively participates in academic conferences and workshops. He is committed to mentoring students, guiding research projects, and contributing to curriculum development. His dedication to academic excellence and innovation makes him a valuable asset to the institution.

Preethiya T is currently serving as an Assistant Professor in the Department of Networking and Communications at SRM Institute of Science and Technology. She holds a Ph.D. in Computer Science from Kalasalingam Academy of Research and Education and has over 10 years of academic experience. She is a dedicated academic and researcher in Computer Science and Engineering and her research interests include Mobile Wireless Sensor Networks, Software-Defined Networking (SDN), NLP, and AI-driven data analytics. She has published extensively in reputed journals and conferences, contributing to secured data transmission, energy-efficient routing, and network optimization. Proficient in MATLAB, Python, R, and NS-2 simulations, she actively mentors students and collaborates on innovative research projects. She is a life member of ISTE and a member of IAENG and IACSIT, reflecting her commitment to academic and professional excellence.

Index

A

B

C

D

E

H

I

M

P

R

S

T

V

www.ingramcontent.com/pod-product-compliance
Lightning Source LLC
LaVergne TN
LVHW080904300926
849162LV00003B/549